Diagnostic Criteria for Cardiovascular Pathology

Acquired Diseases

DIAGNOSTIC CRITERIA FOR CARDIOVASCULAR PATHOLOGY

Acquired Diseases

Editor

Sherman Bloom, M.D.
Professor of Pathology
Chairman, Department of Pathology
University of Mississippi Medical Center
Jackson, Mississippi

Associate Editors

J. T. Lie, M.D.
Professor and Director
Division of Anatomic Pathology
University of California Davis Medical Center
Sacramento, California

Malcolm D. Silver, M.D., Ph.D.
Professor of Pathology
University of Toronto
Senior Staff Pathologist
The Toronto Hospital
Toronto, Ontario, Canada

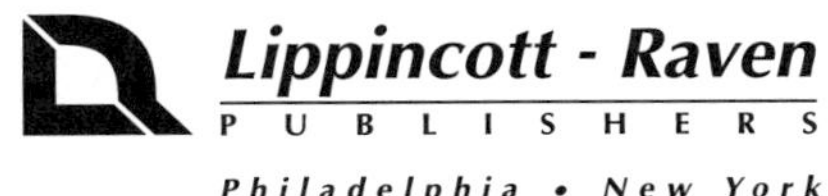

Lippincott - Raven
PUBLISHERS
Philadelphia • New York

Acquisitions Editor: Vickie Thaw
Developmental Editor: Anne Snyder
Manufacturing Manager: Dennis Teston
Production Manager: Larry Bernstein
Production Editor: Loretta Cummings
Cover Designer: Ed Schultheis
Indexer: Nancy Newman
Compositor: Lippincott–Raven Electronic Production
Printer: Maple Press

9 8 7 6 5 4 3 2 1

Library of Congress Cataloging-in-Publication Data

Diagnostic criteria for cardiovascular pathology : acquired diseases / editor, Sherman Bloom; associate editors, J.T. Lie, Malcolm D. Silver.
   p. cm.
Includes bibliographical references and index.
ISBN 0-397-51630-4
1. Cardiovascular system—Diseases—Diagnosis. I. Bloom, Sherman. II. Lie, J.T.
III. Silver, Malcolm D.
[DNLM: 1. Heart Diseases—pathology. 2. Heart Diseases—diagnosis. 3. Vascular Diseases—pathology. 4. Vascular Diseases—diagnosis. WG 210 D536 1997]
RC670.D53 1997
616.1′071—dc20
DNLM/DLC
for Library of Congress

---

*To our colleagues and students,
whose questions and suggestions prompted this book*

Contents

Contributing Authors

H. Thomas Aretz, M.D. *Associate Professor of Pathology, Department of Pathology, New England Deaconess Hospital, One Deaconess Road, Boston, Massachusetts 02215*

Michael D. Bell, M.D. *Clinical Assistant Professor, Department of Pathology, University of Miami School of Medicine, and Associate Medical Examiner, Dade County Medical Examiner Office, Number One Bob Hope Road, Miami, Florida 33136*

Margaret E. Billingham, M.B., B.S., F.R.C.Path. *Professor of Pathology, Emerita, Department of Cardiothoracic Surgery, Stanford University School of Medicine, Falk Cardiovascular Research Building, Stanford, California 94305–5247*

Sherman Bloom, M.D. *Professor of Pathology, Chairman, Department of Pathology, University of Mississippi Medical Center, 2500 North State Street, Jackson, Mississippi 39216–4505*

Allen P. Burke, M.D. *Associate Chairman, Department of Cardiovascular Pathology, Armed Forces Institute of Pathology, 14 Street and Alaska Avenue NW, Washington, DC 20306-6000*

Jagdish W. Butany, M.B.B.S., M.S., F.R.C.P.C. *Associate Professor, Department of Pathology, University of Toronto, and Staff Pathologist, The Toronto Hospital-General Division, EC4-305, 200 Elizabeth Street, Toronto, Ontario, Canada M5G 2C4*

David A. Chiasson, M.D. *Assistant Professor, University of Toronto, and Chief Forensic Pathologist, Office of the Chief Coroner, 26 Grenville Street, Toronto, Ontario, Canada M7A 1Y6*

Stephen M. Factor, M.D. *Professor of Pathology and Medicine, Department of Pathology, Albert Einstein College of Medicine, 1300 Morris Park Avenue, Bronx, New York 10461*

Avrum I. Gotlieb, M.D., C.M. *Professor of Pathology and Clinical Biochemistry, University of Toronto, and Director, Vascular Research Laboratory, The Toronto Hospital, 200 Elizabeth Street, Toronto, Ontario, Canada M5G 2C4*

J. T. Lie, M.D., F.A.C.C., F.A.C.A., F.A.C.R., F.C.C.P. *Professor and Director, Division of Anatomic Pathology, University of California Davis Medical Center, 2315 Stockton Boulevard, Sacramento, California 95817*

Francesca V. Lobo, M.D., F.R.C.P.C.   *Associate Professor of Pathology, McMaster University, and Staff Pathologist, Hamilton Civic Hospitals, General Division, 237 Barton Street East, Hamilton, Ontario, Canada L8L 2X2*

Elizabeth A. Montgomery, M.D.   *Associate Professor of Pathology, Department of Pathology, Georgetown University, 3900 Reservoir Road NW, Washington, DC 20007*

Alan G. Rose, M.D., F.R.C.Path.   *Jesse E. Edwards Registry of Cardiovascular Disease, United Hospital and Saint Paul Heart and Lung Institute, and Clinical Professor of Pathology, University of Minnesota, St. Paul, Minnesota 55102*

Robert J. Siegel, M.D.   *Associate Professor, Department of Pathology and Laboratory Medicine, Emory University School of Medicine, and Director, Pathology Laboratories, Crawford Long Hospital, 550 Peachtree Street NE, Atlanta, Georgia 30365*

Malcolm D. Silver, M.D., Ph.D., F.R.C.P.A., F.R.C.P.C.   *Professor of Pathology, Faculty of Medicine, University of Toronto; Senior Staff Pathologist, The Toronto Hospital; and Department of Pathology, Banting Institute, 100 College Street, Toronto, Ontario, Canada M5G 1L7*

John P. Veinot, M.D.   *Assistant Professor, Department of Pathology and Laboratory Medicine, Ottawa Civic Hospital, University of Ottawa, 1053 Carling Avenue, Ottawa, Ontario, Canada K1Y 4E9*

Renu Virmani, M.D.   *Chairman, Department of Cardiovascular Pathology, Armed Forces Institute of Pathology, 6825 16th Street NW, Washington, DC 20306*

Virginia M. Walley, M.D., F.R.C.P.C.   *Cardiovascular Pathologist, University of Ottawa Heart Institute; Professor, Department of Pathology and Laboratory Medicine, University of Ottawa; Chief, Anatomical Pathology; and Chief, Department of Laboratory Medicine, Ottawa Civic Hospital, 1053 Carling Avenue, Ottawa, Ontario, Canada K1Y 4E9*

Preface

This book is an exposition of the diagnostic criteria used by recognized specialists in acquired cardiovascular pathology. These criteria may be of value to the general medical community, cardiologists, cardiovascular surgeons, and especially to pathologists who do not regularly work with cardiovascular diseases.

The text is divided into six sections, corresponding to settings in which pathology is observed at the time of diagnosis. This categorization facilitates finding information needed to explain a particular set of morphological observations. Each section consists of entries arranged alphabetically by diagnosis and composed of statements that may include synonyms, the definition, gross findings, microscopic findings, special procedures needed for diagnosis, differential diagnosis, key diagnostic criteria, and potential pitfalls. The key diagnostic criteria explicitly describe the features to be considered in establishing the diagnosis. The Systematized Nomenclature of Human and Veterinary Medicine (SNOMED) codes relevant to cardiovascular diseases appear in the Appendix of the book.

Each entry is prepared by an entry author and reviewed by the section editor. In addition, each entry was reviewed by at least one other editor or, in some cases, additional authors. This relatively large number of participants enabled the authors to come as close as possible to a consensus document. Each entry, however, reflects the views of its author. In some cases there may be controversial aspects to the criteria. We have tried to indicate when this is the case, and to provide some indication of its nature. References are sometimes given to clarify the issues. In some cases separate entries are given for a single diagnosis and for virtually identical diagnoses, so that authors with conflicting opinions could express their views.

There is discussion of mechanisms, epidemiology, and other interesting aspects of the diseases as they relate to establishing diagnoses. The focus, however, is on establishing a morphological diagnosis for the reader for a specific case of immediate concern.

The range of conditions covered is intended to be broad—to span almost all of acquired cardiovascular pathology as it is seen in human medicine. Nevertheless, not every possible diagnostic entity is represented. In addition, there is no attempt to deal with the lesions seen in veterinary or experimental pathology, even when these are important in human medicine.

There may be disagreement among experienced pathologists as to some of the criteria. This is to be expected and encouraged as a stimulus to further inquiry. It is our intention to provide information to the general pathologist, and other interested physicians, that would be useful in their daily work. It is not our intention to prepare criteria that might be used for legal purposes. Some criteria will change over time and others are not necessarily complete or infallible. This text is a guidebook, not a definitive encyclopedia intended to resolve disputes.

Many of the conditions described are commonplace. Others are rare, but important when encountered. We hope that this guide will increase the confidence of the generalist in dealing with this special area of pathological practice.

The actual contents of this work was largely determined by the individual authors. They determined which entries were to be included, which criteria would be applied to each condition, how detailed their entries would be, and whether or not bibliographic documentation would be given.

Acknowledgments

Sherian Purvis provided organizational insight, editorial skills, and long hours of work combined with continuous good humor, which greatly facilitated production of this book. Vickie Thaw of Lippincott-Raven Publishers was a patient and insightful advisor.

Diagnostic Criteria for Cardiovascular Pathology

Acquired Diseases

Section 1

Diseases of the Myocardium

Section Editor: Sherman Bloom
Entry Authors: H. Thomas Aretz, Margaret E. Billingham, Sherman Bloom, Stephen M. Factor, Robert J. Siegel, and Renu Virmani

AMYLOIDOSIS

Entry Author: Renu Virmani

DEFINITION: Amyloidosis describes many disease processes that have the common feature of deposition of an extracellular protein characterized by a β-pleated sheet conformation. Several major types of amyloidosis have been described. These include: AA, AF, AL, ASc, and light chain disease. Cardiac deposits are frequent in most types of amyloid and produce congestive heart failure, arrhythmias, restrictive cardiomyopathy, and may induce valvular or ischemic heart disease.

AMYLOID AA: AA amyloid (reactive or secondary) is most often associated with chronic inflammatory states, including familial Mediterranean fever, rheumatoid arthritis, tuberculosis, and osteomyelitis. The amyloid is derived from a serum precursor known as *serum-associated protein* (SAA). It is a non-immunoglobulin protein that is synthesized in the liver and circulates in association with the HDL_3 subclass of lipoproteins. Deposits in AA amyloid lose their affinity for Congo red after treatment with KMn04, while those in other forms of amyloidosis retain their stainability.

AMYLOID, AF: The hereditary amyloidoses, including familial Mediterranean fever (related to AA protein in which the deposits are derived from SAA), and the familial amyloid polyneuropathy (in which the amyloid is derived from mutant forms of transthyretin). Four types of the latter syndrome are recognized: type 1 (Andrade or Portuguese type); type 2 (Rukovina type); type 3 (Van Allem type); type 4 (Meretoja type).

AMYLOID, AL: Amyloid AL occurs in primary amyloidosis and multiple myeloma. Both disorders are characterized by proliferation of plasma cells that produce whole immunoglobulin light chains or fragments (lambda light chain). Proteins are found in plasma and/or urine and are the source of amyloid deposits.

AMYLOID, ASc: In senile amyloidosis the involved protein is known as *senile amyloid* (ASc) protein. Three forms of senile cardiovascular amyloid have been recognized: (a) senile aortic amyloid, (b) isolated atrial amyloid, and (c) systemic senile amyloidosis with cardiovascular involvement. The isolated atrial amyloid corresponds to deposits derived from atrial natriuretic factor. The other two forms of amyloid are derived from transthyretin, a plasma protein that migrates electrophoretically in the prealbumin fraction.

GROSS FINDINGS: The myocardium with clinically significant amyloid deposits is firm and rubbery. The atrial endocardium shows a focal granular, waxy appearance. The atria are dilated, and the ventricular cavity is normal or small. Valvular deposits are also waxy and glistening, but the valve usually functions normally.

MICROSCOPIC FINDINGS: Amyloid is seen in the thickened endocardium of the atrium, surrounding individual myocytes and as focal deposits. Involved blood vessel walls have focal or diffuse deposits which have a homogenous appearance, with or without luminal compromise. The pattern of amyloid deposits can be helpful in predicting the type of amyloid deposits, i.e., pericellular and focal myocardial deposits are more frequent in senile amyloidosis, whereas vascular deposits are more common in familial amyloidosis. Amyloid has distinct staining characteristics, with a homogenous hyaline or fluffy appearance on hematoxylin and eosin, green (dichroic) birefringence after staining with congo red, metachromasia with methyl violet, ultraviolet fluorescence with thioflavin T, and green staining with sulfated alcian blue stain.

SPECIAL PROCEDURES NEEDED FOR DIAGNOSIS: The identity of deposits as amyloid must be confirmed by histochemical stains and the subtypes determined by immunohistochemical methods. However, some amyloid will not stain with the usual stains and electron microscopy may be required for confirmation. The diagnosis of amyloidosis is usually straightforward by histochemical and/or immunohistochemical methods, with electron microscopy as a last resort.

DIFFERENTIAL DIAGNOSIS: Hyalinized collagen can resemble amyloid on hematoxylin and eosin stain, but the distinction is clear after histochemical staining.

KEY DIAGNOSTIC CRITERIA: Amyloid deposits may be focal, pericellular (around individual myocytes), or within blood vessel walls as a pink homogenous material on hematoxylin and eosin stain and further confirmed by immunohistochemical stains for the subtypes. Amyloid fibrils on electron microscopy show unbranching straight or bent structure, randomly arranged, with a diameter of 10 nm. Fibrillin deposits may be confused with amyloid in H&E stains but are Congo red negative and are distinct from either amyloid or light chain by electron microscopy and immunohistochemistry.

POTENTIAL PITFALLS: Hyalinized collagen can be mistaken on H&E for amyloid deposits and vice versa.

ANEURYSM, VENTRICULAR

Entry Author: Robert J. Siegel

DEFINITION: Protrusion or out-pouching of a segment of a ventricular wall.

GROSS FINDINGS: External examination reveals a dome-shaped protrusion, usually of the left ventricle. In a chronic aneurysm, the myocardial wall is thin, often fibrotic, and occasionally calcified. Laminated mural thrombus often adheres to the endocardial surface. The endocardium may be pearly white and the trabeculae carneae absent. An acute aneurysm contains myocardium and little or no fibrous tissue. Aneurysmal segments excised surgically often have this appearance, because the clinical diagnosis of aneurysm can be made before chronic changes occur.

MICROSCOPIC FINDINGS: Because ventricular aneurysm usually occurs in the setting of previous myocardial infarct, the changes of healed infarct typically are seen in the aneurysmal area.

REMARKS: Ventricular aneurysm results from stretching of an akinetic segment of ventricular wall with thinning and outward expansion.

KEY DIAGNOSTIC CRITERIA: The gross appearance just described is distinctive.

POTENTIAL PITFALLS: False aneurysm. This is a sac-like out-pouching of a ventricle produced when its wall is ruptured (as may occur after a myocardial infarction), but its escaping blood is contained by the surrounding tissues which may form a fibrous sac superficially resembling an aneurysm of the (ventricular) wall.

Reference

1. Cabin HS, Roberts WC. True left ventricular aneurysm and healed myocardial infarction. Clinical and necropsy observations including quantification of degrees of coronary artery narrowing. *Am J Cardiol* 1980;46:754–763.

CARCINOID HEART DISEASE

Entry Author: Renu Virmani

DEFINITION: Carcinoid heart disease presents, pathologically, as endocardial plaques usually on the right side of the heart (rarely on the left). The plaques are composed of proliferating smooth muscle cells in a matrix rich in proteoglycans. They are found in patients who have the carcinoid syndrome, characterized by cutaneous flushing, diarrhea, and bronchoconstriction. The carcinoid syndrome is found in patients with malignant carcinoid tumors that have metastasized. The primary tumor is located in the appendix in 60–90% of cases but may be located in the ileum, stomach, duodenum, rectum, or a bronchus. Carcinoid tumors secrete various vasoactive substances, such as bradykinin, serotonin (5-hydroxytryptamine), and histamine which are usually inactivated in liver, lungs, and brain. In cases with hepatic metastasis large quantities of vasoactive mediators reach the heart without being inactivated. These induce lesions in the right heart. Left heart lesions are rare and are usually associated with carcinoid tumor in the lung. Such left heart lesions, when they do occur, are minor and of little hemodynamic significance.

GROSS FINDINGS: The carcinoid endocardial lesions appear as white plaques superimposed on the endocardium of the right atrium and ventricle, atrial aspect of the tricuspid valve and pulmonic aspect of the pulmonary valve (rarely mitral and aortic valves). The fibrous plaques cause leaflet fusion and retraction resulting in pulmonary stenosis. Tricuspid regurgitation and mild stenosis may also be present, but pure tricuspid stenosis is rare.

MICROSCOPIC FINDINGS: Carcinoid plaques are composed of smooth muscle cells with thickened reduplicated basement membrane in a stroma rich in proteoglycans and some collagen. Typically, there are no elastic fibers present. Carcinoid plaques do not infiltrate underlying structures, e.g., valve tissue or myocardium. The pathogenesis of carcinoid plaques is unknown but may be related to endothelial injury from vasoactive amines.

SPECIAL PROCEDURES NEEDED FOR DIAGNOSIS: Chest x-ray shows an enlarged heart. Electrocardiogram shows nonspecific findings except low voltage is often present. Echocardiography may reveal evidence of tricuspid and/or pulmonary valve thickening along with right atrial and ventricular dilation. Symptoms of carcinoid syndrome along with elevated urinary 5-hydroxyindole acetic acid do not help differentiate patients with or without carcinoid heart disease.

DIFFERENTIAL DIAGNOSIS: Endomyocardial fibrosis (Davies' disease, EMF) typically is concentrated at the apex and around the papillary muscle but usually does not involve the atrial surface of the tricuspid valve, and involvement of the pulmonic valve has not been reported. Furthermore, it is usually found in the tropics, whereas carcinoid heart disease has no geographic localization.

Fibroplastic cardiomyopathy (fibroelastosis) is a disease of infants and children, whereas carcinoid heart disease is only seen in adults. Fibroelastosis is also different in that the endocardial scarification contains prominent elastin filaments and is diffuse except for the sparing of valves.

Irradiation usually produces pericardial fibrosis along with endocardial fibrosis, most marked in the right ventricle. It may be accompanied by pulmonic and tricuspid valve thickening which is focal and not diffuse.

KEY DIAGNOSTIC CRITERIA: Gross and microscopic findings are specific.

CARDIAC ALLOGRAFT REJECTION, ACUTE

Entry Author: Margaret Billingham

SYNONYM: Cellular rejection.

DEFINITION: Cardiac rejection is the immunological process of sloughing off the foreign tissue (cardiac allograft) by the recipient. Severity, which is of great clinical importance, can be specified in a number of ways, such as "mild," "moderate," and "severe."

GROSS FINDINGS: In severe cases, the donor (graft) heart is edematous, stiff (loss of compliance), dark plum in color, and has endocardial hemorrhages in a "tigroid" pattern. These gross abnormalities end abruptly at the suture lines. In mild acute rejection there may be no clear gross changes.

MICROSCOPIC FINDINGS: (a) In mild acute rejection there is a perivascular infiltrate of activated T-lymphocytes. (b) In moderate acute rejection there is an interstitial and perivascular infiltrate of activated T-lymphocytes with occasional eosinophils. Early, focal myocyte damage may be seen. (c) Severe rejection is diagnosed when there is myocyte damage and marked mixed interstitial infiltrate of neutrophils, lymphocytes, eosinophils, plasma cells, and histiocytes. There may be vasculitis with interstitial hemorrhage.

SPECIAL PROCEDURES NEEDED FOR DIAGNOSIS: Myocardial tissue including blood vessels should be fresh frozen (cover with Tissue Tec in a Beem capsule) for immunohistochemistry, *in situ* hybridization, immunofluorescence, or elution of antibodies if required. Special stains may be required to rule out organisms.

DIFFERENTIAL DIAGNOSIS: Acute inflammatory myocarditis, lymphoma, "Quilty" effect, ischemic granulation tissue, pressor agent effect.

KEY DIAGNOSTIC CRITERIA: Myocardial inflammation, predominantly lymphocytic and usually focal, that is not due to ischemia, infection, or lymphoma.

CARDIAC ALLOGRAFT REJECTION, CHRONIC

Entry Author: Margaret Billingham

SYNONYMS: Graft vascular disease; graft coronary disease.

GROSS FINDINGS: The cardiac allograft may show yellow-orange cord-like epicardial coronary vessels. The lumen of these vessels is seen, on cut surface, to be filled with yellow material which extends into the small intramyocardial branches.

MICROSCOPIC FINDINGS: Sections of epicardial coronary arteries and their intramyocardial branches as well as sections of the graft portion of the great vessels and their adventitia show *concentric* intimal proliferation. The elastica is mostly intact with minor breaks. The intima contains modified smooth muscle cells, foamy macrophages, fibroblasts, and sometimes, lymphocytes. Perivascular lymphocytes may be present, but frank vasculitis is rare and atherosclerotic plaque occurs rarely in long-term recipients (5 to 15 years).

SPECIAL PROCEDURES NEEDED FOR DIAGNOSIS: Elastic stains should be done.

DIFFERENTIAL DIAGNOSIS: Preexisting atherosclerotic coronary artery disease of the donor.

KEY DIAGNOSTIC CRITERIA: Concentric intimal proliferation affecting small branch vessels.

CARDIAC ALLOGRAFT REJECTION, HUMORAL

Entry Author: Margaret Billingham

SYNONYM: "Vascular" rejection.

DEFINITION: An immune response directed against a cardiac allograft where circulating antibodies present in the recipient react with the cardiac allograft producing acute injury.

GROSS FINDINGS: Large, edematous heart with dilated ventricles.

MICROSCOPIC FINDINGS: The myocardium shows marked interstitial edema with *sparse* inflammatory cells (neutrophils, plasma cells, red cells) and fibrin deposits. Swollen endothelial cells and a capillaritis may be present.

SPECIAL PROCEDURES NEEDED FOR DIAGNOSIS: Immunohistochemistry performed on fresh frozen tissue shows plasma protein deposition on the endothelium of intramural vessels (IgG, IgM, C3, fibrinogen, etc.).

DIFFERENTIAL DIAGNOSIS: Acute cellular rejection (i.e., cardiac allograft rejection, acute).

KEY DIAGNOSTIC CRITERIA: Positive immunohistochemical reactions indicating presence of immunoactive substances on vascular endothelium.

POTENTIAL PITFALLS: False-positive immunofluorescence occurs with ischemia and infections.

CARDIAC ALLOGRAFT REJECTION, HYPERACUTE

Entry Author: Margaret Billingham

SYNONYM: Immediate diffuse rejection.

DEFINITION: Hyperacute rejection is the immediate result of preformed cytotoxic antibodies, usually those against MHC or A, B blood group antigens.

GROSS FINDINGS: The heart (donor graft) is heavy, swollen, edematous, and hemorrhagic in color.

MICROSCOPIC FINDINGS: The myocardium shows *global* interstitial edema and hemorrhage. Myocytes may show contraction bands. Capillaries and small vessel may show fibrin thrombi or "sludged" red cells.

SPECIAL PROCEDURES NEEDED FOR DIAGNOSIS: Freeze tissue for antibody studies.

DIFFERENTIAL DIAGNOSIS: Right ventricular failure due to pulmonary hypertension in the recipient. Damaged heart from donor accident. Massive myocardial infarct from inadvertent coronary damage at transplantation.

KEY DIAGNOSTIC CRITERIA: Positive immunohistochemical reaction demonstrating antibodies in the myocardium of the transplanted heart.

CARDIAC ALLOGRAFT REJECTION, "QUILTY" EFFECT

Entry Author: Margaret Billingham

SYNONYM: Endocardial lymphocytic infiltrate in allografts.

DEFINITION: The "Quilty" lesions are aggregates of lymphocytes found on the endocardial surface of the ventricles in cardiac allografts. The term *Quilty* is from the patient in whom it was first observed.

GROSS FINDINGS: At autopsy, there is a pale geographic outline seen in the affected ventricular endocardium.

MICROSCOPIC FINDINGS: There is an accumulation of lymphocytes (predominantly T cells but with foci of B cells) within the endocardium, although "spillover" may occur, with some lymphocytes distributed among subendocardial myocytes. These lymphocytic aggregates have a distinctive vascular pattern of small vessels within them and a characteristic linear, streaming pattern of the lymphocytes at the edge of the lesion.

REMARKS: The etiology of these lesions is unknown. Their presence or absence provides no clue as to the long-term outcome of the cardiac allograft. There has been an attempt to distinguish "Type A" Quilty lesions from "Type B" lesions, the latter being examples in which there is some apparent myocyte necrosis. However, it has been found that there is no significance to this distinction in terms of reflecting prognosis.

DIFFERENTIAL DIAGNOSIS: Old biopsy sites with entrapped lymphocytes, lymphomatous nodules. Lymphoproliferative disease.

KEY DIAGNOSTIC CRITERIA: Endocardial location and vascular pattern.

CARDIAC DILATION

Entry Author: Robert J. Siegel

SYNONYM: Dilatation.

DEFINITION: Increased volume of any cardiac chamber or combination of chambers, usually leading to an increased size of the heart, and caused by a variety of pathological entities. Thus, chamber dilation may be global in dilated cardiomyopathy (see *Cardiomyopathy, idiopathic dilated*), right-sided in cor pulmonale, left atrial in mitral stenosis, left ventricular in aortic regurgitation, and so on. Cardiac dilation is one of the two causes of cardiomegaly, the other being myocardial hypertrophy.

GROSS FINDINGS: When all chambers are dilated, a characteristic globe-shaped heart is apparent. Single dilated chambers also tend to assume a more spherical shape. Hypertrophy often accompanies dilation, and is a crude indicator of duration of the process that produced dilation. Because chamber volume is difficult to determine, quantitative criteria for dilation have not been firmly established. For example, among adult hearts, said to be morphologically normal, left ventricular volumes ranged from 5 to 140 ml. It has been presumed that some of this variation is due to the degree of myocardial contraction.

MICROSCOPIC FINDINGS: Histologic findings in cardiac dilation are those of the underlying disease process and do not usually reflect dilation per se. If dilation is severe, myocardial fibers may be noticeably thinned and stretched.

REMARKS: Accurate measurement of cardiac chamber volumes at autopsy requires standardized methods of perfusion fixation. Volumes may be estimated by displacement of plastic beads, wax or silastic casts, or more simply, by measuring the volume of water a chamber will hold. Various formulas have been offered for estimating ventricular volumes from opened hearts, generally assuming a conical shape.

DIFFERENTIAL DIAGNOSIS: Once dilation is recognized, the important differential diagnosis then becomes its etiology. Cardiac chambers generally dilate because of volume overload (e.g., LV dilation in aortic insufficiency), obstruction to outflow (e.g., LA dilation in mitral stenosis), or myocardial disease (e.g., dilated cardiomyopathy or myocarditis). Thus, assessment of cardiac valves, histologic examination of myocardium, and clinical correlation are necessary to define the cause.

KEY DIAGNOSTIC CRITERIA: Dilation is present when chamber volume exceeds normal predicted values.

POTENTIAL PITFALLS: The vagaries of volume measurements make recognition of increased chamber size difficult.

Reference

1. Hutchins GM, Anaya OA. Measurement of cardiac size, chamber volumes and valve orifices at autopsy. *Johns Hopkins Med J* 1973;133:96–106

CARDIOMEGALY

Entry Author: Robert J. Siegel

SYNONYM: Cardiac enlargement.

DEFINITION: Heart size larger than normal. A nonspecific term, often used by clinicians to refer to increased cardiac silhouette (cardiothoracic ratio) on CXR. May be caused by dilation, hypertrophy, myocardial infiltrations, or any combination of these factors. Refer to individual entries for details.

CARDIOMYOPATHY, ALCOHOL-ASSOCIATED

Entry Author: Stephen M. Factor

SYNONYMS: Alcoholic cardiomyopathy, nutritional heart disease; beri-beri heart disease, (thiamine deficiency).

DEFINITION: Cardiac hypertrophy and myocardial damage due to the effects of chronic alcohol abuse (usually >10 years). May be secondary to the direct effects of alcohol on the heart, or indirectly due to associated malnutrition (e.g., protein and vitamin deficiency as in beri-beri).

GROSS FINDINGS: Hypertrophy and dilation, both right- and left-sided, ventricles more than atria. Mural thrombi common, with endocardial plaques related to organized thrombi. Areas of myocardial fibrosis may be visible. Heart may be "flabby," and myocardium may have a greasy feel. Chordae tendineae of mitral valve may be focally thickened and fused.

MICROSCOPIC FINDINGS: Myocellular hypertrophy. Interstitial, replacement, and perivascular fibrosis. Small vessel sclerosis. Occasional interstitial edema (particularly with beri beri but may be seen in well-nourished alcoholics), with increased interstitial inflammation. Increased myocellular lipid on either oil red O stain or electron microscopy.

REMARKS: Diagnosis of exclusion. However, presence of hypertrophy, dilation, mural thrombi, and myocardial scarring in a chronic alcoholic should suggest diagnosis. Contribution of hypertension and tobacco use, frequently associated with chronic alcoholism, difficult to assess. Diagnosis may be made in the absence of other features of chronic alcoholism (e.g., hepatic cirrhosis or pancreatitis). Acute effects of alcohol (e.g., binge drinking) can lead to myocardial damage and may cause acute, fatal arrhythmias.

DIFFERENTIAL DIAGNOSIS: Other causes of cardiomyopathy.

KEY DIAGNOSTIC CRITERIA: Dilation of all chambers, increased myocellular lipid, mural thrombi, increased interstitial inflammation (may be difficult to discriminate from borderline myocarditis, on endomyocardial biopsy).

POTENTIAL PITFALLS: There may be a spectrum of disease, from overt cardiac hypertrophy and dilation with severe congestive heart failure, to mild cardiomegaly with no clinical dysfunction. Actual nutritional heart disease (beri-beri and protein deficiency) is relatively rare, although occasional cases may be seen in "street people."

Reference

1. Stout LC, Boor PJ, Whorton EB Jr. Myofibroblastic proliferation on mitral valve chordae tendineae: A distinctive lesion associated with alcoholic liver disease. *Hum Pathol* 1988;19:720-725.

CARDIOMYOPATHY, AMIODARONE-ASSOCIATED

Entry Author: Stephen M. Factor

DEFINITION: Cardiac toxicity directly or indirectly related to chronic amiodarone administration.

GROSS FINDINGS: No specific abnormality. The myocardium may have a chocolate brown color from excessive lipofuscin pigment deposition ("brown atrophy").

MICROSCOPIC FINDINGS: Increased myocellular lipofuscin pigment. May be apparent on light microscopy, or it may require electron microscopy to demonstrate.

REMARKS: A difficult diagnosis. Amiodarone may exacerbate arrhythmias in the absence of any gross or microscopic myocardial injury. Cardiac dysfunction associated with either thyrotoxicosis or hypothyroidism (recognized side effects of chronic amiodarone administration) also must be excluded. Interstitial pneumonitis, another side effect, may cause right ventricular strain and injury independent of any direct effect of the drug on the heart.

DIFFERENTIAL DIAGNOSIS: Other causes of cardiomyopathy associated with arrhythmias.

KEY DIAGNOSTIC CRITERIA: Increased lipofuscin pigment.

POTENTIAL PITFALLS: Lack of specificity of increased lipofuscin pigment, particularly in older age groups.

CARDIOMYOPATHY, AMPHETAMINE-ASSOCIATED

Entry Author: Stephen M. Factor

DEFINITION: Myocardial injury secondary to chronic amphetamine abuse. The major morphologic features are hypertrophy and multiple foci of myocyte necrosis leading to fibrosis.

GROSS FINDINGS: Concentric hypertrophy of left ventricle during the compensated stage, with chamber dilation and mural thinning during decompensation. Presence of small punctate scars. Mural thrombi may be present during the decompensated stage. If amphetamines are being used at the time of death, focal myocytolysis may be recognized grossly.

MICROSCOPIC FINDINGS: The microscopic changes depend on the amount of drug taken, when it was taken, and the vulnerability of the recipient. There may be myocellular hypertrophy, focal replacement scars, areas of myocytolysis in different stages of organization, and/or acute multifocal contraction band necrosis. Small vessel sclerosis may be seen.

REMARKS: May be difficult to ascribe diagnosis specifically to amphetamine use, particularly if multiple agents are being employed for weight loss. Pathological features may be secondary to concurrent hypertension.

DIFFERENTIAL DIAGNOSIS: Any state associated with elevated catecholamines, such as pheochromocytoma, thyrotoxicosis or cocaine-associated cardiomyopathy.

KEY DIAGNOSTIC CRITERIA: Multifocal myocardial injury and ventricular hypertrophy in a patient chronically abusing amphetamines.

POTENTIAL PITFALLS: Absence of specificity.

Reference

1. Smith HJ, Roche AHG, Jagusch MF, Herdson PB. Cardiomyopathy associated with amphetamine administration. *Am Heart J* 1976;91:792–797.

CARDIOMYOPATHY, ANTHRACYCLINE-ASSOCIATED

Entry Author: Stephen M. Factor

SYNONYMS: Adriamycin cardiomyopathy, daunorubicin cardiomyopathy.

DEFINITION: The development of cardiac hypertrophy and myocardial damage, generally associated with clinical congestive heart failure in a patient receiving anthracycline chemotherapy.

GROSS FINDINGS: In the full-blown disease, the heart is enlarged, pale, flabby, with ventricular dilation. Mural thrombi may be present. A spectrum of less severe cardiomyopathic changes may be seen if death ensues due to an arrhythmia or the underlying neoplasm.

MICROSCOPIC FINDINGS: Interstitial edema, myocyte vacuolization or necrosis, and fibrosis may be seen on light microscopy. Specific diagnosis is made by electron microscopy. There are a decreased number of myofibrillar bundles, myofibril lysis, and abnormal or distorted Z-bands. Myocytes with vacuolar change and loss of myofilaments are found adjacent to apparently normal myocytes. Dilation of T tubules may be evident.

REMARKS: The condition is generally related to the cumulative dose of the drug, with 500 mg/M^2 being the threshold level. However, disease may be seen at lower doses, particularly if radiotherapy and/or other chemotherapeutic agents have been administered.

DIFFERENTIAL DIAGNOSIS: Effects of mediastinal radiation and other chemotherapeutic agents must be considered.

KEY DIAGNOSTIC CRITERIA: Ultrastructural features are relatively specific in the appropriate clinical setting. EM changes are similar to those seen in DCM, that there is no hypertrophy and some cells show loss of myofibrils plus dilation of T tubules.

POTENTIAL PITFALLS: The 500 mg/M^2 dose level should not be viewed as an absolute cutoff, below which damage does not occur and above which damage always ensues. There is a continuum of injury that may only be recognized on endomyocardial biopsy prior to the development of overt clinical disease.

CARDIOMYOPATHY, CARNITINE-DEFICIENCY-ASSOCIATED

Entry Author: Renu Virmani

SYNONYM: Fatty acid metabolism disorder.

DEFINITION: The reduced contractile function and morphologic changes of the heart muscle associated with carnitine deficiency. The primary form of this condition is due to an autosomal recessive inborn error of metabolism, while inadequate intake is responsible for the secondary form. This cardiomyopathy is usually of the dilated type but hypertrophy may be present.

GROSS FINDINGS: In a majority of cases, the heart is dilated, with or without hypertrophy. In some cases, there is hypertrophy with no obvious dilation. In cases with dilation, there may be endocardial fibroelastosis.

MICROSCOPIC FINDINGS: Myocytes are enlarged and contain vacuoles that stain positively for lipid. Ultrastructurally, there is disruption of the myofibrils and aggregation of mitochondria which often have bizarre shapes and twisted cristae set in circular array. They often contain electron-dense crystalline inclusions.

REMARKS: Carnitine is an essential cofactor for entry of long-chain fatty acids into mitochondria where oxidation takes place. Carnitine deficiency leads to depressed mitochondrial oxidation of fatty acids and accumulation of fat in myocyte cytoplasm.

SPECIAL PROCEDURES NEEDED FOR DIAGNOSIS: Plasma carnitine levels are low.

DIFFERENTIAL DIAGNOSIS: Plasma carnitine levels and electron microscopic examination of biopsy material are most helpful in distinguishing this condition from idiopathic dilated cardiomyopathy or endocardial fibroelastosis in infancy.

KEY DIAGNOSTIC CRITERIA: Low plasma carnitine levels in a child with biventricular heart failure and biopsy evidence of lipid accumulation, myofibrillar disruption, and bizarre mitochondria in cardiac myocytes.

POTENTIAL PITFALLS: May be difficult to distinguish from idiopathic dilated cardiomyopathy on morphological grounds alone, but lipid accumulation is not a feature of this latter condition.

CARDIOMYOPATHY, CATECHOLAMINE-ASSOCIATED

Entry Author: Stephen M. Factor

SYNONYMS: Subtypes: isoproterenol-induced myocardial necrosis (ISO-MN), epinephrine-induced myocardial necrosis (EPI-MN).

DEFINITION: Cardiac muscle disease secondary to the effects of catecholamines, either administered or endogenously produced. Acute effect is focal myocyte necrosis with resulting inflammation and fibrosis, whereas chronic effect is myocyte hypertrophy. The condition has been studied extensively in experimental animals.

GROSS FINDINGS: In chronic exposure to low doses, there may be biventricular hypertrophy, concentric in character. Focal myocardial scars may be observed. Acute exposure to high doses produces focal myocardial necrosis, particularly in the apical and subendocardial location. These appear as small, pale, or hemorrhagic areas.

MICROSCOPIC FINDINGS: In acute injury there is focal contraction band necrosis of myocytes, various stages of myocytolysis, and focal replacement and interstitial fibrosis. With chronic exposure there may be myocyte hypertrophy. Rarely, significant damage to muscular arteries may be observed. The inflammatory response is characterized by lymphocytes and monocytes, with a paucity of polymorphonuclear leukocytes.

REMARKS: Damage is associated with nonreceptor selective adrenergic agonists, although beta agonists may cause focal injury. A reversible cardiomyopathy has been described with pheochromocytoma that leads to a restoration of cardiac function after the tumor is removed. This has been interpreted as the absence of significant myocardial necrosis and scarring but may reflect cessation of ongoing toxicity. See entry, Myocarditis, catecholamine-induced.

DIFFERENTIAL DIAGNOSIS: Cocaine cardiomyopathy can mimic all of the features of catecholamine injury. Patients with cardiomyopathy due to other causes and with cardiogenic shock, may have additive catecholamine-induced damage secondary to administered agents. Patients with congestive heart failure also have chronically elevated catecholamine levels that may contribute to myocardial injury. The diagnosis of catecholamine-associated cardiomyopathy should be reserved for cardiac disease secondary only to catecholamines without other known cause.

KEY DIAGNOSTIC CRITERIA: The presence of contraction band necrosis and myocytolysis are indicative of catecholamine-induced injury.

POTENTIAL PITFALLS: Difficulty in separating catecholamine effects from other causes of myocardial damage.

References

1. Bloom S, Cancilla PA. Myocytolysis and mitochondrial calcification in rat myocardium after low doses of isoproterenol. *Am J Pathol* 1969;54:373–392.
2. Rona G. Editorial review: Catecholamine cardiotoxicity. *J Mol Cell Cardiol* 1985;17:291–306.
3. Imperato-McGinley J, Gautier T, Ehlers K, Zullo MA, Goldstein DS, Vaughan ED, Jr. Reversibility of catecholamine-induced dilated cardiomyopathy in a child with a pheochromocytoma. *N Engl J Med* 1987;316:793–797.

CARDIOMYOPATHY, COBALT-ASSOCIATED

Entry Author: Stephen M. Factor

SYNONYM: Beer-drinker's heart.

DEFINITION: Development of severe dilated cardiomyopathy following the ingestion of beer-containing cobalt. Cobalt intoxication following industrial exposure or from therapeutic administration of cobalt salts rarely may lead to a similar syndrome.

GROSS FINDINGS: Dilated, hypertrophied, and flabby heart with mural thrombi common. Often associated with pericardial effusion. Areas of myocardial necrosis may be visible, occasionally even resembling myocardial infarction.

MICROSCOPIC FINDINGS: Multifocal and extensive myocellular necrosis and degeneration. Hyaline necrosis and vacuolar change of myocytes. Interstitial edema, focal inflammation, and fibrosis. Edema of small muscular blood vessels. Electron microscopy shows characteristic cobalt profiles.

REMARKS: Clinical condition virtually disappeared after removal of cobalt (as a foam stabilizer) from beer after outbreaks were described in 1960s from Quebec and Omaha, among other areas. Preconditioning of human subjects by protein deficiency appears to be necessary for the full-blown disease.

DIFFERENTIAL DIAGNOSIS: Alcoholic cardiomyopathy.

KEY DIAGNOSTIC CRITERIA: Dilated cardiomyopathy with extensive acute and subacute damage following the ingestion of cobalt salts (with associated protein deficiency).

POTENTIAL PITFALLS: May mimic other toxic cardiomyopathies, particularly that related to chronic alcohol ingestion.

CARDIOMYOPATHY, COCAINE-ASSOCIATED

Entry Author: Stephen M. Factor

SYNONYM: "Crack heart."

DEFINITION: Acute or chronic myocardial damage secondary to the direct or indirect effects of illicit cocaine use.

GROSS FINDINGS: Complex and variable. The heart may be concentrically hypertrophied with multifocal areas of necrosis or scarring. Segmental myocardial infarction or scars may be present. Coronary arteries may have focal atherosclerotic lesions, more severe or extensive than anticipated by age or gender of the patient. Coronary thrombosis may be superimposed on plaques.

MICROSCOPIC FINDINGS: Contraction band necrosis, acutely. Multifocal myocytolysis in various stages of healing. Segmental scars if coronary artery disease is severe. Small vessel thickening. Rarely, focal active myocarditis (see Myocarditis, cocaine-induced).

REMARKS: Condition may mimic ischemic heart disease or it may lead to a dilated cardiomyopathy, similar to catecholamine-associated cardiomyopathy (see *Cardiomyopathy, catecholamine-associated*). Diagnosis occasionally can be made by endomyocardial biopsy, if focal ischemic (myocytolytic) lesion is sampled.

DIFFERENTIAL DIAGNOSIS: Catecholamine-associated cardiomyopathy, ischemic heart disease, hypertensive heart disease, idiopathic sudden arrhythmic death.

KEY DIAGNOSTIC CRITERIA: Hypertrophied ventricle with multifocal scars, with or without coronary artery disease. Contraction band necrosis and myocytolysis are characteristic lesions. Presence of cocaine or cocaine derivatives in blood and tissues, or a documented clinical history of prior cocaine abuse.

POTENTIAL PITFALLS: In absence of cocaine in system or history of cocaine abuse, may be difficult to differentiate from hypertensive or ischemic heart disease, or other conditions associated with high levels of catecholamines.

SEE ALSO: Myocarditis, cocaine-associated.

CARDIOMYOPATHY, DIABETIC

Entry Author: Stephen M. Factor

DEFINITION: Development of myocardial disease out of proportion to the degree of coronary atherosclerosis (if any) in patients with insulin- or noninsulin-dependent diabetes mellitus, usually of greater than 10 years duration, and often in association with systemic hypertension.

GROSS FINDINGS: Cardiomegaly, with a firm, somewhat pale concentrically hypertrophied left ventricle and a small left ventricular cavity. Infrequently, the ventricle may be dilated. Right ventricle may be hypertrophied and dilated. Small, focal scars may be seen. Significant coronary artery atherosclerotic plaques may be present or absent.

MICROSCOPIC FINDINGS: Marked myocellular hypertrophy. Diffuse interstitial fibrosis, and multifocal replacement and perivascular fibrosis. Myocytolysis in various stages of organization. Extensive small muscular artery disease. Microaneurysms of the coronary microcirculation may be demonstrated with perfusion studies.

REMARKS: Relatively rare to see full-blown picture of diabetic cardiomyopathy in the absence of hypertension. Extensive interstitial scarring contributes to myocardial stiffness and gives rise to diastolic and systolic dysfunction. Microcirculation abnormal.

DIFFERENTIAL DIAGNOSIS: Ischemic heart disease, hypertensive heart disease.

KEY DIAGNOSTIC CRITERIA: Cardiomegaly with marked concentric hypertrophy and extensive myocardial fibrosis out of proportion to the degree of coronary artery disease in a patient with chronic diabetes mellitus and hypertension.

POTENTIAL PITFALLS: May be difficult to separate effects of diabetes mellitus from those of ischemic heart disease, hypertension, or other complications of diabetes mellitus (e.g., chronic renal failure).

CARDIOMYOPATHY, DUCHENNE MUSCULAR DYSTROPHY-ASSOCIATED

Entry Author: Renu Virmani

DEFINITION: Duchenne muscular dystrophy is a sex-linked recessive disorder, transmitted by the mother to one half of her sons as overt disease and to one half of her daughters who are carriers. The incidence is believed to be 1:5,000 male births in the general population. The defective gene is located on the X chromosome. Dystrophin, a high molecular weight protein, normally present in the sarcolemma of skeletal muscle, is absent in patients with Duchenne dystrophy. Patients with this condition have an abnormal electrocardiogram with short P-R interval. The QRS shows an anterior shift in right precordial leads and deep but narrow Q-waves in leads I, AVL, and V4-6.

GROSS FINDINGS: Biventricular dilation and hypertrophy more marked on the left side. There is scarring of the posterobasal and lateral wall of the left ventricle.

MICROSCOPIC FINDINGS: Severe subepicardial fibrosis of the left ventricle but the subendocardium also shows areas of fibrosis with interspersed myocytes. No inflammation is found in areas of fibrosis. Ultrastructurally, there is myofibrillar loss, with disorganized Z-band material and preservation of transverse tubules. The epicardial coronary arteries are normal, but intramural coronary arteries may show luminal narrowing.

SPECIAL PROCEDURES NEEDED FOR DIAGNOSIS: The electrocardiogram is fairly specific for cardiac involvement. Female carriers show some abnormalities when compared to normal women, with R/S ratio larger in leads V1-2 in the carrier group. Noninvasive positron emission tomography and echocardiography may show segmental abnormalities of the LV wall, with accelerated exogenous glucose (^{18}F fluorodeoxyglucose) utilization in the posterobasal and contiguous lateral wall of the left ventricle.

DIFFERENTIAL DIAGNOSIS: Idiopathic dilated cardiomyopathy or other muscular dystrophies must be considered, but absence of dystrophin in skeletal muscle biopsies is diagnostic.

KEY DIAGNOSTIC CRITERIA: The absence of dystrophin establishes the diagnosis of Duchenne muscular dystrophy. Cardiac involvement is established pathologically by a dilated and enlarged heart, ultrastructural findings of myofibrillar loss, disorganized Z-band material, and preservation of transverse tubules.

CARDIOMYOPATHY, ELECTRIC SHOCK-ASSOCIATED

Entry Author: Stephen M. Factor

DEFINITION: Acute myocardial damage associated with electrical trauma (e.g., electrocution or lightening), or chronic damage. Rarely associated with electroconvulsive therapy (ECT).

MICROSCOPIC FINDINGS: Acutely, contraction band necrosis and myocytolysis (see entry) with scarification if there is survival. Segmental myocardial infarction. Necrosis of smooth muscle of coronary arteries may be observed. Multifocal scars with ECT.

REMARKS: Direct effects of electrical injury on myocardium with acute electrocution, or indirect effects due to coronary artery spasm or injury leading to thrombosis. Elevated catecholamines may contribute to myocardial injury in cases with repeated ECT events.

DIFFERENTIAL DIAGNOSIS: Coronary artery disease, acute ischemic heart disease, catecholamine-induced injury.

KEY DIAGNOSTIC CRITERIA: Unequivocal evidence of acute electrical injury (e.g., witnessed event, superficial burn). In cases with ECT as the purported etiology of injury, there should be no other potential cause for observed pathology, such as coronary atherosclerosis.

POTENTIAL PITFALLS: In presence of coronary artery disease, and in the absence of history of electrical burn, it may be impossible to say with certainty that electric shock led to sudden death or chronic myocardial injury.

CARDIOMYOPATHY, HEAT STROKE-ASSOCIATED

Entry Author: Stephen M. Factor

DEFINITION: Myocardial injury following prolonged exposure to high ambient temperatures leading to body temperature of more than 40°C. Alternatively, may be seen with severe exertion. In either case, electrolyte abnormalities are common, and in exertional heat-stroke there may be generalized rhabdomyolysis.

GROSS FINDINGS: When severe, the heart may be dilated and flabby. Otherwise, there may be no notable gross abnormalities.

MICROSCOPIC FINDINGS: Multifocal hyaline degeneration of myocytes (presence of eosinophilic protein droplets in sarcoplasm) and coagulative necrosis. Myocytolysis may be seen also. Intramyocardial small vessel thrombi focally.

REMARKS: Diagnosis, particularly in elderly with associated coronary artery disease, is dependent on demonstration of high ambient temperatures and elevation of core temperature.

DIFFERENTIAL DIAGNOSIS: Coronary artery disease, in appropriate age group.

KEY DIAGNOSTIC CRITERIA: Elevated core temperature.

POTENTIAL PITFALLS: Absence of significant elevation of core temperature makes diagnosis unlikely.

CARDIOMYOPATHY, HIV-ASSOCIATED

Entry Author: Renu Virmani

SYNONYMS: AIDS-associated dilated cardiomyopathy, AIDS cardiomyopathy.

DEFINITION: Severe congestive heart failure due to myocardial dysfunction associated with infection by the human immunodeficiency virus. Not distinguishable from idiopathic dilated cardiomyopathy either clinically or morphologically. This diagnosis should not normally be made in the presence of an opportunistic infection of the heart.

GROSS FINDINGS: The heart is enlarged but not excessively. The most impressive finding is dilation of all four chambers (ventricles more than atria). There may be thrombi in any or all of the chambers.

MICROSCOPIC FINDINGS: Myocarditis is most often seen but is usually mild to moderate with myocyte necrosis. To diagnose dilated cardiomyopathy there should be absence of opportunistic infections, but often such infection is not marked enough to explain the clinical picture of severe congestive heart failure. There is some myocyte hypertrophy, but it is usually not impressive. Interstitial fibrosis is sometimes present.

SPECIAL PROCEDURES NEEDED FOR DIAGNOSIS: Clinically, echocardiography may be useful in identifying global left ventricular dysfunction as the cause of the dyspnea, as opposed to primary lung disease, which must be ruled out.

DIFFERENTIAL DIAGNOSIS: Severe septicemia terminally can lead to global left ventricular dysfunction and must be excluded before diagnosing HIV-associated cardiomyopathy. Also, specific opportunistic infections of the myocardium, such as CMV, toxoplasmosis, and fungal infections must be ruled out.

KEY DIAGNOSTIC CRITERIA: None of the morphologic or clinical findings are specific for HIV-associated cardiomyopathy.

POTENTIAL PITFALLS: Dilated cardiomyopathy from any specific causes in a patient with HIV disease may be mistakenly diagnosed as HIV-associated cardiomyopathy.

CARDIOMYOPATHY, HYPERPARATHYROIDISM-ASSOCIATED

Entry Author: Stephen M. Factor

SYNONYM: Hypercalcemic heart disease

DEFINITION: Cardiac damage due to the effects of either primary or secondary hyperparathyroidism.

GROSS FINDINGS: No specific features. If there is associated hypertension due to primary hyperparathyroidism or secondary to renal failure, then left ventricular hypertrophy will be present. If renal failure is the cause, then there also may be acute or chronic fibrinous pericarditis. Gritty white foci of myocardial calcification may be seen but rarely. When present, may be detected by scraping scalpel blade along cut surface of myocardium. Valvular or annular calcification may be present.

MICROSCOPIC FINDINGS: Foci of single or grouped myocytes with calcification. Intramyocardial vessels and epicardial coronary arteries may have calcification of their elastic laminae with extension into medial smooth muscle. If there is associated hypertension, then myocellular hypertrophy and myocardial fibrosis will be observed.

REMARKS: Unclear if the etiology of focal calcification is elevated calcium that causes myocellular necrosis with dystrophic deposition in dead cells. Experimental evidence suggests that this occurs.

DIFFERENTIAL DIAGNOSIS: Hypercalcemia due to other causes (e.g., metastatic or metabolic bone disease).

KEY DIAGNOSTIC CRITERIA: Dystrophic calcification in the heart associated with either primary or secondary elevation of parathormone.

POTENTIAL PITFALLS: Rarely, calcification of necrotic myocytes can occur in the absence of abnormal calcium metabolism. Annular and valvular calcification occurs commonly, unrelated to elevated parathormone levels.

CARDIOMYOPATHY, HYPERTROPHIC

Entry Author: Robert J. Siegel

SYNONYMS: Idiopathic hypertrophic subaortic stenosis (IHSS), asymmetric septal hypertrophy (ASH), hypertrophic obstructive cardiomyopathy, and many more. Hypertrophic cardiomyopathy (HCM) is the preferred term.

DEFINITION: A primary disorder of heart muscle leading to myocardial hypertrophy, often asymmetric and primarily involving interventricular septum. Characteristically associated with myocyte disarray, microvascular sclerosis, and focal scarification.

GROSS FINDINGS: Classically, the basal portion of the interventricular septum (IVS) is hypertrophic and bulges into the left ventricular outflow tract. This alters hemodynamics in such a way that the anterior leaflet of the mitral valve may slap against the septal endocardium, causing thickening of this leaflet and a corresponding (mirror image) fibrotic endocardial patch at the point of contact with the interventricular septum. ASH is said to be present if the ratio of interventricular septum thickness to that of the posterior left ventricular wall is greater than 1.5. However, hypertrophic cardiomyopathy may instead cause concentric hypertrophy (see entry), or asymmetric hypertrophy, in the apical or mid-ventricular regions. Hypertrophy of the septal band in the right ventricular outflow tract also may occur.

MICROSCOPIC FINDINGS: The hallmark is myocardial fiber disarray noted in the hypertrophic area. In the septal hypertrophy type, a horizontal section at the mid-portion of the IVS should be examined. Disarray is characterized by a disorganized, whorled, or tangled orientation of myocardial fibers that are multipolar rather than bipolar (i.e., branching may be prominent). This abnormality should occupy at least 5% of the cross sectional area. Myocyte hypertrophy and interstitial fibrosis (see entry), are present. The fibrosis associated with fiber disarray has a haphazard arrangement referred to as *plexiform.* Intramyocardial arterioles typically are thick-walled.

REMARKS: Mutations in the beta-cardiac myosin gene have been found in cases of phenotypically classic HCM as well as in asymptomatic family members, suggesting that the genetic abnormality is causative. HCM may be inherited as an autosomal dominant condition with variable penetrance, although sporadic cases are common.

DIFFERENTIAL DIAGNOSIS: Asymmetric septal hypertrophy may occur in elderly individuals and in others who do not demonstrate the full clinical and pathologic features of HCM. It is unclear whether these patients have HCM or an acquired cardiac disorder with overlapping morphologic features. In children and elderly patients, HCM may present as dilated cardiomyopathy. HCM is an important cause of sudden death, particularly in young adults.

KEY DIAGNOSTIC CRITERIA: Unexplained hypertrophy, most commonly asymmetric septal, occurring in young individuals. In this form the interventricular septum thickness should be at least 1.5 times that of the posterior left ventricular wall and myocardial fiber disarray should occupy more than 5% of the area in the affected zone.

POTENTIAL PITFALLS: Small areas of disarray occur in normal hearts, especially at the junction of IVS and RV.

References

1. Maron BJ, Roberts EC. Quantitative analysis of cardiac muscle cell disorganization in the ventricular septum of patients with hypertrophic cardiomyopathy. *Circ* 1979;59:689–706.
2. Shapiro LM. Hypertrophic cardiomyopathy in the elderly. *Br Heart J* 1990;67:265–266.
3. Watkins H, Seidman CE, MacRae C, Deidman JG, McKenna W. Progress in familial hypertrophic cardiomyopathy: Molecular genetic analyses in the original family studied by Teare. *Br Heart J* 1992;67: 34–38.

CARDIOMYOPATHY, IDIOPATHIC DILATED

Entry Author: Renu Virmani

SYNONYMS: Congestive cardiomyopathy, Cardiomyopathy NOS.

DEFINITION: Contractile dysfunction of the myocardium resulting in decreased ejection fraction, dilation of all cardiac chambers, and diffuse ventricular hypokinesis with no demonstrable etiology such as systemic hypertension, coronary artery disease, valvular disease, congenital heart disease, or intrinsic pulmonary disease. There may be secondary mitral and/or tricuspid valve regurgitation.

GROSS FINDINGS: The heart is globular in shape and increased in weight. All four cardiac chambers are dilated, ventricles more than atria. There may be focal myocardial and/or patchy endocardial fibrosis. Mural thrombi are present in the dependent parts of the atria or ventricles in 50% of cases.

MICROSCOPIC FINDINGS: Findings are nonspecific, with or without interstitial or focal fibrosis and myocyte hypertrophy (best appreciated as nuclear hypertrophy) with myofibrillar loss or myocyte atrophy. Lipofuscin deposition and basophilic degeneration may be pronounced. Mild chronic lymphocytic inflammation is present in over 50% of cases.

SPECIAL PROCEDURES NEEDED FOR DIAGNOSIS: Because this is a diagnosis of exclusion, it is necessary to rule out many conditions that can lead to congestive heart failure with a gross picture similar to that of idiopathic dilated cardiomyopathy. These include systemic hypertension, coronary atherosclerosis with healed myocardial infarction, valvular heart disease, congenital heart disease, and intrinsic lung diseases. Over 75 specific heart diseases may cause dilated cardiomyopathy, including myocarditis, storage diseases, amyloidosis, hemochromatosis, toxic cardiomyopathy, sarcoidosis, post partum cardiomyopathy, alcoholism, and HIV infection. Endomyocardial biopsy is performed to help rule out the presence of specific diseases.

DIFFERENTIAL DIAGNOSIS: Any condition that gives rise to congestive heart failure may be confused with idiopathic cardiomyopathy. During life, echocardiography and cardiac catheterization procedures help exclude presence of valvular abnormalities, congenital heart disease, coronary heart disease.

KEY DIAGNOSTIC CRITERIA: Enlarged heart with ventricles dilated more than atria in the absence of any specific condition that may cause congestive heart failure. Myocardial hypertrophy (heart weight >350 g for women, >400 g for men). Endomyocardial biopsy is important to help exclude specific conditions that can present as dilated cardiomyopathy. Typical diagnosis on endomyocardial biopsy report from a case of dilated cardiomyopathy will read "myocyte hypertrophy, focal myofibrillar loss, focal and interstitial fibrosis. In the absence of coronary, valvular, and hypertensive heart disease, the findings are consistent with dilated cardiomyopathy."

POTENTIAL PITFALLS: Always know detailed clinical history and rule out specific conditions that can cause congestive heart failure. Focal diseases, such as sarcoidosis, can be difficult to demonstrate by morphological means during life.

CARDIOMYOPATHY, IRON TOXICITY-ASSOCIATED

Entry Author: Stephen M. Factor

SYNONYMS: Cardiomyopathy of hemochromatosis ("bronze diabetes"), hemosiderosis.

DEFINITION: Abnormal deposition of iron in the myocardium regardless of the etiology. Such deposition is associated with autosomal recessive hemochromatosis or the increased iron load (hemosiderosis) due to chronic transfusion therapy for anemia (e.g., thalassemia or sickle cell anemia) and rarely to chronic ingestion of iron salts.

GROSS FINDINGS: Moderate cardiomegaly with predominant left ventricular hypertrophy and dilation. Myocardium has a chocolate brown color and may be firm or flabby. Fibrosis may be visible and may be preferentially in the subepicardium with relative sparing of the subendocardium.

MICROSCOPIC FINDINGS: Intramyocellular iron deposition, confirmed by iron stain, electron microscopy, and biochemical analysis. Iron and myocellular degeneration are more prevalent in subepicardium of ventricle than the subendocardium. Atria and conduction system are relatively spared. Iron deposition may occasionally be observed in histiocytes within fibrous tissue. Interstitial and replacement multifocal fibrosis may be extensive in the ventricle but is often not as severe as the iron deposition.

REMARKS: Because of the increased subepicardial localization of iron and fibrosis, endomyocardial biopsy may not provide a representative sample of myocardium.

SPECIAL PROCEDURES NEEDED FOR DIAGNOSIS: Iron stains should be carried out, whenever iron deposition is suspected, to rule out presence of other confounding golden pigment in myocytes (e.g., lipofuscin).

DIFFERENTIAL DIAGNOSIS: Increased lipofuscin pigment ("brown atrophy") in the elderly, in cachexia, and in amiodarone cardiotoxicity may resemble iron pigment. Iron stain will be negative with lipofuscin. Increased iron also may accumulate in the myocardium of patients with copper toxicity (Wilson's disease).

KEY DIAGNOSTIC CRITERIA: Presence of iron in myocytes in association with hemochromatosis affecting the skin, pancreas, and liver, or in conjunction with an acquired increased iron load.

POTENTIAL PITFALLS: Underestimation of severity because of reliance on endomyocardial biopsy when deposits and fibrosis are most severe in the subepicardium. Confusion of lipofuscin with iron is also a possibility.

CARDIOMYOPATHY, ISCHEMIC

Entry Author: Renu Vermani

SYNONYMS: End-stage coronary heart disease with congestive heart failure.

DEFINITION: Burch and colleagues coined the term to describe patients in whom coronary artery disease resulted in severe myocardial dysfunction leading to heart failure. Morphologically healed myocardial infarction, dilated ventricles, and severe coronary atherosclerosis.

GROSS FINDINGS: There is myocardial fibrosis (subendocardial or transmural) reflecting prior multiple infarcts, left ventricular dilation, and signs of congestive heart failure. Diffuse focal fibrosis may also be present reflecting global ischemia. Patient also has severe coronary atherosclerosis often with complete occlusion of one or more major arteries. There is no evidence of acute myocardial infarction. Patients with ventricular aneurysms are usually not considered to have ischemic cardiomyopathy.

MICROSCOPIC FINDINGS: There may be one large healed transmural or subendocardial infarct or multiple infarcts widely distributed in the left ventricle. Diffuse interstitial fibrosis not grossly apparent may be seen histologically. Myocytes adjacent to areas of scarification are usually hypertrophied but may show evidence of acute ischemia.

SPECIAL PROCEDURES NEEDED FOR DIAGNOSIS: Coronary arteries must be examined.

DIFFERENTIAL DIAGNOSIS: Idiopathic dilated cardiomyopathy is ruled out when severe coronary atherosclerosis is found.

KEY DIAGNOSTIC CRITERIA: Presence of severe coronary atherosclerosis, left ventricular myocardial scarring (healed infarcts), with ventricular dilation.

POTENTIAL PITFALLS: The term *ischemic cardiomyopathy* is not universally accepted, and many consider it misleading because it indicates a primary coronary arterial disease and a secondary myocardial disease. From this perspective, it would be better called congestive heart failure secondary to severe coronary atherosclerosis and myocardial infarction.

CARDIOMYOPATHY, MYOTONIC DYSTROPHY-ASSOCIATED

Entry Author: Renu Virmani

SYNONYM: Steinert's disease.

DEFINITION: An autosomal dominant (locus on chromosome 19) multisystem disorder that results in weakness of the flexor muscle of the neck, atrophy of the sternocleidomastoid muscles, and presence of myotonia (delayed relaxation after contraction) after voluntary, mechanical, or electrical stimulation. The nonmyopathic features include cataracts, testicular atrophy, premature baldness, mental deterioration, and involvement of smooth muscle (esophagus, colon, uterus). Cardiac manifestations are most prevalent in the conduction system, rather than the "working" myocardium. The most common electrocardiographic abnormalities are prolonged P–R interval, left anterior fascicular block, and increased QRS duration. These reflect His-Purkinje disease.

GROSS FINDINGS: Most hearts appear normal. However, some show hypertrophy, dilation, or both, and focal fibrosis. Coronary arteries are normal.

MICROSCOPIC FINDINGS: The most frequent histopathologic findings are in the conduction system. These consist of fibrosis, fatty infiltration, and atrophy of the sinus node, AV node, His bundle, and bundle branches. The remainder of the myocardium may be unremarkable, but patchy interstitial fibrosis, fatty infiltration, and hypertrophy have been described in a small proportion of individuals.

SPECIAL PROCEDURES NEEDED FOR DIAGNOSIS: The electrocardiogram is a sensitive determinant of conduction system involvement.

DIFFERENTIAL DIAGNOSIS: Myotonia congenita (Thompsen's disease) and paramyotonia congenita must be differentiated from myotonic muscular dystrophy. Thompsen's disease is characterized by myotonia but not dystrophy, and is a benign disease with normal longevity and no cardiac involvement. Paramyotonia congenita is a rare autosomal dominant condition characterized by prolonged myotonic reaction to cold. There is no cardiac involvement described.

KEY DIAGNOSTIC CRITERIA: There are no diagnostic changes to be found in the cardiac morphology. The diagnosis is established by clinical criteria given in the definition.

POTENTIAL PITFALLS: A diagnosis of myotonic dystrophy cardiomyopathy should not be made without supportive clinical information.

CARDIOMYOPATHY, MYXEDEMA-ASSOCIATED

Entry Author: Stephen M. Factor

SYNONYM: Hypothyroid heart disease.

DEFINITION: Cardiac damage specifically related to the effects of hypothyroidism.

GROSS FINDINGS: Diffuse cardiomegaly, with ventricular hypertrophy and dilation of all four chambers. Myocardium has been described as pale and flabby. Protein-rich pericardial effusion is common. There is accelerated atherosclerosis.

MICROSCOPIC FINDINGS: Myocardial hypertrophy. Many myocytes have sarcoplasmic basophilic inclusions ("basophilic degeneration") that stain brilliantly magenta with PAS and are diastase resistant. These are not a specific finding. Electron microscopy reveals electron dense, granular material that is not glycogen and resembles Lafora bodies. Intramyocardial muscular arteries are thick walled. Interstitial fibrosis may be present focally. Ischemic damage may occur if coronary disease is severe.

REMARKS: Often a difficult disease to diagnose, particularly in elderly with coronary artery disease and hypertension. Presence of basophilic inclusions is often a helpful clue. The accelerated atherosclerosis is secondary to altered lipid metabolism characteristic of hypothyroidism.

DIFFERENTIAL DIAGNOSIS: The presence of hypothyroidism, which is an absolute requirement for this diagnosis, is important in separating this from ischemic heart disease, hypertensive heart disease, basophilic degeneration of the elderly, familial cardiomyopathy (Lafora body disease).

KEY DIAGNOSTIC CRITERIA: Presence of cardiac disease out of proportion to degree of coronary artery atherosclerosis, and in association with clinical hypothyroidism, including abnormal thyroid function tests (low T_4 and elevated TSH).

CARDIOMYOPATHY, POTASSIUM DEPLETION-ASSOCIATED

Entry Author: Stephen M. Factor

SYNONYM: Hypokalemic cardiomyopathy.

DEFINITION: Myocardial injury secondary to the effects of systemic depletion of potassium (hypokalemia).

GROSS FINDINGS: No specific features.

MICROSCOPIC FINDINGS: Multifocal or generalized swelling, pallor, and vacuolization of myocytes of all chamber walls. In experimental animals, there is myocytolytic necrosis involving all chambers progressing to organization and focal interstitial fibrosis. Similar changes occur in patients whose condition is complicated by factors other than hypokalemia (as is often the case), such as dehydration or complex electrolyte abnormalities.

REMARKS: Serum potassium level is only a rough guide for intracellular potassium. Thus, a direct correlation between serum potassium level and the development of pathology is not possible. In general, however, pathological changes may be observed when serum levels are below 3.0 mEq/L for prolonged periods of time. Severe hyperkalemia (serum potassium usually exceeding 7.0 mEq/L) is also cardiotoxic, causing arrhythmia, but this is not associated with any morphologic change.

DIFFERENTIAL DIAGNOSIS: Myocytolytic necrosis may be seen in conditions associated with severe hypokalemia (e.g., dehydration and electrolyte imbalance due to vomiting or diarrhea).

KEY DIAGNOSTIC CRITERIA: Widespread myocellular swelling and vacuolization in patient with hypokalemia.

POTENTIAL PITFALLS: Difficulty in assessing cause of myocytolytic damage in complex disease states associated with hypokalemia because other possible etiologies are often present.

CARDIOMYOPATHY, RADIATION-ASSOCIATED

Entry Author: Stephen M. Factor

DEFINITION: Cardiac damage secondary to the effects of ionizing radiation directed at the mediastinum and surrounding structures.

GROSS FINDINGS: No specific features. Because radiation leads to a pancardiac injury there may be pericardial and epicardial fibrosis, particularly over the anterior surfaces of the heart. Coronary arteries may show fibrous plaques in their proximal segments. Radiation may induce atherosclerosis in coronary arteries of young people. Myocardium may have segmental or focal scarring. Valves may be thickened and, rarely, insufficient.

MICROSCOPIC FINDINGS: Acute damage may lead to myocardial edema, hemorrhage, and acute neutrophilic inflammation. Acute valvulitis and fibrinous pericarditis may be seen. Chronically, myocardial scarring associated with vascular sclerosis (more in the right than left ventricle) is characteristic.

REMARKS: Cardiac damage may be delayed several years after completion of radiotherapy. Radiation-induced damage is also potentially additive to that of chemotherapeutic agents that affect the heart (see *Cardiomyopathy, anthracycline-associated*).

DIFFERENTIAL DIAGNOSIS: Tumor involving the pericardium and myocardium. Hypothyroidism (see *Cardiomyopathy, myxedema-associated*) due to mediastinal radiation. Ischemic heart disease secondary to pre-existing coronary artery atherosclerosis or due to radiation-induced coronary artery damage.

KEY DIAGNOSTIC CRITERIA: Mediastinal radiation. Fibrosis of the pericardium and myocardium, with greater damage of the right ventricle than the left (unless there is significant coronary artery disease). Microscopic scarring with hyperplastic, atypical fibroblasts, and thickened small vessels with prominent endothelial cells.

POTENTIAL PITFALLS: May be difficult to separate the effects of direct radiation injury from those of other anti-neoplastic agents or underlying ischemic heart disease.

CARDIOMYOPATHY, RESTRICTIVE

Entry Author: Robert J. Siegel

SYNONYMS: Obliterative, restrictive-obliterative, infiltrative, nondilated cardiomyopathy.

DEFINITION: Heart dysfunction manifested by impairment of ventricular filling (decreased compliance, diastolic dysfunction). This definition encompasses (a) fibrosing disorders of the endomyocardium, such as endomyocardial fibrosis (EMF), Loeffler's endocardial fibrosis (LE), and endocardial fibroelastosis (EFE)]; (b) infiltrative disorders such as amyloidosis and neoplastic infiltrates; (c) intracellular accumulations, such as iron or glycogen storage products;

(d) other disorders with excessive myocardial scarring. (Also, see entries: *Endomyocardial fibrosis, tropical* and *Myocarditis, eosinophilic, hypereosinophilia syndrome*).

GROSS FINDINGS: In EMF and the fibrotic stage of LE, a plaque-like endocardial fibrotic patch typically involves the inflow tract and has a rolled edge. Mural thrombus is often present. In LE, a pearly-white rubbery thickening of the endocardium affects mainly the left ventricle. EFE is grossly similar to EMF but is limited to infants and small children. Neoplastic heart involvement may be detected grossly as streaky white infiltrates or nodular tumor masses. Significant biatrial dilation is typical of the restrictive disorders.

MICROSCOPIC FINDINGS: In EMF, a dense acellular collagen layer is seen on the endocardial surface. Late stages of LE are histologically similar, but infiltrates of eosinophils with myocyte necrosis and eosinophil-rich thrombi characterize earlier stages. The hallmark of EFE is the elastin-rich endocardial fibrosis. Infiltrative disorders are identified by the particular abnormal intercellular or intracellular component.

REMARKS: Endomyocardial biopsy has a relatively high diagnostic yield in this group of disorders.

DIFFERENTIAL DIAGNOSIS: The main clinical differential is constrictive pericarditis.

KEY DIAGNOSTIC CRITERIA: Obliterative endocardial fibrosis, myocardial infiltrates or accumulations.

References

1. Edwards WD. In: Virmani R, Atkinson J, Fenoglio J. *Major Problems in Pathology: Cardiovascular Pathology,* WB Saunders Co., 1991;23:282–292.
2. Wilmshurst PT, Katritsis D. Restrictive cardiomyopathy. *Br Heart J* 1990;63:323–324.

CARDIOMYOPATHY, SELENIUM DEFICIENCY-ASSOCIATED

Entry Author: Stephen M. Factor

SYNONYMS: Keshan disease, white muscle disease (of swine).

DEFINITION: Multifocal myocardial necrosis with inflammation followed by healing with scar formation, associated with chronic dietary deficiency of selenium (and possibly vitamin E). Particularly associated with the Keshan district of China where the condition was apparently widespread until the introduction of selenium supplements to the diet.

GROSS FINDINGS: Acutely, the heart may be dilated, edematous, and flabby with mural thrombi. Chronically, the heart is enlarged, hypertrophied, and dilated, with multifocal scarring.

MICROSCOPIC FINDINGS: Acutely, interstitial edema and focal areas of contraction band necrosis. In chronic deficiency there is contraction band necrosis, myocytolysis, and various stages of healing leading to replacement scars.

REMARKS: It is uncertain if selenium deficiency alone can be responsible for cardiac damage, or if vitamin E deficiency along with malnourishment is also required. Supplemental selenium in the diet of individuals living in Keshan, China, appears to have prevented cardiac disease. Deficiency of selenium and other anti-oxidants may occur in severely malnourished patients with cancer or AIDS leading to development of cardiomyopathy similar to Keshan disease.

DIFFERENTIAL DIAGNOSIS: Stress, high catecholamine states, and other types of malnutrition can lead to the multifocal damage characteristic of selenium deficiency.

KEY DIAGNOSTIC CRITERIA: Multifocal damage with contraction band necrosis and myocytolysis with decreased levels of tissue selenium.

POTENTIAL PITFALLS: Etiology may be multifactorial. Selenium deficiency alone does not produce damage experimentally unless vitamin E is also deficient. May be a cause of cardiomyopathy associated with severe cachexia but often not a diagnostic consideration.

CARDIOMYOPATHY, SERUM SICKNESS-ASSOCIATED

Entry Author: Stephen M. Factor

SYNONYMS: Hypersensitivity, type III; Immune complex hypersensitivity; antigen-antibody complex disease.

DEFINITION: Cardiac injury in the presence of endogenous or exogenous antigens that elicit an antibody response, with the antigen-antibody complex depositing in, and damaging, tissue.

GROSS FINDINGS: No specific features in the heart.

MICROSCOPIC FINDINGS: No changes unique to the heart. There may be a necrotizing vasculitis involving small intramyocardial vessels. Interstitial edema and hemorrhage, acute inflammation, and myocyte necrosis (e.g., changes diagnostic of myocarditis) are all features that may be observed.

REMARKS: The heart may be damaged as part of a systemic condition. Acute changes may lead to significant cardiac injury; more prolonged injury may occur with chronic antigen release (as in systemic lupus erythematosus). The chronically affected heart may show evidence of hypertrophy and multifocal scarring. Coronary artery vasculitis may cause ischemic necrosis.

DIFFERENTIAL DIAGNOSIS: Causes of vasculitis and myocarditis in the absence of antigen-antibody complexes must be considered.

KEY DIAGNOSTIC CRITERIA: Microscopic changes as described with either a strong clinical history of an event that may be associated with serum sickness (e.g., immunization or penicillin treatment) or the demonstration of tissue localized or circulating immune complexes.

POTENTIAL PITFALLS: Unless immune complexes are identified, the pathological changes are not specific.

CARDIOMYOPATHY, STEROID-ASSOCIATED

Entry Author: Stephen M. Factor

SYNONYMS: Glucocorticoid cardiomyopathy; Cushing's syndrome and cardiomyopathy; anabolic steroid cardiomyopathy.

DEFINITION: Development of cardiac disease in association with either exogenous chronic administration or elevated endogenous levels of glucocorticoids or anabolic steroids.

GROSS FINDINGS: Diffuse cardiomegaly, with concentric hypertrophy of the left ventricle. Adipose tissue may be prominent in the epicardium of patients with Cushing's syndrome. There is also evidence that adipose tissue is increased in the interstitium of the right ventricle, thereby appearing similar to arrhythmogenic right ventricular dysplasia (see entry). Focal scarring may be found in the left or right ventricle.

MICROSCOPIC FINDINGS: No specific feature. Myocyte hypertrophy, interstitial and focal fibrosis, and small vessel sclerosis with either glucocorticoid excess or anabolic steroid excess. Myocyte necrosis has been described.

REMARKS: Controversy exists over whether either type of steroid independently leads to cardiac damage. With glucocorticoids, the marked increased prevalence of hypertension, and the associated electrolyte abnormalities (see entry: *Potassium toxicity-associated*) of chronically elevated steroids can damage the heart secondarily. The increased adipose tissue may play no direct role in cardiac dysfunction unless abnormal right ventricular contractility and arrhythmias can be demonstrated. There is some theoretical support for the concept that damage to cardiac connective tissue due to steroid use may lead to contractile dysfunction. With anabolic steroids (e.g., used by weight lifters and other athletes), some reports have suggested that there is an associated cardiomyopathy because cases of sudden death have been observed. Anabolic steroids also have been linked to the development of a peripheral myopathy.

KEY DIAGNOSTIC CRITERIA: Presence of Cushing's syndrome or demonstrated chronic anabolic steroid use with cardiac changes as described.

POTENTIAL PITFALLS: Lack of specificity for the cardiac changes.

COAGULATIVE NECROSIS

Entry Author: Robert J. Siegel

SYNONYMS: Coagulation necrosis, infarct necrosis.

DEFINITION: The type of myocardial necrosis associated with infarction without reperfusion, in which myocytes retain their overall shape but undergo karyolysis and demonstrate a glassy, eosinophilic cytoplasm.

GROSS FINDINGS: The myocardium is pale in early stages. Subsequently yellow with hyperemic border.

MICROSCOPIC FINDINGS: Myocytes are hypereosinophilic and lack cytoplasmic detail, although "ghosts" or cross striations may persist. The cells retain their shape but may be stretched or wavy. Nuclei typically disappear in the first 24 hours.

DIFFERENTIAL DIAGNOSIS: Should be distinguished from the other major types of myocyte necrosis, namely contraction band necrosis and myocytolysis, although the latter may not reflect true necrosis (irreversible injury). These have different pathophysiologic implications but may coexist in ischemic heart disease.

KEY DIAGNOSTIC CRITERIA: Hypereosinophilic myocardial fibers without cytoplasmic detail, contraction bands, or nuclei.

POTENTIAL PITFALLS: Very early coagulative necrosis may be difficult to distinguish from regional variation in staining of tissue sections.

Reference

1. Baroldi G, Falzi G, Mariani F. Sudden coronary death. A postmortem study in 208 selected cases compared to 97 "normal" subjects. *Am Heart J* 1979;98:20–31.

CONTRACTION BAND ARTEFACT

Entry Author: Robert J. Siegel

SYNONYM: Contraction band change.

DEFINITION: Transverse eosinophilic bands in myocyte cytoplasm which occur as an artefact in a high proportion of endomyocardial biotome biopsies.

MICROSCOPIC FINDINGS: The myocardial fibers show transverse eosinophilic bands in the cytoplasm, indistinguishable from those seen in contraction band necrosis, except that myocyte nuclei in the latter are pyknotic. (see entry).

REMARKS: This histologic finding may occur in biopsies of normal hearts. Therefore, contraction band change is not an indicator of ischemic or reperfusion injury in endomyocardial biopsies.

DIFFERENTIAL DIAGNOSIS: Because contraction band change cannot be distinguished morphologically from contraction band necrosis, other features of the endomyocardial biopsy must be evaluated to identify true myocardial injury.

KEY DIAGNOSTIC CRITERIA: Eosinophilic bands in myocyte fibers.

POTENTIAL PITFALLS: Erroneous interpretation of contraction band change as evidence of *in vivo* myocyte injury when observed in an endomyocardial biopsy.

Reference

1. Edwards SW. Pathology of endomyocardial biopsy. In: Waller BF, ed. *Contemp issues in surgical pathol, vol. 12: Pathology of the heart and great vessels.* 1988:191–275.

CONTRACTION BAND NECROSIS

Entry Author: Robert J. Siegel

SYNONYMS: CBN, coagulative myocytolysis, Zenker necrosis, catecholamine necrosis.

DEFINITION: Transverse hypereosinophilic bands, known as *contraction bands*, within myocardial fibers, recognized in routine light microscopic preparations.

GROSS FINDINGS: No specific gross appearance indicates to CBN, but it is usually seen at the periphery of grossly recognized infarcts, where it is associated with reperfusion.

MICROSCOPIC FINDINGS: Dense transverse eosinophilic bands, often alternating with pale zones, are seen in the cytoplasm of myocardial fibers. Myocyte nuclei often are pyknotic. The finding may be focal, limited to isolated fibers or small groups of fibers or extensive. Commonly seen at the periphery of infarcts. Typically, there is no apparent relationship to blood vessels. The changes of CBN may be observed before an inflammatory reaction has developed. Ultra-structurally, there is hypercontraction, with fusion of adjacent Z-discs forming the contraction bands and disrupting the normal sarcomeric pattern.

REMARKS: CBN is the morphologic pattern associated with reperfusion injury or certain toxic states, such as catecholamine or cocaine-associated toxicity but may also occur in a variety of unrelated conditions. The change is thought to reflect a high level of intracellular calcium (calcium-mediated hypercontraction with Z-disc fusion) which occurs both in reperfusion of necrotic myocytes, catecholamine toxicity, and any situation where there is a strong inotropic stimulus.

DIFFERENTIAL DIAGNOSIS: Contraction bands are a common artefact in endomyocardial biopsies and should not be interpreted as evidence of necrosis unless there is corroborating evidence (see entry: *Contraction band change*). Pyknotic myocyte nuclei in CBN may be useful in distinguishing artefact from necrosis.

KEY DIAGNOSTIC CRITERIA: The transverse eosinophilic bands are characteristic in routine H&E sections.

POTENTIAL PITFALLS: Contraction band artefact in endomyocardial biopsies; see above.

References

1. Karch SB, Billingham ME. Myocardial contraction bands revisited. *Hum Pathol* 1986;17:9–13.
2. Baroldi G, Falzi G, Mariani F. Sudden coronary death. A postmortem study in 208 selected cases compared to 97 "control" subjects. *Am Heart J* 1979;98:20–31.

COR BOVINUM

Entry Author: Robert J. Siegel

SYNONYM: Massive myocardial hypertrophy.

DEFINITION: Outdated descriptive term for very large hearts, historically applied to hearts with massive hypertrophy and/or dilation such as occurs in volume overload (e.g., aortic insufficiency).

GROSS FINDINGS: See entries for myocardial hypertrophy and myocardial hypertrophy, volume overload.

REMARKS: Antiquated term. Included here because it unfortunately remains in use. More specific terms are preferred, such as massive myocardial hypertrophy or (if appropriate) massive four chamber dilation.

COR PULMONALE

Entry Author: Robert J. Siegel

DEFINITION: Right ventricular hypertrophy and/or dilation due to pulmonary hypertension.

GROSS FINDINGS: Enlargement (some degree of hypertrophy and/or dilation) of the right ventricle and occasionally the right atrium are present (see entries: *Myocardial hypertrophy* and *Cardiac dilation*). In the acute form, for example, associated with massive pulmonary embolism, only dilation is present. Right ventricular hypertrophy causes a characteristic straightening of the IVS. In some patients, unexplained LVH accompanies cor pulmonale.

MICROSCOPIC FINDINGS: The right ventricular myocardium shows myocardial hypertrophy (see entry).

REMARKS: The most common cause is chronic obstructive pulmonary disease, but other causes include pulmonary vascular diseases and structural or neuromuscular chest wall abnormalities. Increased pulmonary artery pressure appears to be the common denominator.

DIFFERENTIAL DIAGNOSIS: Other causes of right heart enlargement include valvular heart disease (tricuspid, pulmonic) and congenital heart disease (e.g., atrial septal defect). Right heart enlargement also may accompany disorders of left heart function.

KEY DIAGNOSTIC CRITERIA: Right ventricular enlargement in the presence of lung disease without other identifiable etiology.

Reference

1. Enson T. Pulmonary heart disease: Relation of pulmonary hypertension to abnormal lung structure and function. *Bull NY Acad Med* 1977;53:551–566.

CYSTICERCOSIS OF THE HEART

Entry Author: H. Thomas Aretz

SYNONYMS: Larval taeniasis; bladder worm infestation.

DEFINITION: A systemic infestation caused by the larval stage of the tapeworm *Tenia solium*.

GROSS FINDINGS: In a severe case, there may be multiple fluid-filled cysts containing the larva within the myocardium.

MICROSCOPIC FINDINGS: The intact cyst is lined by fibrous tissue and there is only scant inflammatory response. When the larva degenerates, it elicits a granulomatous inflammatory response. The larva itself shows the characteristic cyst wall and scolex with its sucker and hooklets, which permits identification.

DIFFERENTIAL DIAGNOSIS: If there is a single degenerated cyst, it may be impossible to distinguish this from other parasitic infestations or granulomatous diseases.

KEY DIAGNOSTIC CRITERIA: Characteristic cyst morphology.

POTENTIAL PITFALLS: Degeneration of larva with resultant granulomatous inflammation that may mimic other diseases.

ENDOMYOCARDIAL FIBROSIS, TROPICAL

Entry Author: Renu Virmani

SYNONYMS: Endomyocardial fibrosis (EMF), Davies' disease, EMF of tropics and subtropics.

DEFINITION: Endomyocardial fibrosis is characterized by fibrous endocardial thickening of the inflow portions of the right or left ventricle, or both, often with involvement of the atrioventricular valves which produces regurgitation. It occurs most frequently in Africa, especially Uganda in the Rwandan tribe and in people of low socioeconomic status in the tropical and subtropical regions of India, Brazil, Columbia, and Sri Lanka. Rare in whites.

GROSS FINDINGS: Heart is mildly enlarged or of normal size. Often a serous pericardial effusion is present. The atria are enlarged, especially the right atrium, and the right ventricle shows an indentation in the right heart border cephalad to the apex due to endocardial scarring of the apex. There is extensive, dense, endocardial thickening in inflow portions of the right and left ventricles with extension into the apex, with involvement of the papillary muscles and chordae tendinea. On the right side, the tricuspid valve is pulled down and distorted. On the left side the posteromedial papillary muscle is usually involved along with the posterior mitral leaflet. The anterior mitral leaflet is spared. There may be thrombi present in the apices of both ventricular cavities and in the atria. These are in various stages of organization.

MICROSCOPIC FINDINGS: The endocardial thickening is composed of dense collagen close to the myocardium whereas toward the cavity there is granulation tissue and thrombus. Fibrous septae extend into the myocardium along with granulation tissue. Portions of the mitral and tricuspid valve show fibrous adhesion to the underlying myocardium with or without organizing thrombus.

SPECIAL PROCEDURES NEEDED FOR DIAGNOSIS: Diagnosis is based on clinical and laboratory features along with appropriate geographic location. Endocardial biopsy may be helpful but is contraindicated because of the danger of embolizing a mural thrombus.

DIFFERENTIAL DIAGNOSIS: At one time Löffler endocarditis was considered a separate disease but now both are considered a spectrum of one disease. Löffler's endocardial fibrosis is a disease of temperate countries with patients typically presenting with hypereosinophilia (≥ 1500 eosinophils/mm^3) for at least 6 months or until death and biventricular cardiac involvement, mural apical thrombi with endocardial thickening in the inflow portion of the ventricles and mitral and/or tricuspid valve thrombi. Histologically, there is eosinophilic myocarditis and varying stages or organization of the mural thrombus that is rich in eosinophils.

KEY DIAGNOSTIC CRITERIA: None, but the diagnosis is based on clinical and morphologic findings.

POTENTIAL PITFALLS: Endomyocardial fibrosis can occur from many conditions, e.g., radiation, glycogen storage disease, dilated cardiomyopathy.

SEE ALSO: Myocarditis, eosinophilic, hypereosinophilia syndrome.

GLYCOGEN STORAGE DISEASE

Entry Author: Renu Virmani

DEFINITION: An inborn error of metabolism usually found in infants or children and characterized by the accumulation of glycogen as a result of a deficiency in one or more of the enzymes involved in either the biosynthesis or degradation of glycogen. There are a number of forms of glycogen storage disease, corresponding to various enzyme deficiency states. The heart is almost always involved in type II (Pompe's disease), whereas in type III (Cori's disease) and type IV (Anderson's disease) glycogen storage disease there is variable involvement of the heart. In cases of cardiac involvement, especially type II, the excessive myocardial glycogen deposition within the myocardium is uniformly distributed within the myocytes. This leads to cardiac failure because of mechanical factors.

SEE ALSO: Entries for specific glycogen storage diseases.

GLYCOGEN STORAGE DISEASE, TYPE II

Entry Author: Renu Virmani

SYNONYM: Pompe's disease.

DEFINITION: Type II glycogen storage disease is the result of deficiency of a lysosomal α-1,4-glycosidase or acid maltase. It is transmitted through a single recessive gene. The classic form, Pompe's disease, is the infantile form with marked cardiac manifestations. There are also juvenile and adult forms. In these, the disease progresses slowly and is primarily a skeletal muscle disease.

GROSS FINDINGS: The heart in Pompe's disease is grossly enlarged, with thickening of all four walls but especially the left ventricular free wall and papillary muscles. Usually there is a small left ventricular cavity. The muscle is rubbery and pale pink. In 20% of cases there is accompanying endocardial fibroelastosis.

MICROSCOPIC FINDINGS: On histologic examination, there is diffuse central myocyte vacuolization with peripheral myofibril displacement giving a lace-work appearance caused by extensive glycogen deposition. Glycogen deposition is also seen in conduction system, endothelial cells and vascular smooth muscle cells.

SPECIAL PROCEDURES NEEDED FOR DIAGNOSIS: The glycogen is deposited within lysosomes and can be demonstrated by electron microscopy (Thiery stain) or by periodic acid Schiff stains with diastase on frozen sections from unfixed tissue or following methanol fixation. Myocardial glycogen content is increased and may constitute up to 9% of wet tissue weight.

DIFFERENTIAL DIAGNOSIS: Usually should not pose any problems, as marked diffuse cardiac myocyte vacuolization in an infant is almost diagnostic of glycogen storage disease. Focal vacuolization is seen in rhabdomyomas, but this gives the myocytes a "spider cell" appearance with a central cytoplasmic mass and strands of cytoplasm that extend to the cell membrane. The intercalated disks are located around the periphery of the rhabdomyoma.

KEY DIAGNOSTIC CRITERIA: The diagnosis of glycogen storage disease should not be based only on the demonstration of increased glycogen content in the myocardium but must be confirmed by analysis of glycogen structure and by demonstration of the specific enzymatic defect. The latter can be accomplished using leukocytes or cultured skin fibroblasts.

POTENTIAL PITFALLS: Rhabdomyomas (see Section 5, entry for *Rhabdomyoma*) may be mistaken for glycogen storage disease if the diagnosis is based on microscopic criteria without biochemical confirmation of abnormal glycogen structure and enzyme deficiency.

GLYCOGEN STORAGE DISEASE, TYPE III

Entry Author: Renu Virmani

SYNONYM: Cori's disease.

DEFINITION: Glycogen storage disease, type III is caused by deficiency of amylo-1,6-glucosidase or debrancher enzyme. Cardiac involvement is common but is usually less severe than in type II. Only 23% of patients have been found to have cardiomegaly and morphologic findings have only rarely been described. The myocytes show vacuolar changes, but these may be limited to the deeper (i.e., the subendocardial) layers of the heart. The glycogen is biochemically abnormal, with short outer branches, but it appears unremarkable by electron microscopy and is found free within the cytoplasm.

GLYCOGEN STORAGE DISEASE, TYPE IV

Entry Author: Renu Virmani

SYNONYM: Anderson's disease.

DEFINITION: Glycogen storage disease, type IV, is caused by deficiency of brancher enzyme or α-1,4-glucan: α-1,4-glucan 6-glucosyl transferase. Clinical manifestations of heart disease are variable. Most commonly encountered in neonates, but a juvenile form of the disease has also been described.

GROSS FINDINGS: The heart is often enlarged and extensive deposits of glycogen are present in myocytes.

MICROSCOPIC FINDINGS: With hematoxylin and eosin staining the glycogen deposits appear as basophilic areas within myocytes that are resistant to amylase digestion. The glycogen is biochemically abnormal, with long outer branches. Ultrastructurally, it shows a fibrillar structure. The fibrils are 5 to 6 nm thick and are free in the cytoplasm.

SPECIAL PROCEDURES NEEDED FOR DIAGNOSIS: Biochemical demonstration of structurally abnormal glycogen in the heart as well as the deficiency of brancher enzyme in leukocytes or skin fibroblast cultures.

DIFFERENTIAL DIAGNOSIS: Same as type II. Can be distinguished from rhabdomyoma as described in the entry for type II glycogen storage disease.

KEY DIAGNOSTIC CRITERIA: Presence of abnormal glycogen (long outer branches) within tissues and deficiency of the brancher enzyme, α-1,4-

glucan: α-1,4-glucan, 6-glucosyl transferase. Ultrastructural demonstration of fibrillar glycogen is not diagnostic because similar changes are found in cardiac myocytes in Lafora type of myoclonic epilepsy and in basophilic degeneration of the heart.

POTENTIAL PITFALLS: Failure to rule out presence of Lafora-type myoclonic epilepsy or basophilic degeneration of hypothyroidism.

INTERSTITIAL MYOCARDIAL FIBROSIS, FOCAL SCAR

Entry Author: Robert J. Siegel

SYNONYMS: Replacement fibrosis, microscopic scar, patchy fibrosis, focal fibrosis.

DEFINITION: Fibrous tissue replacing areas of myocardium.

GROSS FINDINGS: Ranges from inapparent grossly to a grossly firm, gray-white area within myocardium. (See also: *Myocardial infarct, healed.*)

MICROSCOPIC FINDINGS: Groups of myocardial fibers are replaced by scar tissue in one or several areas.

REMARKS: Scarring fibrosis represents fibrous replacement in damaged foci of myocardium, whether on an ischemic basis or secondary to a previous inflammatory lesion (e.g., healed Aschoff body, abscess, granuloma) or trauma. Scarring fibrosis also occurs in progressive systemic sclerosis (scleroderma).

DIFFERENTIAL DIAGNOSIS: Amyloid, by special stains. Fibrous plaques from organization of mural thrombi may need to be distinguished from myocardial scars.

KEY DIAGNOSTIC CRITERIA: Patches of fibrous tissue replace myocardium.

INTERSTITIAL MYOCARDIAL FIBROSIS, INTERFIBER

Entry Author: Robert J. Siegel

SYNONYMS: Diffuse interstitial fibrosis, interfibrosis, pericellular fibrosis, intercellular fibrosis.

DEFINITION: Increased collagen deposited between myocytes.

GROSS FINDINGS: Usually not apparent grossly.

MICROSCOPIC FINDINGS: The usually delicate pericellular collagen is exaggerated and individual myocytes are surrounded and separated by fibrous connective tissue. A "honeycomb" pattern may result.

REMARKS: This is a relatively common, nonspecific finding. To some extent, it seems to be a manifestation of aging. Along with perivascular fibrosis, it is characteristically seen in dilated cardiomyopathy, especially in the subendocardial area. Interfiber fibrosis also occurs in hypertensive heart disease and after radiation to the heart.

DIFFERENTIAL DIAGNOSIS: Marked interstitial fibrosis (especially interfiber type) may be confused with amyloid deposition, from which it may be distinguished by appropriate special stains.

KEY DIAGNOSTIC CRITERIA: Collagen deposition between myocardial fibers.

INTERSTITIAL MYOCARDIAL FIBROSIS, PERIVASCULAR

Entry Author: Robert J. Siegel

DEFINITION: Increased collagen deposited around intramyocardial blood vessels.

GROSS FINDINGS: Usually not apparent grossly.

MICROSCOPIC FINDINGS: Periadventitial collagen of intramyocardial blood vessels is exaggerated and groups of myocardial fibers may appear to be encircled by fibrovascular septa.

REMARKS: Perivascular fibrosis often accompanies interfiber fibrosis in the conditions listed under that entry.

KEY DIAGNOSTIC CRITERIA: Fibrous tissue encircling intramyocardial vessels.

INTERSTITIAL MYOCARDIAL FIBROSIS, PLEXIFORM

Entry Author: Robert J. Siegel

DEFINITION: Increased collagen in a haphazard arrangement, especially between fibers showing myocyte disarray in hypertrophic cardiomyopathy.

GROSS FINDINGS: Usually not apparent grossly.

MICROSCOPIC FINDINGS: Seen characteristically in association with myofiber disarray (see *Hypertrophic cardiomyopathy*). Irregular coarse bundles of collagen fill the spaces between the disarrayed myocardial fibers.

REMARKS: Plexiform fibrosis is characteristic of hypertrophic cardiomyopathy but not entirely specific.

KEY DIAGNOSTIC CRITERIA: Collagen deposition within myocardium in characteristic patterns just described.

References

1. Anderson KR, Sutton MG, Lie JT. Histopathological types of cardiac fibrosis in myocardial disease. *J Pathol* 1979;128:79–85.
2. Sugihara N, Genda A, Shimizu M, Suematu T, Kita Y, Horita Y, Takeda R. Quantitation of myocardial fibrosis and its relation to function in essential hypertension and hypertrophic cardiomyopathy. *Clin Cardiol* 1988;11:771–778.
3. Klima M, Burns TR, Chopra A. Myocardial fibrosis in the elderly. *Arch Pathol Lab Med* 1990;114: 938–942.

LIGHT CHAIN DEPOSITS

Entry Author: Renu Virmani

DEFINITION: Light chain disease is a variant of multiple myeloma where only kappa or lambda light chains are synthesized. Light chain deposit disease is characterized by progressive renal failure, congestive heart failure, restrictive cardiomyopathy, hepatic failure, and polyneuropathy.

GROSS FINDINGS: With clinically significant deposits the heart is likely to be firm and rubbery, but deposits may be present with no significant abnormality.

MICROSCOPIC FINDINGS: Deposits are myocytic and amorphous, as well as being subendothelial in arterioles and muscular arteries. They do not stain as amyloid. By electron microscopy, with uranyl acetate and lead citrate stains, the deposits appear electron-dense and amorphous. They lack the fibrillar character of amyloid.

DIFFERENTIAL DIAGNOSIS: To rule out true amyloid fibrillar material, Congo red stain or other amyloid stains and immunohistochemical stains for kappa and lambda light chain should be performed along with electron microscopy. Fibrillin deposits are Congo red negative. They appear similar to amyloid by light microscopy but are distinct from amyloid and light chain deposits both by electron microscopy and immunohistochemistry.

KEY DIAGNOSTIC CRITERIA: Histologic confirmation by lack of staining by the usual amyloid stains, positive immunohistochemical staining by kappa or lambda light chain with electron-dense granular material seen on electron microscopy adjacent to the plasma membrane of cardiac myocytes, arteriolar endothelial and smooth muscle cells, and neural elements.

POTENTIAL PITFALLS: Deposits can be missed if electron microscopy or staining for kappa and lambda light chain has not been carried out.

MUCOPOLYSACCHARIDOSIS

Entry Author: Renu Virmani

SUBTYPES: Mucopolysaccharidosis I, II, III, IV, and VI (see entries).

DEFINITION: A family of hereditary diseases characterized by the accumulation of mucopolysaccharides due to deficiency in a lysosomal enzyme normally responsible for the degradation of this mucopolysaccharide. The mucopolysaccharides involved include heparan sulfate, dermatan sulfate, and keratin sulfate. In these conditions, there are anatomic changes, apparently related to effects of the acid mucopolysaccharides on collagen, in the cardiac valves, skin, cartilage, and bone.

MUCOPOLYSACCHARIDOSIS I

Entry Author: Renu Virmani

SUBTYPES: Hurler syndrome, Scheie syndrome, and intermediate Hurler-Scheie syndrome.

DEFINITION: A form of mucopolysaccharidosis in which there is reduced activity of the enzyme α-L-iduronidase and excessive urinary secretion of dermatan sulfate and heparan sulfate. Three distinct subtypes have been described.

Type I-H: Hurler syndrome. This syndrome is characterized by coarse facial features, hepatosplenomegaly, severe skeletal abnormalities, and progressive neurologic deterioration which come to medical attention in the first 2 years of life. Death occurs before the age of 10 years in most cases. A majority of children have multiple valvular lesions and severe coronary artery narrowing.

Type I-S: Scheie syndrome is a variant of Hurler syndrome. The same enzyme, α-L-iduronidase, is deficient as a result of allelic mutation. Manifestations of Scheie syndrome are mild, and the condition is never diagnosed in infancy, typically remaining undiagnosed until adulthood. Several features of Scheie syndrome are similar to those of Hurler syndrome, including progressive clouding of the cornea, joint contractures, and valvular disease. Individuals have normal intelligence and longevity.

Type I-H-S: Hurler-Scheie syndrome is phenotypically intermediate between Hurler and Scheie syndromes and may represent an individual who is a compound heterozygote for the two allelic disorders. The disease is usually diagnosed during childhood with a more prolonged survival than Hurler's syndrome. Cardiac involvement consists of thickening of the valve leaflets with aortic and mitral regurgitation.

GROSS FINDINGS: The cardiovascular lesions in Hurler syndrome involve valves, endocardium, myocardium, coronary arteries, and large systemic arteries. The valves are thickened, especially the mitral valve. Right-sided valves are less severely affected than left-sided ones. Commissures are not fused. Chordae tendinea of the mitral valve are both thickened and shortened. Calcification occurs deep to the base of the posterior mitral leaflet (mitral annular calcification) and on the aortic surface of the aortic cusps. The endocardium is diffusely thickened, more on the left than right side of the heart. Large epicardial coronary arteries are rigid and thickened with severe luminal narrowing (>75%). The aorta and large systemic arteries have raised intimal plaques. In Scheie syndrome, both aortic stenosis and regurgitation have been reported clinically. In Hurler-Scheie syndrome, mitral stenosis and regurgitation and aortic regurgitation with calcification occur.

MICROSCOPIC FINDINGS: The valves, endocardium, myocardium, coronary arteries, and aorta contain large, oval, or rounded connective tissue cells (Hurler cells) filled with numerous clear vacuoles containing acid mucopolysaccharide material. Also, small granular cells have been described that contain membrane-bound electron-dense material associated with fragments of collagen fibrils. There is also increased fibrous connective tissue. Cardiac myocytes and intimal and medial smooth muscle cells of coronary arteries also contain deposits of glycolipid material that appear in the form of concentric or parallel lamellae. In myocytes, these are perinuclear and occupy only a small fraction of the cell volume, whereas coronary smooth muscle cells have much more extensive deposits.

SPECIAL PROCEDURES NEEDED FOR DIAGNOSIS: The activity of α-L-iduronidase can be determined in cultured fibroblasts. This activity correlates with disease severity. Molecular genetic investigation reveals the gene defect is localized to the short arm of chromosome 4, region 16.3 (4p 16.3).

DIFFERENTIAL DIAGNOSIS: Dysplasia of the ventricular arterial and atrioventricular valves must be differentiated from Hurler's syndrome. In the former, the proteoglycans are distributed in the interstitium and not within cells. Coronary artery disease in adults with atherosclerosis is an eccentric disease with large areas of necrotic core and foam cells. Whereas in the latter, Hurlers cells are uniformly distributed in the intima and the lesions tend to be concentric with central lumens.

KEY DIAGNOSTIC CRITERIA: Presence of Hurler cells in the intima and media of coronary arteries, valves, and endocardium. By electron microscopy the foam cells contain electron-lucent, membrane-limited vacuoles thought to be lysosomes. None of these findings are diagnostic or specific. Key criteria are biochemical and genetic studies.

POTENTIAL PITFALLS: Other storage diseases may be mistaken for Hurler syndrome. Enzyme and genetic studies should always be carried out for confirmation.

MUCOPOLYSACCHARIDOSIS II

Entry Author: Renu Virmani

SYNONYM: Hunter syndrome.

DEFINITION: Hunter syndrome is characterized by an enzymatic defect in iduronate 2-sulfatase, the gene which is located on the X-chromosome (locus 1 27.3). There is a recessive mode of inheritance. A severe and a mild form are recognized. In the severe form, usually diagnosed before 4 years of age, there is corneal clouding, kyphoscoliosis, mental retardation, and death before 15 years of age. In the mild form corneal clouding and kyphoscoliosis are absent. There is moderate skeletal and respiratory involvement with survival into adulthood with little or no intellectual impairment. Cardiovascular disease is present in a high proportion of patients with either form of Hunter's syndrome. Cardiac valve involvement may cause congestive heart failure, the leading cause of death in affected individuals.

GROSS FINDINGS: The mitral valve may show diffuse micronodular thickening, especially around the line of closure, with mild thickening and shortening of chordae tendinea and resultant mitral regurgitation. The aortic valve in older individuals has been described to have calcified micronodules ("waxed droppings") located along the line of closure and most pronounced in the central third of each leaflet.

MICROSCOPIC FINDINGS: The valve contains large clear cells similar to those in patients with Hurler syndrome as well as small sudanophilic cells. There is also increased fibrous tissue. Clear cells are also present in the myocardium and endocardium but not in coronary arteries. Myocytes do not contain abnormal material.

SPECIAL PROCEDURES NEEDED FOR DIAGNOSIS: Patients with Hunter's syndrome excrete excessive amounts of dermatan sulfate and heparan sulfate in the urine. It is possible to separate Hurler and Hunter syndrome by means of the ratio of dermatan sulfate to heparan sulfates, which is 70:30 in Hurler and 50:50 in Hunter. The primary defect, iduronate-2-sulfatase, can be demonstrated in cultured fibroblasts. Molecular genetic investigations reveal the gene defect to be located on the X-chromosome region q27.3.

DIFFERENTIAL DIAGNOSIS: Similar to mucopolysaccharide type I.

KEY DIAGNOSTIC CRITERIA: Morphologic criteria are not diagnostic or specific. Both clinical findings and biochemical and genetic studies are essential for establishing the diagnosis.

MUCOPOLYSACCHARIDOSIS III

Entry Author: Renu Virmani

SYNONYMS: Sanfilippo syndrome, heparan sulfaturia.

DEFINITION: Sanfilippo syndrome is characterized by deficiency of any one of the following lysosomal enzymes: heparan N-sulfatase (III A), α-N-acetylglucosaminidase (III B), acetyl-CoA: α-glucosaminide N-acetyltransferase (III C), or N-acetylglucosamine 6-sulfatase. This autosomal recessive disorder is characterized by the excretion of large amounts of heparan sulfate in urine and the accumulation of excessive amounts of heparan sulfate glycosaminoglycan in lysosomes. There are few stigmata other than severe progressive mental retardation. Clinical cardiac signs and symptoms are rare in Sanfilippo syndrome.

GROSS FINDINGS AND MICROSCOPIC FINDINGS: The heart is morphologically involved. There is mitral valve deformity, rigidity, thickening of the leaflets, and shortening of chordae tendinea secondary to diffuse fibrosis and intra- and extra-cellular deposits of acid mucopolysaccharide material. Grossly, the valve involvement is similar to that found in the other forms of mucopolysaccharidosis. Intracellular deposits are localized in small granular cells, but large clear Hurler-like cells have not always been described.

KEY DIAGNOSTIC CRITERIA: Morphologic criteria are not diagnostic or specific. Clinical findings, biochemical, and genetic studies are essential for establishing the diagnosis.

MUCOPOLYSACCHARIDOSIS IV

Entry Author: Renu Virmani

SYNONYMS: Morquio syndrome, keratan sulfaturia.

DEFINITION: A syndrome with two biochemically distinct forms, both of which are inherited as autosomal recessive traits: Morquio syndrome, type A (galactose 6-sulfatase deficiency) and Morquio syndrome, type B (β-galactosidase deficiency). The affected children are dwarfed, barrel chested, and have corneal clouding, thin tooth enamel, and progressive spinal cord damage.

GROSS FINDINGS: Cardiac involvement is well recognized. There is cardiac hypertrophy and thickening and nodularity, with or without annular calcification, of the mitral, aortic, tricuspid, and pulmonic valves. There is also thickening of the endocardium, aorta, pulmonary trunk, and coronary arteries. The myocardial hypertrophy is secondary to the valvular disease, primarily aortic insufficiency.

MICROSCOPIC FINDINGS: Ultrastructural studies show vacuoles consistent with lysosomes in the cytoplasm of smooth muscle cells.

SPECIAL PROCEDURES NEEDED FOR DIAGNOSIS: The feature that distinguishes Morquio syndrome from other mucopolysaccharides is ineffective keratan sulfate catabolism. The type IV A disease results from defective lysosomal galactose 6-sulfatase, whereas for type IV B there is deficiency of β-galactosidase enzymatic activity.

KEY DIAGNOSTIC CRITERIA: Morphologic criteria are not diagnostic or specific. Clinical, biochemical, and genetic studies are essential for establishing the diagnosis.

MUCOPOLYSACCHARIDOSIS VI

Entry Author: Renu Virmani

SYNONYMS: Maroteaux-Lamy syndrome, polydystrophic dwarfism.

DEFINITION: An autosomal recessive hereditary disorder due to a deficiency of N-acetylgalactosamine 4-sulfate and characterized by clinical features similar to those of Hurler syndrome. These include extreme short stature, kyphoscoliosis, normal intelligence, and corneal clouding. Dermatan sulfate is the preponderant urinary mucopolysaccharide. Aortic stenosis and regurgitation, presenting in adolescence or later, are the most important lesions clinically.

GROSS FINDINGS: Endocardial thickening, with mitral and aortic valve calcification have been reported.

MICROSCOPIC FINDINGS: There is infiltration by foam cells which may be fibroblasts or macrophages and ultrastructurally show either parallel electron-dense lamellae or flocculent material.

SPECIAL PROCEDURES NEEDED FOR DIAGNOSIS: Increased urinary excretion of glycosaminoglycan with dermatan sulfate accounting for 70–95% and the remainder being heparan sulfate. The gene has been localized to the short arm of chromosome 5, bands 11 to 13 (5 q11-q13).

DIFFERENTIAL DIAGNOSIS: Similar to mucopolysaccharidosis type I.

KEY DIAGNOSTIC CRITERIA: Morphologic criteria are not diagnostic or specific. Clinical findings, biochemical, and genetic studies are essential for establishing the diagnosis.

MYOCARDIAL ABSCESS

Entry Author: H. Thomas Aretz

DEFINITION: A localized myocardial collection of acute (and chronic) inflammatory cells associated with necrosis and destruction of the myocardium typical of a suppurative process. These lesions may be single and contiguous to an infected focus (e.g., bacterial endocarditis). They may be multiple as a result of a miliary infectious process (endocarditis, Chagas' disease) or they may be present in the setting of other forms of myocardial necrosis (e.g., myocardial infarct).

GROSS FINDINGS: The gross appearance depends on the underlying etiology and duration of the inflammatory process. Acutely, there is an area of liquefactive necrosis containing purulent material. With time, larger abscesses may become cystic and a fibrous wall may form which occasionally calcifies. In the case of miliary small abscesses, there may be numerous yellow to slightly hemorrhagic foci scattered throughout the myocardium. Depending on the size of the abscesses and their location, they may heal as small scars or leave a cystic space (sometimes communicating with the chambers) lined by fibrous tissue which may contain calcification. Myocardial abscesses involving the aortic valve annulus constitute a special case. These may extend into the pericardium via a sinus tract which is sometimes grossly demonstrable. If the abscess extends into the membranous septum, a careful examination of the conduction system should be carried out.

MICROSCOPIC FINDINGS: Single or multiple well-defined foci of suppurative myocardial inflammation, resulting in myocardial necrosis and tissue destruction. With healing, organization will be seen at the edge of the lesion. Depending on the etiology and stage of infection, microorganisms may be readily visible by H&E staining. This is the case, for example, in Chagas' disease, bacterial endocarditis, staphylococcal or fungal infections. In cases of aortic valve annular abscesses, microscopic examination may reveal a purulent pericarditis or involvement of the conduction system, in particular the bundle of His.

REMARKS: Myocardial abscesses should always be investigated by appropriate special stains to detect microorganisms. Even the absence of demonstrable microorganisms does not exclude an infectious etiology, as lesions associated with less virulent organisms may fail to demonstrate stainable organisms. The distinction of microabscesses from the frequently seen microinfarcts (the so-called Bracht-Wachter bodies) may not always be possible, but the latter should not contain microorganisms. In cases of angioinvasive fungi, such as aspergillus, a mixture of abscesses and infarcted myocardium may be seen.

DIFFERENTIAL DIAGNOSIS: The pathology is fairly distinct when the entire heart is available for examination. Confusion may arise in a myocardial biopsy, where microabscesses can mimic ischemic or toxic injury.

KEY DIAGNOSTIC CRITERIA: Localized suppurative lesion with myocardial destruction.

POTENTIAL PITFALLS: Failure to identify microorganisms that may lead to the diagnosis of a noninfectious process.

MYOCARDIAL ATROPHY

Entry Author: Robert J. Siegel

DEFINITION: Decrease in heart size. The reduction in mass of myocardium through reduced mass of individual cells. Seen in elderly individuals, often in association with generalized wasting.

GROSS FINDINGS: Firm criteria are not established but the heart is smaller than expected for body size. The aortic root appears inappropriately large compared to the left ventricular outflow tract. Often accompanied by so-called "gelatinous transformation" or "serous atrophy" of epicardial fat, in which the fat has an edematous, gelatinous appearance. Myocardium may be darker brown than usual. Coronary arteries are tortuous because their original length is now accommodated to a smaller heart.

MICROSCOPIC FINDINGS: Myocytes have a reduced transverse diameter, which averages around 11 microns in normal hearts, and myocardial nuclei appear closer together. Lipofuscin accumulation within myocytes may be increased, producing a dark brown gross appearance descriptively termed *brown atrophy* or *mahogany heart.*

REMARKS: These changes are most commonly a manifestation of chronic, wasting diseases or malnutrition, rather than a direct result of aging. The functional significance is uncertain.

KEY DIAGNOSTIC CRITERIA: Decreased heart weight and myocyte diameter.

Reference

1. Gould SE. *Pathology of the heart and blood vessels, 3rd ed.* Charles Thomas, Springfield, IL; 1968:520–521.

MYOCARDIAL CALCIFICATION

Entry Author: Robert J. Siegel

DEFINITION: Deposition of calcium salts within the myocardium that are demonstrable grossly, microscopically, or ultrastructurally. Encompasses both interstitial and intracellular (myocyte) deposition, which occur under different conditions.

GROSS FINDINGS: Extracellular deposits are most commonly seen in scar tissue. Extensive calcification, for example, in old infarcts, may be grossly visible as chalky white areas with the characteristic hard consistency of calcium deposits. Such calcification also may be present in the walls of ventricular aneurysms. Intracellular deposits are usually not grossly demonstrable. (See also: *Mitral valve annulus, calcification*, in Section 2.)

MICROSCOPIC FINDINGS: Calcium deposits are recognized as dark blue-purple basophilic amorphous to granular material within cardiac myocytes or in fibrotic areas of healed infarcts. In myocytes, usually at the edge of an infarct, the deposits have the form of finely granular basophilic material, which electron microscopy shows to be located either in mitochondria or as hydroxyapatite crystals within Z-disks. Within scar tissue, the deposits are basophilic by light microscopy and composed of hydroxyapatite by electron microscopy.

SPECIAL PROCEDURES NEEDED FOR DIAGNOSIS: The von Kossa stain is generally used to verify that a basophilic material is calcium. However, this stain is not specific for calcium because it actually stains the anionic component of the calcium deposits (primarily phosphate). Demonstration of very fine needle-like crystals by electron microscopy is highly suggestive of hydroxyapatite, but this too is not absolutely specific. If greater certainty is required, it is necessary to use electron microprobe analysis.

REMARKS: The most common form of myocardial calcification is the dystrophic type in which there is deposition of calcium salts in necrotic (usually infarcted) tissue or in a postnecrotic scar. "Metastatic" calcification, associated with marked hypercalcemia (see *Cardiomyopathy, hyperparathyroidism-associated*), also may occur.

KEY DIAGNOSTIC CRITERIA: Basophilic intracellular or extracellular material that stains positive with the von Kossa stain. Absolute proof requires a definitive test such as electron microprobe analysis.

References

1. Lockard VG, Bloom S. Morphological features and nuclide composition of infarction-associated mineralization in humans. *Am J Path* 1991;139:565–572.
2. Catellier MJ, Chua GT, Youmans G, Waller BF. Calcific deposits in the heart. *Clin Cardiol* 1990;13:287–294.

MYOCARDIAL HYPERTROPHY

Entry Author: Robert J. Siegel

SYNONYMS: Myocyte hypertrophy. Related terms: left ventricular hypertrophy (LVH), right ventricular hypertrophy (RVH), biventricular hypertrophy.

DEFINITION: Increased cardiac muscle mass due to an increased size, rather than number, of myocytes. Depending on the stimulus, hypertrophy may be generalized or limited to one or more cardiac chambers. Because hypertrophy of the myocardium reflects pressure or volume loads, it can be used for diagnostic purposes. In the left ventricle, hypertrophy may become so pronounced as to interfere with mechanical function of the heart through increased myocardial stiffness.

GROSS FINDINGS: Heart weight is a more accurate reflection of muscle mass at autopsy and is more reliable than the often used ventricular wall thickness. This is because dilation may cause thinning of a hypertrophied ventricular wall.

Three morphologic patterns of LVH can be recognized: concentric, in which the wall is thickened but chamber volume is reduced (see *Myocardial hypertrophy, concentric*); hypertrophy with an increased ventricular volume, in which chamber dilation accompanies hypertrophy (see *Myocardial hypertrophy, eccentric*); and asymmetric, in which disproportionate hypertrophy occurs, particularly in the interventricular septum (see *Myocardial hypertrophy, asymmetric, septal*).

MICROSCOPIC FINDINGS: Hypertrophic muscle fibers are increased in thickness. In one study, normal myocytes had a transverse diameter of approximately 11 microns, whereas in hypertrophy, mean diameters of 15 microns were encountered (1). They have enlarged nuclei that are often "box-car" shaped. The actual amount of basophilic material in the nuclei of hypertrophied cardiac myocytes has been found to be increased. Morphometric analysis of Feulgen-stained sections indicate that most normal myocardial nuclei are 4n (tetraploid) and that the ploidy tends to increase with heart weight (2). An increase in interstitial tissues often accompanies hypertrophy.

REMARKS: Cardiac dilation and hypertrophy often occur together and dilation may be an etiologic factor in hypertrophy. When both are present, cardiac weight is still a valid indicator of hypertrophy but wall thickness is not.

Because myocardial mass varies with physiologic demands, larger people have heavier hearts. A convenient rule of thumb is that the normal heart weight is 0.4–0.5% of the body weight, or 300 and 350 g, respectively, for women and men, and a heart weight of 50 g more than this is taken to reflect hypertrophy. Whereas myocardial mass also varies with athletic activity, there is no convention for this source of variation in the diagnosis of myocardial hypertrophy. Tables for predicted heart weight based on body weight have been published (3,4).

Accurate assessment of ventricular mass at autopsy requires chamber partition techniques. After removal of the atria and great vessels, the right ventricle is cut away at its intersection with the IVS. The septum can be removed and weighed separately or left in continuity with the LV. In either case, LV weight should include the weight of the IVS. Published figures for ventricular weights considered indicative of LVH in adults range from 177 to 225 g, and in RVH 65 to 80 g (5). Data segregated by gender are sparse, but ventricular weights in women are on the order of 15–20% less than corresponding weights in men. Total heart weights are an insensitive measurement of individual ventricular hypertrophy, particularly for the RV because significant RVH may be masked by a normal total heart weight. Epicardial fat is another source of error in determination of myocardial mass.

DIFFERENTIAL DIAGNOSIS: Microscopic examination will differentiate myocyte hypertrophy from other causes of increased cardiac chamber mass, particularly from the infiltrative disorders. Because myocardial hypertrophy is a common compensatory phenomenon in many types of heart disease, the differential diagnosis of the etiology is complex. Causes of LVH include systemic arterial hypertension (associated with concentric hypertrophy), valvular heart disease (particularly aortic stenosis, also causing concentric hypertrophy, and aortic insufficiency, causing hypertrophy with dilation), cardiomyopathy, and ischemic heart disease. RVH is seen secondary to severe lung disease (cor pulmonale), and may accompany LVH in the disorders listed above.

KEY DIAGNOSTIC CRITERIA: Objective criteria for LVH and RVH should be based on isolated ventricular chamber weights, corroborated by microscopic examination.

POTENTIAL PITFALLS: Reliance on RV and LV thickness or total heart weight rather than individual chamber weights at autopsy will lead to inappropriate overdiagnosis and underdiagnosis of ventricular hypertrophy.

References

1. Ishikawa S, Fattal GA, Popiewicz J, Wyatt JP. Functional morphometry of myocardial fibers in cor pulmonale. *Amer Rev Respir Dis* 1972;105:358–367.
2. Sandritter W, Scomazzoni G. Desoxyribonucleic acid content (Feulgen photometry) and dry weight (interference microscopy) in normal and hypertrophied heart muscle fibers. *Nature* 1964;202: 100–101.
3. Scholz DG, Kitzman DW, Hagen PT, Ilstrup DM, Edwards WD. Age-related changes in normal human hearts during the first 10 decades of life. Part I (Growth): A quantitative anatomic study of 200 specimens from subjects from birth to 19 years old. *Mayo Clin Proc* 1988;63:126–136.
4. Kitzman DW, Scholz DG, Hagen PT, Ilstrup DM, Edwards WD. Age-related changes in normal human hearts during the first 10 decades of life. Part II (Maturity): A quantitative anatomic study of 765 specimens from subjects 20–99 years old. *Mayo Clin Proc* 1988;63:137–146.
5. Urbanova D. Assessment of left and right ventricular hypertrophy by various macroscopic techniques. *Cor Vasa* 1983;25:450–458.

MYOCARDIAL HYPERTROPHY, ASYMMETRIC, SEPTAL

Entry Author: Robert J. Siegel

SYNONYMS: Asymmetric septal hypertrophy (ASH), idiopathic hypertrophic subaortic stenosis (IHSS), hypertrophic cardiomyopathy.

DEFINITION: A subset of hypertrophic cardiomyopathy (see separate entry for cardiomyopathy, hypertrophic) in which there is disproportionate hypertrophy of the interventricular septum, with ratio of interventricular septum to posterior left ventricular wall thickness of 1.5 or more. This finding is a feature of hypertrophic cardiomyopathy but does not in itself define that condition.

GROSS FINDINGS: The interventricular septum, or more usually a portion of it, bulges into the left ventricular outflow tract. This focal area of hypertrophy is usually just below the aortic valve, opposite the anterior leaflet of the mitral valve. A fibrotic patch on the endocardium of this hypertrophied area, reflecting the impact of the anterior mitral leaflet on the endocardium, may be found. However, the hypertrophic area may be located anywhere in the septum: anterior, posterior, basal, mid-ventricular, or apical.

MICROSCOPIC FINDINGS: Myocyte hypertrophy is present. In cases of hypertrophic cardiomyopathy, myocyte fiber disarray must be present (see discussion under that entity).

REMARKS: Asymmetric septal hypertrophy does not always imply hypertrophic cardiomyopathy and may be seen in hypertensive left ventricular hypertrophy, aortic stenosis, and in aging hearts.

DIFFERENTIAL DIAGNOSIS: Hypertrophic cardiomyopathy; see discussion in differential diagnosis for that entity. An enlarged interventricular septum also may be seen with tumors (fibroma) and other infiltrative processes involving the septum. In elderly individuals, a "sigmoid" shape of the interventricular septum may produce a bulge into the left ventricular outflow tract that mimics asymmetric septal hypertrophy. Prominence of the right ventricle in newborns similarly may give the appearance of septal hypertrophy.

KEY DIAGNOSTIC CRITERIA: Ratio of interventricular septum to posterior left ventricular wall thickness of 1.5 or more.

MYOCARDIAL HYPERTROPHY, CONCENTRIC

Entry Author: Robert J. Siegel

DEFINITION: Increased left ventricular (LV) muscle mass distributed uniformly over the LV wall giving the appearance of reduction in cavity size.

GROSS FINDINGS: LV wall thickness is increased uniformly, often in the 2–3 cm range, and the left ventricular cavity appears small. Isolated LV weight is increased and total heart weight usually is increased (see entry for *Myocardial hypertrophy*).

MICROSCOPIC FINDINGS: Myocytes are increased in diameter and have enlarged nuclei with "boxcar" or bizarre shapes. Some degree of interstitial fibrosis (see entry) is often present.

DIFFERENTIAL DIAGNOSIS: Ventricular wall thickening grossly resembling hypertrophy may occur in infiltrative disorders. Light microscopy of routine histologic sections is sufficient to distinguish these. Concentric LVH is characteristic of systemic arterial hypertension and aortic stenosis but is occasionally seen in patients with ischemic heart disease and no (known) history of hypertension.

KEY DIAGNOSTIC CRITERIA: Uniform increase in LV wall thickness at the apparent expense of LV cavity size.

POTENTIAL PITFALLS: A normal-sized heart fixed in systolic configuration may have increased LV wall thickness and apparently reduced chamber size. Mistaking an infiltrative disorder, such as amyloidosis or some tumor infiltrates, for concentric hypertrophy may occur if an examination is limited to gross.

MYOCARDIAL HYPERTROPHY, ECCENTRIC

Entry Author: Robert J. Siegel

SYNONYM: Volume overload hypertrophy.

DEFINITION: Increased myocardial mass together with dilation of a cardiac chamber usually secondary to increased stroke volume. Although it may affect any chamber, this condition is most common and most striking in cases of aortic insufficiency or arteriovenous shunt, and for many pathologists the diagnosis is essentially limited to such left ventricular volume overload lesions.

GROSS FINDINGS: Some of the largest hearts, to which the descriptive term *cor bovinum* has been applied, are seen in this group. Heart weights over 1,000 g may be seen. The heart is globally enlarged, with increased total heart weight and isolated left ventricular weight, and the LV cavity is enlarged and concave. With aortic insufficiency, patches of endocardial fibrosis representing "jet lesions" may be observed in the LV outflow region.

MICROSCOPIC FINDINGS: Findings of myocardial hypertrophy are present, usually accompanied by significant interstitial myocardial fibrosis (see entry).

DIFFERENTIAL DIAGNOSIS: Aortic insufficiency is a common cause of left ventricular volume overload hypertrophy. Increased myocardial muscle mass combined with dilation also may be seen in long-standing dilated cardiomyopathy and in late hypertensive heart disease where cardiac failure reflected by left ventricular dilation is superimposed on concentric hypertrophy (see *Myocardial hypertrophy, concentric*).

KEY DIAGNOSTIC CRITERIA: Combined hypertrophy and dilation of left ventricle is present.

Reference

1. Murphy ML, White HJ, Meade J, Straub KD. The relationship between hypertrophy and dilatation in the postmortem heart. *Clin Cardiol* 1988;11:297–302.

MYOCARDIAL INFARCT, ACUTE

Entry Author: Robert J. Siegel

DEFINITION: Ischemic necrosis of myocardium usually caused by coronary artery disease, especially atherosclerosis.

GROSS FINDINGS: Acute myocardial infarcts may be regional, following the distribution of a major coronary artery, or subendocardial. The latter either focally or circumferentially involves the inner myocardium. Regional infarcts extending from endocardium to epicardium involving at least two thirds of the wall thickness are designated *transmural*, and those that do not are called *nontransmural*. In transmural infarcts, finding a thrombotic occlusion of a severely atherosclerotic coronary artery supplying the infarcted area is usual. Infarcts "at a distance" occur in myocardium distal to the expected distribution of an occluded coronary artery, in an area supplied by collaterals.

Infarcts less than 24 hours old may be difficult to recognize, but the cut surface is often pale and dry as early as 12–18 hours after onset of symptoms. Subsequently, the infarcted region may appear hyperemic, followed by development of a distinct yellow center with hyperemic border over the first week. In the second and third weeks, a red-purple peripheral zone of granulation tissue enlarges at the expense of the yellow-brown center. Gradually, this granulation tissue is replaced by scar.

MICROSCOPIC FINDINGS: Hypereosinophilic "wavy" fibers may be visible within the first few hours after infarction, and within the first 12 hours, signs of coagulative necrosis (see entry) should be seen. Contraction band necrosis may occur at the periphery of an infarct or if reperfusion has occurred. Intercellular edema and infiltration by neutrophils also commence after several hours, but neutrophils are not conspicuous until about 24 hours with the maximal neutrophilic exudation at 2–3 days. In small infarcts, dissolution of necrotic myocytes and phagocytosis by macrophages is complete and formation of granulation tissue is under way by the end of the first week. In large infarcts this takes longer, and necrotic myocytes may remain "mummified" for extended periods. Lymphocytes and plasma cells appear and may persist for weeks or months. Collagen is progressively deposited, with healing normally complete in 6–7 weeks. Timing of these stages is approximate and depends on infarct size and other factors.

REMARKS: Although usually caused by coronary atherosclerosis, other forms of coronary artery disease (e.g., vasculitis, anomalous origin) should be considered as should other causes of myocardial ischemia in the absence of abnormal coronary arteries.

Special enzymatic stain techniques (e.g., triphenyl tetrazolium chloride) can improve the gross recognition of early infarcts.

DIFFERENTIAL DIAGNOSIS: The infiltrate of neutrophils sometimes needs to be distinguished from infectious exudative processes involving the myocardium (myocardial abscess, myocardial extension of infectious endocarditis, etc.). A combination of gross, clinical, and bacteriologic data readily separates these conditions.

KEY DIAGNOSTIC CRITERIA: Gross: discrete area of pale, hyperemic, or yellow-brown myocardium in typical distribution; Microscopic: wavy eosinophilic fibers, coagulative necrosis, infiltrate of neutrophils, organization into scar by granulation tissue.

Reference

1. Fishbein MC, Maclean D, Maroko PR. The histopathologic evolution of myocardial infarction. *Chest* 1978;73:843–849.

MYOCARDIAL INFARCT, HEALED

Entry Author: Robert J. Siegel

SYNONYMS: Myocardial scar, healed infarction; myocardial infarct, old.

DEFINITION: Regional myocardial scarring resulting from organization of an acute myocardial infarct (AMI) (see entry).

GROSS FINDINGS: Healed infarcts are recognized by white areas of scarring replacing the myocardium. Occasionally, calcification may occur in these areas (see entry, *Myocardial calcification*). As in acute infarcts, these most commonly involve the left ventricle and may be regional (following the distribution of a major coronary artery) or subendocardial. The left ventricle most commonly is affected, followed by right ventricle and rarely right or left atrium. Large healed transmural infarcts may be complicated by ventricular aneurysm formation (see entry, *Aneurysm, ventricular*). Scars of very small infarcts may be recognized only microscopically.

MICROSCOPIC FINDINGS: The process of organization of an AMI results in gradual replacement of necrotic myocytes by scar tissue (replacement fibrosis). In completely healed infarcts, dense hypocellular collagen replaces the myocardium, with few or no inflammatory cells or remaining myocytes. At the periphery, residual myocytes, commonly hypertrophic, interdigitate with the scar tissue. In more recently healed infarcts, the scar is more vascular and contains more inflammatory cells, particularly lymphocytes, plasma cells, and hemo-siderin-containing histiocytes.

DIFFERENTIAL DIAGNOSIS: Areas of myocardial scarring may result from processes other than infarction (abscess, trauma, etc.). Distribution and relation to diseased coronary arteries are helpful differentiating features. The etiology of small, microscopic scars may, however, be obscure.

KEY DIAGNOSTIC CRITERIA: Replacement of myocardium by scar tissue, variable chronic inflammatory cells, hemosiderin-containing histiocytes.

Reference

1. Fishbein MC, Maclean D, Maroko PR. The histopathologic evolution of myocardial infarction. *Chest* 1978;73:843–849.

MYOCARDIAL INFARCT WITH RUPTURE

Entry Author: Robert J. Siegel

SYNONYMS: Myocardial infarct with tear, perforation.

DEFINITION: Transmural tear through myocardium in which there is a subendocardial infarct or a transmural infarct. In subendocardial infarction there may be an endocardial tear with dissecting hemorrhage. In either case, if the free wall is involved, blood escapes into the pericardial cavity leading to tamponade.

GROSS FINDINGS: Usually, the rupture is within a transmural acute myocardial infarct (AMI) (see *Myocardial infarct, acute*) in its first or second week. In free wall rupture, this leads to massive hemopericardium which is usually rapidly fatal. If the rupture involves the interventricular septum, it produces a ventricular septal defect with left to right shunting and severe congestive heart failure. Sudden death due to rupture of a myocardial infarct leading to tamponade may occur with no premonitory signs, and may be due to early rupture or to silent infarction with consequences of rupture as the first overt sign. The infarct associated with papillary muscle rupture often is nontransmural. The important point here is that the tear traverses the infarcted area.

MICROSCOPIC FINDINGS: The perforation may not be easy to trace microscopically. When it is traced, changes of acute myocardial infarction are usually found accompanied by hemorrhage around the perforating tract. In some cases, the myocardium around the tract may reveal changes of a healing, rather than acute, myocardial infarct.

REMARKS: Rupture in the setting of AMI most commonly occurs in the left ventricular free wall, followed by the interventricular septum and papillary muscle (usually posterior). Patients often are elderly, female, and experiencing their first myocardial infarct. In surgical specimens of mitral valve replacement for papillary muscle rupture, the jagged edge of papillary muscle should be examined microscopically for evidence of infarct. Rarely, rupture of an atrial or right ventricular wall is encountered.

KEY DIAGNOSTIC CRITERIA: Tear through recently infarcted myocardium.

Reference

1. Vlodarer Z, Edwards SE. Rupture of ventricular septum or papillary muscle complicating myocardial infarction. *Circ* 1977;55:815–822.

MYOCARDITIS, BACTERIAL

Entry Author: H. Thomas Aretz

DEFINITION: Myocardial necrosis and inflammation caused by direct bacterial infection, such that bacteria are demonstrable in the myocardium.

GROSS FINDINGS: In many cases, the myocardium is quite unremarkable grossly, unless there is abscess formation. Bacteria that cause granulomatous inflammation produce grossly conspicuous lesions. As bacterial myocarditis is often associated with bacterial endocarditis and sepsis, endocardial and pericardial abnormalities may be present.

MICROSCOPIC FINDINGS: Multiple microabscesses, i.e., foci of myocyte necrosis with an infiltrate of polymorphonuclear neutrophiles, are common. Bacterial organisms can usually be demonstrated when the offending organisms are cocci, which is often the case. If larger abscesses are present, bacterial colonies may be readily apparent. Calcification may be seen in chronic abscesses.

REMARKS: Gram stain should always be done, along with fungal stains, as fungal myocarditis may present similar lesions.

DIFFERENTIAL DIAGNOSIS: Fungal microabscesses and sterile emboli may yield similar lesions.

KEY DIAGNOSTIC CRITERIA: Microabscesses with demonstrable bacteria.

POTENTIAL PITFALLS: Failure to obtain special stains for bacteria and fungi.

MYOCARDITIS, CATECHOLAMINE-INDUCED

Entry Author: H. Thomas Aretz

SYNONYM: Pressor lesions.

DEFINITION: Toxic myocarditis caused by catecholamine compounds, resulting in myocardial necrosis and inflammation.

GROSS FINDINGS: Possible dilation but not very apparent changes. May have mottled discoloration due to pallor associated with inflammatory cell infiltrates. Lesions tend to be apical and subendocardial.

MICROSCOPIC FINDINGS: Multiple foci of myocyte necrosis, often less than 10 myocytes, associated with a sparse inflammatory infiltrate usually containing mononuclear cells.

REMARKS: Clinical history is needed to make the diagnosis in most cases, but the morphological changes can be so pronounced that the diagnosis may be supported based on the histology alone. In myocardial biopsies in particular, a modified trichrome stain can help to identify the necrotic myocytes.

DIFFERENTIAL DIAGNOSIS: Myocardial necrosis due to ischemia, emboli, bacterial myocarditis, other toxic substances.

KEY DIAGNOSTIC CRITERIA: Multifocal myocyte necrosis with sparse mononuclear infiltrate.

POTENTIAL PITFALLS: Absence of drug history or clinically occult catechol-producing neoplasm.

SEE ALSO: Cardiomyopathy, catecholamine-associated.

MYOCARDITIS, CHAGAS' DISEASE, ACUTE

Entry Author: H. Thomas Aretz

DEFINITION: Myocarditis caused by the parasite *Trypanosoma cruzi*.

GROSS FINDINGS: Chagas' disease leading to acute death usually causes dilated chambers. The myocardium is soft, focally hemorrhagic, and yellow in areas. There may be pericarditis and endocarditis.

MICROSCOPIC FINDINGS: There is a prominent plasmalymphocytic infiltrate associated with myocyte necrosis. The organisms, usually in the amastigote form, are present within myocytes, which may rupture leading to abscess formation. There is marked interstitial edema and alteration of capillaries, possibly immune-mediated. The organisms may be present in noninflamed myocardium, which may be a pitfall.

REMARKS: Serological tests, clinical correlation, and history are all important in making this diagnosis. The intracellular organisms may be distinguished from Toxoplasma organisms by PAS staining, which is positive for Toxoplasma and negative for trypanosomes. Ultrastructural studies are helpful in identifying the organisms.

DIFFERENTIAL DIAGNOSIS: Other forms of lymphocytic myocarditis, particularly that due to *Toxoplasma*.

KEY DIAGNOSTIC CRITERIA: The demonstration of organisms in the myocardium.

POTENTIAL PITFALLS: Failure to examine noninflamed areas of the myocardium and lack of clinical information.

MYOCARDITIS, CHLAMYDIAL

Entry Author: H. Thomas Aretz

SYNONYM: "Psittacosis."

DEFINITION: Myocarditis caused by *Chlamydia psittaci* or, rarely, another species of *Chlamydia*. Occurs in patients with systemic *C psittaci* infection.

GROSS FINDINGS: Pancarditis with fibrinous pericarditis may be present.

MICROSCOPIC FINDINGS: Lymphocytic myocarditis.

REMARKS: Serologic correlation is extremely important because patients exposed to birds may also be afflicted with hypersensitivity myocarditis.

DIFFERENTIAL DIAGNOSIS: Any cause of lymphocytic myocarditis.

KEY DIAGNOSTIC CRITERIA: Serologic correlation and history, together with lymphocytic myocarditis.

POTENTIAL PITFALLS: Insufficient history, so that exposure to birds may not be recognized.

MYOCARDITIS, COCAINE-ASSOCIATED

Entry Author: H. Thomas Aretz

DEFINITION: Myocardial inflammation secondary to cocaine use and reflecting either toxicity, hypersensitivity, or ischemia.

GROSS FINDINGS: The gross appearance varies with nature of the lesions. Toxic or hypersensitivity myocarditis may show no conspicuous changes if mild, or the myocardium may be flabby or boggy and edematous. Ischemic lesions, if present, are those of myocardial infarction.

MICROSCOPIC FINDINGS: The toxic myocarditis resembles the changes seen with catecholamines with contraction bands possibly very prominent (see entries for *Cardiomyopathy, catecholamine-associated* and *Myocarditis, catecholamine-induced*). Eosinophiles may be prominent and may represent a hypersensitivity-type reaction. Because cocaine is a strong vasoconstrictor and may cause arteritis, myocardial ischemia may be prominent.

REMARKS: Toxicologic studies and history of drug abuse are extremely important. Lesions due to ischemia may reflect coronary artery spasm with no, or little, underlying atherosclerosis. Coronary thrombosis may be present (see entry, *Cardiomyopathy, cocaine-associated*).

DIFFERENTIAL DIAGNOSIS: Ischemic lesions may be due to coronary atherosclerosis unrelated to cocaine use, even in a young person. A toxic myocarditis could be due to some other substance or a combination of substances. If eosinophiles are prominent, there may be eosinophilic myocarditis (see entries for *Myocarditis, eosinophilic*). In almost any myocarditis, sepsis or endocarditis should be considered.

KEY DIAGNOSTIC CRITERIA: Supportive history and presence of multifocal lesions with contraction bands.

POTENTIAL PITFALLS: Failure to recognize cocaine because of insufficient history given the various morphological expressions of the drug effect.

MYOCARDITIS, COLLAGEN VASCULAR DISEASE-ASSOCIATED

Entry Author: H. Thomas Aretz

SYNONYMS: Subtypes include lupus carditis, polymyositis heart, scleroderma heart.

DEFINITION: Myocarditis associated with collagen vascular diseases, which include systemic lupus erythematosus, scleroderma, mixed connective tissue disease, dermatomyositis.

GROSS FINDINGS: The group of diseases encompassed under this rubric vary greatly in their manifestations. The gross findings include endocarditis, pericarditis, vasculitis, and ischemic lesions.

MICROSCOPIC FINDINGS: Lupus classically causes fibrinoid necrosis, often perivascular, associated with a lymphocytic or mixed myocarditis. When vasculitis is present, it may be found in the heart as well as elsewhere, as can be infarcts, either secondary to coronary arteritis or microvascular thrombosis. Dermatomyositis is associated with a lymphocytic myocarditis. Scleroderma may acutely cause a lymphocytic myocarditis as well but chronically causes extensive subendocardial fibrosis.

REMARKS: Clinical correlation is extremely important, as is a thorough drug history, because some drugs may cause similar changes.

DIFFERENTIAL DIAGNOSIS: Among the conditions that might show some of the changes of this group of conditions are: ischemic lesions due to coronary atherosclerosis, lymphocytic myocarditis of other etiology, drug-related myocarditis, vasculitis unrelated to collagen vascular disease, and thrombotic thrombocytopenia purpura, which may mimic the microvascular thrombosis of antiphospholipid antibody syndrome.

KEY DIAGNOSTIC CRITERIA: History and serologic tests are absolutely necessary.

POTENTIAL PITFALLS: Insufficient history and clinical correlation.

MYOCARDITIS, COXSACKIE VIRUS-ASSOCIATED

Entry Author: H. Thomas Aretz

SYNONYMS: Viral myocarditis, not otherwise specified, is the term used when a specific diagnosis is not possible. Coxsackie virus is thought to be the etiologic agent in a large proportion of such cases.

DEFINITION: A primary inflammatory condition of the heart caused by a member of the Coxsackie virus family, which exhibits both myocyte necrosis and an associated inflammatory infiltrate, thus fulfilling the criteria for myocarditis (see *Myocarditis, NOS*).

GROSS FINDINGS: The gross appearance varies from almost normal to marked dilation of the cardiac chambers. Pericarditis may be present. In cases with extensive myocardial necrosis, there may be multiple foci of yellow myocardium with or without endocardial thrombi, and the myocardium may be "flabby." Chronic cases may show the typical findings of dilated cardiomyopathy.

MICROSCOPIC FINDINGS: Lymphocytic myocarditis fulfilling the criteria of myocarditis. In animals and pediatric patients, there may be extensive necrosis, sometimes with calcification, associated with an inflammatory infiltrate that is scant in proportion to the extent of necrosis. Chronic cases may show the changes of dilated cardiomyopathy (see *Cardiomyopathy, idiopathic dilated*).

REMARKS: Identification of the virus responsible for the pathology observed in a particular patient has been a longstanding problem. The techniques of molecular diagnosis have been applied to this problem with mixed and controversial results, and are therefore not presently practical for routine diagnostic use. Serologic tests are useful in the setting of a known epidemic or when a rising titer can be demonstrated.

DIFFERENTIAL DIAGNOSIS: Lymphocytic myocardial infiltrates may also be seen in myocarditis that is idiopathic, rickettsial, spirochetal, toxic, autoimmune, or associated with collagen vascular diseases, sarcoidosis, healed infarcts, and lymphomas.

KEY DIAGNOSTIC CRITERIA: Lymphocytic myocarditis with epidemiological, serologic, and/or other evidence of acute Coxsackie virus infection.

POTENTIAL PITFALLS: The major pitfall is lack of information needed for diagnostic specificity or to rule out other conditions.

MYOCARDITIS, DIPHTHERIA-ASSOCIATED

Entry Author: H. Thomas Aretz

SYNONYM: Diphtheritic myocarditis.

DEFINITION: Toxic myocarditis (see *Myocarditis, toxic*) caused by the exotoxin of *Corynebacterium diphtheriae*, seen rarely nowadays.

GROSS FINDINGS: Flaccid, pale myocardium; ventricular dilation.

MICROSCOPIC FINDINGS: In the early stages, there is extensive hyaline degeneration, myocytolysis, and intracellular fat accumulation. Later an interstitial lymphocytic myocarditis, disproportionately mild in comparison to the myocardial damage, develops. Interstitial myocardial fibrosis may develop during healing. Involvement of the conduction system is the rule.

REMARKS: Extensive mitochondrial damage may be evident on electron microscopy. Clinical correlation is essential.

DIFFERENTIAL DIAGNOSIS: Toxic myocarditis, drug-related.

KEY DIAGNOSTIC CRITERIA: Toxic myocardial changes; myocardial degeneration disproportionate to interstitial inflammatory infiltrate.

POTENTIAL PITFALLS: Insufficient clinical/laboratory data to be certain myocardial changes are related to *Corynebacterium diphtheriae* infection.

MYOCARDITIS, DRUG-INDUCED

Entry Author: H. Thomas Aretz

SYNONYMS: Subsets include toxic myocarditis and hypersensitivity myocarditis, as well as necrotizing and nonnecrotizing vasculitis.

DEFINITION: Myocarditis caused by the effects of drugs, therapeutic or illicit, either as a result of direct toxicity or immunological reaction.

MORPHOLOGY: Varies widely with the type of drug and which of the four react classes (see Table 1) is involved.

MYOCARDITIS, EOSINOPHILIC, HYPEREOSINOPHILIA SYNDROME

Entry Author: H. Thomas Aretz

SYNONYMS: Löffler's disease, fibroplastic parietal endocarditis, endomyocardial fibrosis, eosinophilic heart disease, eosinophilic endomyocardial disease.

DEFINITION: A form of myocarditis associated with eosinophilia, regardless of the cause of the eosinophilia. The myocarditis is apparently secondary to injurious effects of cationic proteins derived from eosinophilic granules. The proteins apparently produce myocyte necrosis with a resultant secondary mixed inflammation. In some patients, there is an endomyocarditis, with endocardial damage related to adhesion and degranulation of eosinophiles. This may be especially prominent in the right ventricular outflow tract.

GROSS FINDINGS: The gross changes reflect myocarditis or endomyocarditis. The myocardium may be mottled, edematous, flabby. There may be mural thrombi in the ventricles. At a late stage of the disease, there may be

TABLE 1. *Drugs causing inflammatory myocardial lesions*

Myocarditis		Vasculitis	
Hypersensitivity	Toxic	Nonnecrotizing	Necrotizing
Amphotericin B	Amphetamines	Allopurinol	Arsenic
Horse serum	Anthracyclines	Ampicillin	Bismuth
Isoniazid	Antihypertensives	Bromide	Cyclophosphamide
Methyldopa	Antimony	Carbamazepine	(Cytoxan)
Penicillin	Arsenicals	(Tegretol)	Gold
Phenindione	Barbiturates	Chloramphenicol	Methamphetamine
Phenylbutazone	Caffeine	Chlorothiazide	Sulfonamides
Smallpox vaccine	Catecholamines	Chlorpropamide	
Streptomycin	Cyclophosphamide	Chlortetracycline	
Sulfonamides	Diphtheria toxin	Chlorthalidone	
Sulfonylureas	Emetine hydrochloride	Colchicine	
Tetanus toxoid	Epinephrine (Adrenalin)	Cromolyn sodium	
Tetracyclines	5-Fluorouracil	Dextran	
	Immunosuppresives	Diphenhydramine	
	Lithium carbonate	Diphenylhydantoin	
	Paraquat	(Phenytoin sodium)	
	Phenothiazines	Griseofulvin	
	Plasmocid	Indomethacin (Indocin)	
	Quinidine	Isoniazid	
	Rapeseed oil	Levamisole	
	Theophylline	Methylthiouracil	
		Oxyphenbutazone	
		Penicillin	
		Phenylbutazone	
		Potassium iodide	
		Procainamide	
		Quinidine	
		Spironolactone	
		Sulfonamides	
		Tetracyclines	
		Trimethadione	
		(Tridione)	

Also see hypersensitivity angiitis (Section 3), as well as myocarditis, toxic and myocarditis, hypersensitivity.

endomyocardial fibrosis. The changes reflecting myocarditis, endocarditis, and endomyocardial fibrosis, are thought to develop sequentially.

MICROSCOPIC FINDINGS: Acute myocarditis with prominent myocyte necrosis and eosinophiles forming a large proportion of the inflammatory cells. Degranulation of eosinophiles may be obvious (i.e., eosinophilic granules may be numerous). When present, endocarditis often seen as fibrin on endocardium, sometimes with entrapped eosinophiles. Mural thrombosis may be well developed. This becomes organized and converted to scar.

REMARKS: Giemsa stain may help to identify degranulated eosinophiles.

DIFFERENTIAL DIAGNOSIS: In hypersensitivity myocarditis myocyte necrosis is less prominent, but the inflammatory infiltrate is more prominent.

Unlike necrotizing eosinophilic myocarditis, the myocarditis of this condition is only seen together with peripheral eosinophilia.

KEY DIAGNOSTIC CRITERIA: Eosinophiles with degranulation and myocyte necrosis in a patient with evidence or a history of hypereosinophilia.

POTENTIAL PITFALLS: Insufficient information about eosinophilia. Partial treatment with steroids may interfere with diagnosis by altering the hematologic as well as the histopathologic changes.

SEE ALSO: Endomyocardial fibrosis; myocarditis, eosinophilic, necrotizing.

MYOCARDITIS, EOSINOPHILIC, NECROTIZING

Entry Author: H. Thomas Aretz

DEFINITION: Rapidly fatal necrotizing myocarditis with predominant eosinophilic infiltrate often in the absence of systemic eosinophilia.

GROSS FINDINGS: Heart may appear grossly unremarkable but may be dilated and the myocardium may be mottled.

MICROSCOPIC FINDINGS: Diffuse or multifocal myocyte necrosis with mixed inflammatory infiltrate in which eosinophiles are prominent, and these may show degranulation.

REMARKS: Clinical history of sudden onset in young patients. Giemsa stain may help identify eosinophiles.

DIFFERENTIAL DIAGNOSIS: Myocarditis, hypersensitivity; myocarditis, idiopathic; myocarditis, giant cell; myocarditis, eosinophilic, hypereosinophilia syndrome.

KEY DIAGNOSTIC CRITERIA: Eosinophiles associated with myocyte necrosis often in young patients.

POTENTIAL PITFALLS: Underestimating the importance of the eosinophilic component.

MYOCARDITIS, FUNGAL

Entry Author: H. Thomas Aretz

DEFINITION: Myocarditis caused by a fungus. Generally seen in the setting of immunosuppression, systemic sepsis, or endocarditis.

GROSS FINDINGS: The myocardium may show multiple small foci of necrosis as well as larger abscesses.

MICROSCOPIC FINDINGS: Multiple foci of myocyte necrosis with acute inflammatory infiltrates are seen in candida infections, aspergillosis, and sporothrix. Granulomas are seen with histoplasmosis (showing numerous organisms in macrophages), coccidioidomycosis, actinomycosis (including sulphur granules), blastomycosis, and cryptomycosis. In aspergillosis, the angioinvasive nature of the organism may lead to hemorrhagic necrosis.

REMARKS: Special stains are absolutely necessary to establish the diagnosis. Grocott methenamine silver (GMS) and periodic acid Schiff (PAS) stains will stain most organisms, but the Gram stain will identify actinomyces, and a mucin stain is helpful in demonstrating cryptococci.

DIFFERENTIAL DIAGNOSIS: Myocarditis due to a fungus can be confused with other forms of myocarditis, but demonstration of fungal organisms establishes the diagnosis.

KEY DIAGNOSTIC CRITERIA: Demonstration of causative organisms by special stains.

POTENTIAL PITFALLS: Not recognizing the possible causative agents on regular stains and not doing the special stains.

MYOCARDITIS, GIANT CELL

Entry Author: H. Thomas Aretz

SYNONYMS: Fiedler's myocarditis. While the term "granulomatous myocarditis" has been applied to this condition, these are actually distinct conditions (see *Myocarditis, granulomatous*).

DEFINITION: An often fatal mixed cell myocarditis of unknown etiology with a prominent component of giant cells but no well-formed granulomas.

GROSS FINDINGS: Mottled, flaccid myocardium with a dilated ventricular cavity. Pale areas, generally described as serpiginous, contain inflammatory cells.

MICROSCOPIC FINDINGS: Diffuse or multifocal mixed inflammation, primarily chronic, with single or clustered giant cells and myocyte necrosis that is commonly extensive. Eosinophiles may be abundant. Well-formed granulomas are not characteristic.

DIFFERENTIAL DIAGNOSIS: This condition is to be distinguished from granulomatous myocarditis, hypersensitivity myocarditis, fungal myocarditis, Whipple's disease (endocarditis, infective, of heart valve, Whipple's disease), and acute rheumatic fever, and sarcoidosis-associated myocarditis. See entries in this section, except for Whipple's disease, which is in Section 2 (endocarditis, infective, of heart valve, Whipple's disease).

KEY DIAGNOSTIC CRITERIA: Mixed inflammatory infiltrate with giant cells, myocyte necrosis, and no demonstrable organisms or other etiology.

POTENTIAL PITFALLS: Overlooking specific organisms in look-alikes; sampling error.

MYOCARDITIS, GRANULOMATOUS

Entry Author: H. Thomas Aretz

SYNONYMS: This condition has been referred to as giant cell myocarditis but is distinguished from that condition as indicated below (see entry: *Myocarditis, giant cell*).

DEFINITION: A form of myocarditis, due to any one of several etiologies or of unknown etiology in which there are well-formed granulomas, either between myocytes (i.e., interstitial) or replacing myocytes.

GROSS FINDINGS: Depending on the etiology, the myocardial lesions vary from diffuse mottling to focal necrosis or abscesses. There may be distinct areas of pale, almost "fish-flesh," tissue within the myocardium or forming thick plaques within the endocardium.

MICROSCOPIC FINDINGS: The lesions vary depending on etiology. Granulomas may be interstitial, such as the ones seen in hypersensitivity reactions, or myocardial, as seen in mycobacterial, or fungal infections, and also in sarcoidosis. Granulomas may be necrotizing or nonnecrotizing, depending on the etiology. Necrotizing granulomas are invariably associated with a fungal or bacterial etiology. In hypersensitivity-type reactions, there may be a prominent eosinophilic component.

REMARKS: The term *granulomatous myocarditis* should be reserved for the forms of myocarditis in which there are well-formed granulomas, and should be distinguished from giant cell myocarditis, as etiology and prognosis may differ markedly.

DIFFERENTIAL DIAGNOSIS: Myocarditis, giant cell; myocarditis, fungal; myocarditis, hypersensitivity; myocarditis, bacterial direct; myocarditis, sarcoidosis-associated; myocarditis, foreign body reaction.

KEY DIAGNOSTIC CRITERIA: Myocarditis with well-formed granulomas.

POTENTIAL PITFALLS: Failure to exclude all specific causes.

MYOCARDITIS, HYPERSENSITIVITY

Entry Author: H. Thomas Aretz

DEFINITION: A form of myocarditis (see Myocarditis, NOS) caused by a hypersensitivity reaction, usually to a drug, which therefore may resolve without sequelae upon withdrawal of the offending agent.

GROSS FINDINGS: Varies from normal in color and consistency to mottled and/or flabby. The ventricles may be dilated.

MICROSCOPIC FINDINGS: The hallmark of hypersensitivity myocarditis is a diffuse infiltrate, primarily interstitial, rich in eosinophiles. Myocyte necrosis is seen in a small proportion of cases. This is presumably mediated by the cationic protein released in eosinophilic granules, as is the case in other forms of eosinophilic myocarditis (see entry). Eosinophile degranulation may be seen on high power. In addition to the eosinophiles, there may be occasional giant cells and scattered histiocytes in the interstitium approaching the appearance of a granulomatous myocarditis or giant cell myocarditis. In general, however, the severity of the interstitial infiltrate is disproportionate to the myocyte damage, and complete resolution of the infiltrate and full return to normal function is common. Eosinophilic myocarditis is probably related to the hypersensitivity that is frequently seen in explanted recipient hearts, as these patients usually receive a plethora of drugs. It is possible that the lymphocytic perivascular (perivenular) infiltrate associated with certain drugs is a milder form of hypersensitivity "myocarditis."

REMARKS: A complete history, revealing candidate drugs, is important in establishing this diagnosis (see Table 1 under *Myocarditis, drug-induced*). Special stains, such as the Giemsa stain, may highlight eosinophile granules.

DIFFERENTIAL DIAGNOSIS: Any condition that results in peripheral hypereosinophilia may give rise to an eosinophilic myocarditis (Löffler's) which must be distinguished from the present condition. Parasitic infestation, hematologic malignancies, and generalized allergic states are examples of conditions in which this may occur. Clinical history is therefore extremely important, as the histologic findings may be quite confounding. Mixed forms of myocarditis with or without giant cells often contain a prominent eosinophilic component as does cardiac transplant rejection (cardiac allograft rejection) and the early healing phase of myocardial infarction. In these conditions, the inflammatory infiltrate is generally proportional to the myocardial damage. In hypersensitivity myocarditis there is relatively little necrosis considering the amount of inflammation. There are cases, however, where there is extensive necrosis. Some authors have referred to this as necrotizing eosinophilic myocarditis (see entry).

KEY DIAGNOSTIC CRITERIA: Prominent interstitial eosinophilic inflammatory infiltrate disproportionate to the amount of myocyte damage in the appropriate clinical setting.

POTENTIAL PITFALLS: The major pitfalls relate to differentiation from the conditions outlined in the differential diagnosis.

MYOCARDITIS, LYME DISEASE-ASSOCIATED

Entry Author: H. Thomas Aretz

DEFINITION: Myocarditis caused by the Lyme disease agent, the spirochete *Borrelia burgdorferi*.

GROSS FINDINGS: The gross findings may be quite innocuous and non-specific. Pericarditis may be present but is not specific.

MICROSCOPIC FINDINGS: Lyme carditis is a lymphocytic myocarditis, often with a prominent plasmacytic component. Involvement of the conduction system, particularly the atrioventricular node, may be prominent and correlates with the clinical finding of temporary heart block.

REMARKS: The agent can be demonstrated in autopsy or biopsy tissues by silver impregnation techniques.

DIFFERENTIAL DIAGNOSIS: Lyme disease-associated myocarditis must be distinguished from the numerous other causes of lymphocytic myocarditis.

KEY DIAGNOSTIC CRITERIA: Lymphocytic myocarditis with a prominent plasma cell component together with demonstration of the organism by special stains, or positive serological data or other basis for the diagnosis in the affected patient.

POTENTIAL PITFALLS: Insufficient clinical history.

MYOCARDITIS, METHYLDOPA-ASSOCIATED

Entry Author: Stephen M. Factor

SYNONYMS: Related terms include allergic myocarditis, eosinophilic myocarditis, drug-induced myocarditis.

DEFINITION: An eosinophilic myocarditis that occurs as part of the complex hypersensitivity reaction to methyldopa.

GROSS FINDINGS: No specific feature related to methyldopa independent of the underlying cardiac disease (e.g., hypertension).

MICROSCOPIC FINDINGS: Acute myocarditis with myocyte necrosis and with eosinophiles as a prominent component of the inflammatory infiltrate. See entries: *Myocarditis, eosinophilic, Myocarditis, drug-induced.*

REMARKS: May be difficult to link disease specifically to methyldopa if other drugs are used concurrently. However, methyldopa is a common cause of drug-induced myocarditis.

DIFFERENTIAL DIAGNOSIS: Hypersensitivity to other drugs and other causes for eosinophilic myocarditis.

KEY DIAGNOSTIC CRITERIA: Eosinophilic myocarditis. Inflammation abates with drug withdrawal (and returns with re-challenge, but retreatment is virtually never attempted).

POTENTIAL PITFALLS: There are many causes of eosinophilic myocarditis. In absence of re-challenge it is difficult to ascribe hypersensitivity to methyldopa with absolute certainty.

MYOCARDITIS, NOS

Entry Author: H. Thomas Aretz

SYNONYM: Idiopathic myocarditis.

DEFINITION: According to the Dallas classification, myocarditis is defined as a myocardial inflammatory infiltrate associated with myocyte necrosis or degeneration. There are many causes of myocarditis including infectious, immune-mediated, drug-induced, and idiopathic. There is great variability in the cellular components (lymphocytes, eosinophiles, giant cells, mixed) and the healing process (fibrosis or no fibrosis). It is, therefore, difficult to determine the time course of the disease on first biopsy or at autopsy unless a prior pathologic diagnosis is known and available for comparison to establish a diagnosis of healing or healed myocarditis.

GROSS FINDINGS: The gross appearance may be quite variable as involvement of the myocardium can be very focal, restricted to one or some of the chambers, or global. In diffuse, extensive involvement, often accompanied clinically by congestive failure, the hearts are dilated and flabby and the myocardium appears mottled. Endocardial thrombi are commonly present and the pericardium may be dull and shaggy, as there may be concomitant pericarditis. In the more chronic stages, scattered scars or typical findings of congestive cardiomyopathy (see *Cardiomyopathy, idiopathic dilated*) may be present. Depending on etiology, a variety of extramyocardial lesions may be present. For example, endocarditis and pericarditis may be present, together with myocarditis, in rheumatic fever. The gross changes are therefore quite variable.

MICROSCOPIC FINDINGS: A combination of myocyte damage and an inflammatory infiltrate is required. Myocyte damage may take the form of myocyte drop-out, myocytolysis, irregular myocyte contours, or frank necrosis. Under certain circumstances groups of myocytes may be necrotic and calcified, particularly in coxsackie virus B myocarditis (see *Myocarditis, coxsackie virus-associated*) in early childhood. The interstitium is generally widened, edematous, and filled with inflammatory cells reflecting specific subgroups of myocarditis. These infiltrates may be focal, confluent, or diffuse, judged in biopsy specimens by the involvement of multiple pieces and the extent of infiltration in each fragment. Fibrosis and hypertrophy may be present, which may reflect underlying disease or healing and compensatory processes. The endocardium is often involved and may be heavily infiltrated by inflammatory cells and thrombus may be present, in some forms invariably (e.g., the organizing phase of Löffler's). When sequential biopsies are available, the process may be classified as persistent, healing, or healed, depending on the severity of the infiltrate and the histologic changes of repair. Healed myocarditis may show no residua, or there may be fibrosis, hypertrophy, or residual inflammatory cells, which should be confined to the areas of scarring and myocyte necrosis. There should be no inflammatory cells adjacent to the healed area.

REMARKS: An adequate clinical history and clinicopathological correlation is essential. Infectious agents must be identified and the inflammatory infiltrate clarified. The use of immunologic activation markers to establish the diagnosis of myocarditis in general, particularly in the face of a sparse infiltrate (borderline myocarditis) is under active investigation.

DIFFERENTIAL DIAGNOSIS: Any condition that gives rise to a myocardial inflammatory infiltrate with or without necrosis may be confused with myocarditis. Ischemic changes usually do not involve the immediate subendocardial region and show coagulation necrosis (see entry) followed by healing as classically described (see entries for *Myocardial infarct, acute* and *Myocardial infarct, healed*). The small catecholamine-mediated foci of myocyte necrosis may be particularly troubling, because the contraction bands seen in these lesions are a common artefact in biopsies, but the typical scant inflammatory infiltrate should alert one to this possibility. In biopsies, previous biopsy sites may resemble myocarditis, but they are generally broadly endocardially based with organizing fibrin, early, and are later surrounded by irregular myocyte hypertrophy with myocyte disarray. Dilated cardiomyopathy (see *Cardiomyopathy, idiopathic dilated*) may often show areas of chronic inflammation which should, however, be confined to areas of fibrosis or should be scant in the interstitium. A background of hypertrophied myocytes, interstitial fibrosis, replacement fibrosis and myocyte degeneration is strong evidence that the process is chronic, although a combination of cardiomyopathy and myocarditis can certainly be seen, particularly in patients who relapse. Lymphoproliferative disorders involving the myocardium may very much resemble lymphocytic myocarditis. Although they are often not associated with myocyte necrosis, this can be seen. Cytologic features are often helpful, as are studies for cell markers and clonality. Still, atypical T-cell infiltrates as seen in AIDS may be difficult to distinguish from myocarditis on biopsy. At autopsy the nodular or mass-like involvement of the myocardium becomes more apparent and helps in the differentiation. Cardiac transplant rejection (see *Cardiac allograft rejection*) certainly mimics myocarditis, but clinical history should make this distinction apparent. Nonetheless, myocarditis may arise in transplant patients, particularly parasitic (e.g., toxoplasmosis) or viral (e.g., CMV). Finally, the insertion of catheters and pacemakers into the right ventricle may on occasion give rise to confusion in endomyocardial biopsy specimens, particularly if the intervention preceded the biopsy by a few days, as there may be an endocardial inflammatory infiltrate.

KEY DIAGNOSTIC CRITERIA: Myocyte degeneration/necrosis with an adjacent inflammatory infiltrate not indicative of ischemic damage and occurring in the appropriate clinical setting.

POTENTIAL PITFALLS: Thrombi may be mistaken for necrotic myocytes with inflammatory cells on biopsy. Biopsy artifacts, such as contraction bands or crush artefact and separation of myocytes may be mistaken for myocyte necrosis and interstitial edema. In addition, all the conditions mentioned in the section on differential diagnosis constitute pitfalls in diagnosis.

MYOCARDITIS, PARASITIC, IMMUNOLOGIC

Entry Author: H. Thomas Aretz

DEFINITION: Myocarditis caused by an auto-immune reaction initiated by a parasite resulting in a usually lymphocytic myocarditis. Offending organisms include *Trichinella spiralis* and *Trypanosoma cruzi*.

GROSS FINDINGS: Acute myocarditis may show areas of mottling and necrosis. There may be ventricular dilation.

MICROSCOPIC FINDINGS: The pathology of Chagas' disease is described elsewhere in this work (see *Myocarditis, Chagas' disease*) but is essentially a necrotizing lymphocytic myocarditis. Trichinosis may cause necrosis in reaction to the larval forms, toxic changes, or a hypersensitivity type reaction with prominent eosinophiles.

REMARKS: Clinical history and serology is helpful.

DIFFERENTIAL DIAGNOSIS: Myocarditis, NOS; hypersensitivity myocarditis.

KEY DIAGNOSTIC CRITERIA: Clinicopathological correlation and careful examination of the myocardium for possible organisms.

POTENTIAL PITFALLS: Insufficient history and missing organisms in noninflamed areas of the myocardium.

MYOCARDITIS, PNEUMOCYSTIS CARINII-ASSOCIATED

Entry Author: H. Thomas Aretz

DEFINITION: Myocarditis caused by *Pneumocystis carinii,* virtually always in immunosuppressed patients. Generally an incidental finding at autopsy.

GROSS FINDINGS: The gross findings more often reflect the underlying condition responsible for immunosuppression but which may cause cardiomyopathy itself. Examples of these include AIDS or treatment with drugs such as adriamycin.

MICROSCOPIC FINDINGS: Just as in the lung, the organisms are found in association with a fluffy eosinophilic fibrinous infiltrate, which may replace myocytes. The organisms are extracellular and can be suspected even in an H&E-stained slide by virtue of their characteristic negative staining.

REMARKS: The organisms can be easily demonstrated using the Grocott methenamine silver (GMS) stain.

DIFFERENTIAL DIAGNOSIS: The findings are rather specific, but confusion may arise with myocyte degeneration or focal fibrosis.

POTENTIAL PITFALLS: The major pitfall relates to not thinking of the possibility and therefore not doing the GMS stain to demonstrate the organisms. Confusion with focal fibrosis or myocyte drop-out may arise.

MYOCARDITIS, RHEUMATIC

Entry Author: H. Thomas Aretz

SYNONYMS: Related terms: acute rheumatic fever; rheumatic heart disease.

DEFINITION: The myocarditis that is sometimes a feature of acute rheumatic fever, which, in turn, sometimes follows infection by group A beta-hemolytic streptococci and is caused by an autoimmune reaction triggered by the antigens of this organism that mimic antigens found in the endocardium and elsewhere in the heart. This myocarditis has a characteristic form of inflammation that includes the Aschoff nodule, a form of granuloma pathognomonic for rheumatic myocarditis.

GROSS FINDINGS: In acute rheumatic fever, there may be an endocarditis, pericarditis, myocarditis, or any combination of these three. Whereas the pericardial and endocardial changes may be prominent grossly, the myocardial changes usually are not, even when such lesions are microscopically prominent.

MICROSCOPIC FINDINGS: The particular interstitial granulomatous myocarditis of acute rheumatic fever is highly characteristic and taken as pathognomonic, but this lesion evolves over time. It starts as foci of edema and fibrinoid necrosis of the interstitium. Diffuse inflammatory infiltrates, mainly lymphocytic but occasionally with mixed cell population, may also be seen early. These early lesions develop into the characteristic focal granulomas known as *Aschoff bodies*. These consist of several cell types, including the mononuclear and multinuclear Aschoff cell. This cell has amphophilic cytoplasm and vesicular nuclei with a prominent single mass of chromatin, conferring an "owl's eye" appearance. Other forms of inflammatory cells are also present, including the Anitschkow myocyte. This spindle-shaped cell has pale cytoplasm and a vesicular nucleus with a central wavy line of chromatin. This cell type is seen in many forms of myocardial injury and does not have the diagnostic significance of the Aschoff cell. The Aschoff nodule appears during the acute rheumatic fever period of this disease, and may be found, particularly in the atrial muscle, even in the stages of rheumatic heart disease. Aschoff nodules are slowly replaced by scar tissue, so that active lesions are rarely seen in the ventricles of patients with rheumatic heart disease, although they do persist in the atria for longer periods. The interstitial fibrosis left by healed rheumatic myocarditis is particularly prominent around blood vessels where active lesions are found in the early stages.

REMARKS: The diagnosis is established clinically by application of the well-known "Jones Criteria." The myocardial lesions are also sufficiently characteristic, that, when they are clearly present, a diagnosis of rheumatic myocarditis can be made.

DIFFERENTIAL DIAGNOSIS: Hypersensitivity myocarditis; idiopathic myocarditis (see *Myocarditis, NOS*); giant cell myocarditis; sarcoidosis. Although the Aschoff nodule is pathognomonic, it may be confused with a true granuloma or giant cell infiltrate, but the presence of the characteristic cells should alert one to the true diagnosis. The earlier stages of rheumatic carditis may be more problematic, as foci of fibrinoid necrosis may raise the possibility of collagen vascular disease. The diffuse form of myocardial involvement may be even more problematic, as it may be confused with idiopathic or hypersensitivity myocarditis, but careful clinical history and supporting data should alert one to the correct diagnosis.

KEY DIAGNOSTIC CRITERIA: Aschoff nodules and other data supporting a diagnosis of rheumatic fever/rheumatic heart disease.

POTENTIAL PITFALLS: Mistaken diagnoses are not common, but this disease could be confused with other forms of myocarditis.

MYOCARDITIS, RHEUMATOID

Entry Author: H. Thomas Aretz

DEFINITION: Myocarditis in a patient with rheumatoid arthritis, either nonspecific or granulomatous.

GROSS FINDINGS: Fibrinous pericarditis is common and the left-sided valves may be fibrotic and deformed or contain rheumatoid nodules. The myocardial findings are only prominent if rheumatoid nodules are present. These are well circumscribed and most often located at the bases of the valves. The conduction system is often involved as well.

MICROSCOPIC FINDINGS: A nonspecific myocarditis, usually marked by a mononuclear interstitial infiltrate is common. Necrosis may be present rarely. The hallmark of the disease is the typical rheumatoid nodule, which is a granuloma characterized by central fibrinoid necrosis surrounded by palisading histiocytes, fibroblasts, and often giant cells.

REMARKS: Serologic and other clinical data are necessary to confirm the diagnosis when there is only nonspecific myocarditis.

DIFFERENTIAL DIAGNOSIS: Because the interstitial myocarditis is nonspecific, other causes have to be looked for actively, which may include diseases such as Lyme disease, rickettsial diseases, and viral infections, all of which may mimic rheumatoid disease clinically and histologically. Presence of rheumatoid factor is almost pathognomonic.

KEY DIAGNOSTIC CRITERIA: Rheumatoid nodules. In their absence, clinicopathological correlation is crucial.

MYOCARDITIS, RICKETTSIAL

Entry Author: H. Thomas Aretz

DEFINITION: Myocarditis caused by any *Rickettsiae*, such as *R. tsutsugamushi* (scrub typhus), *R. prowazekii* (epidemic typhus), *R. burnetii* (Q fever), or *R. rickettsii* (Rocky Mountain spotted fever).

GROSS FINDINGS: The myocardium is generally unremarkable but may be flaccid. Ventricular dilation may be present. Endocarditis may be present in Q fever.

MICROSCOPIC FINDINGS: Predominantly perivascular lymphocytic and plasmacytic/histiocytic interstitial infiltrate with interstitial edema. Generally there is no myocyte necrosis. Vasculitis with thrombosis may be prominent and perivascular fibrinoid necrosis and collections of inflammatory cells (typhus nodules) may be present with any of the *Rickettsiae,* except possibly Q fever.

REMARKS: The diagnosis can be established only by demonstrating the organism or a specific indicator of infection, such as a rising antibody titer. Organisms may be revealed in endothelial cells by Giemsa stain. Clinical data are taken as sufficient in the presence of an epidemic.

DIFFERENTIAL DIAGNOSIS: Because there is generally no myocyte necrosis and the infiltrate is mononuclear, other conditions such as Lyme disease, viral myocarditis, especially borderline, and collagen vascular disease enter into the differential. The typhus nodules and a prominent vasculitic component, together with serologic and clinical data, should allow one to differentiate this entity.

KEY DIAGNOSTIC CRITERIA: Scattered interstitial, perivascular lympho-plasmacytic infiltrate without significant myocyte necrosis together with microbiological, serological, or clinical criteria for making the diagnosis of a specific rickettsial infection.

POTENTIAL PITFALLS: Lack of clinicopathological correlation.

MYOCARDITIS, SARCOIDOSIS-ASSOCIATED

Entry Author: H. Thomas Aretz

SYNONYM: Cardiac sarcoidosis.

DEFINITION: Sarcoidosis involving the myocardium. A granulomatous myocarditis that is a manifestation of sarcoidosis. Although this myocarditis may be the first clinical manifestation of sarcoidosis, the diagnosis should not be made in the absence of other evidence of this disease, such as anergy to common fungal antigens and an increased serum ACE (angiotensin converting enzyme) level.

GROSS FINDINGS: Large sharply delineated areas of granulomatous inflammation or scarring may be seen. Zones of active inflammation are pale and firm or even rubbery. Areas of predilection are the papillary muscles, the cephalad portions of the ventricles including the septum, and conduction system and the free walls of the right and left ventricle. After treatment and resultant fibrosis, aneurysms may be present in the free walls of the ventricles and the upper septum may appear markedly thinned.

MICROSCOPIC FINDINGS: Well-formed nonnecrotizing granulomas replacing the myocardium are the rule. Giant cells are usually present and the areas of inflammation may be very large and confluent. The conduction system is often involved. Chronically, especially after treatment with steroids, fibrosis may replace the granulomatous areas.

REMARKS: Special stains are necessary to rule out other causes of granulomatous myocarditis particularly mycobacterial or fungal infections.

DIFFERENTIAL DIAGNOSIS: Any granulomatous disease which can involve the myocardium enters the differential diagnosis, as it does in other organ systems such as the lungs or skin. Sarcoidosis is a diagnosis of exclusion, and specific causes such as mycobacteria, fungi, or foreign materials must be ruled out by the appropriate special studies. Differentiation from giant cell myocarditis may be difficult, but sarcoidosis generally presents with clearly formed granulomas, typical sarcoidal giant cells, and less diffuse myocardial involvement. Fibrosis may also be more prominent in sarcoidal granulomas.

KEY DIAGNOSTIC CRITERIA: Granulomatous myocarditis with no evidence of an infectious origin in a patient with sarcoidosis.

POTENTIAL PITFALLS: Sampling error in myocardial biopsies. Lack of special stains or clinical history, or superimposed effects of treatment.

MYOCARDITIS, SPIROCHETAL

Entry Author: H. Thomas Aretz

DEFINITION: Myocarditis caused by spirochetes such as *Treponema pallidum* (syphilis), *Leptospira sp.* (Weil's disease), *Borrelia recurrentis* (relapsing fever), or *Borrelia burgdorferi* (Lyme disease).

GROSS FINDINGS: The heart may be enlarged and gummas may be present in adult syphilis, predominantly located in the upper septum and the conduction system. These appear as spherical masses of pale material with a firm consistency.

MICROSCOPIC FINDINGS: Leptospirosis will cause interstitial edema, hemorrhage, and a mononuclear cell infiltrate, often involving the conduction system. The organisms may be demonstrable by silver stains. Relapsing fever also shows edema, a lymphoplasmacytic infiltrate in the interstitium and petechial hemorrhages but no myocyte necrosis. Syphilis, in its infantile form, causes an interstitial myocarditis similar to other spirochetes. In the adult form gummas are present. These show a mass of necrotic myocardium surrounded by epithelioid cells, fibroblasts, and, sometimes, giant cells.

REMARKS: Although silver stains may demonstrate the organism, serologic confirmation is the diagnostic procedure of choice.

DIFFERENTIAL DIAGNOSIS: Other forms of interstitial myocarditis, such as rickettsial disease or collagen vascular disease, enter into the differential. The presence of focal hemorrhages, organisms on special silver stains, and serological evidence of infection all help to establish the correct diagnosis. Findings in other organs at autopsy are most helpful.

KEY DIAGNOSTIC CRITERIA: Interstitial edema, focal hemorrhages, and mononuclear infiltrate; gummas for syphilis. Serologic correlation.

POTENTIAL PITFALLS: Lack of clinicopathological correlation.

MYOCARDITIS, TOXIC

Entry Author: H. Thomas Aretz

DEFINITION: Myocardial necrosis/degeneration and the resulting inflammation caused by chemical or biological toxins.

GROSS FINDINGS: The myocardium may be flaccid, mottled, sometimes hemorrhagic, and dilated.

MICROSCOPIC FINDINGS: There is multifocal myocyte degeneration, usually disproportionate to the amount of inflammation which may follow the degenerative process. In the early stages, edema may be prominent. The inflammatory infiltrate may be monomorphic or mixed, with both polymorphonuclear neutrophiles and mononuclear cells. The myocardial lesions are often of various ages, some acute, some healing, and some healed, presumably reflecting repeated exposures.

REMARKS: Toxicologic studies or clinical information indicating involvement of a particular toxic substance are necessary to make the diagnosis with certainty. (See Table 1 in entry for *Myocarditis, drug-induced*).

DIFFERENTIAL DIAGNOSIS: Because myocyte necrosis and an inflammatory infiltrate are associated with toxic myocarditis, other forms of myocarditis, which include most types, enter into the differential diagnosis. The scant inflammatory infiltrate, which is disproportionate to the amount of myocyte damage, and lesions of various ages in chronic toxic injuries, are all clues to this diagnosis. Clinical history and toxicology studies are absolutely necessary to make this diagnosis.

KEY DIAGNOSTIC CRITERIA: Lesions of varying ages; myocyte degeneration; clinical correlation.

POTENTIAL PITFALLS: Lack of toxicologic or positive clinical data.

MYOCARDITIS, TOXOCARA CANIS-ASSOCIATED

Entry Author: H. Thomas Aretz

SYNONYM: Visceral larva migrans.

DEFINITION: Inflammation of the myocardium secondary to infestation by larvae of *Toxocara canis*. This can occur by either of two mechanisms: (a) the direct effect of degenerating larvae that elicit a granulomatous inflammatory reaction, or (b) a secondary effect due to hypereosinophilia (see entry, *Myocarditis, eosinophilic, hypereosinophilia syndrome*).

GROSS FINDINGS: Focal areas of necrosis may be present in the myocardium.

MICROSCOPIC FINDINGS: The degenerating larva incites an intense granulomatous reaction usually marked by a prominent eosinophilic component with palisading histiocytes and scattered giant cells. Fibrosis results chronically. Intact larvae are about 15 to 20 microns in diameter and 400 microns long.

REMARKS: The direct involvement is usually found incidentally, and clinically significant disease is usually related to hypereosinophilia, the pathology of which is discussed in the entry myocarditis, eosinophilic, hypereosinophilia syndrome.

DIFFERENTIAL DIAGNOSIS: The granulomatous lesions may conceivably be confused with rheumatoid nodules, although the history, degenerated larval forms and eosinophilia, should alert one of the correct diagnosis. Other necrotizing granulomatous lesions can be excluded by special stains and history.

KEY DIAGNOSTIC CRITERIA: Granulomatous reaction to larval forms.

POTENTIAL PITFALLS: The major pitfall may be related to not finding or recognizing the degenerating larvae. Visceral larval migrans due to species of other than *T. canis* must be dealt with through a combination of history, immunological tests, and morphology. *T. cati*, in particular, may produce a similar condition.

MYOCARDITIS, TOXOPLASMA GONDII-ASSOCIATED

Entry Author: H. Thomas Aretz

DEFINITION: Myocarditis caused by the intracellular parasitic forms of *Toxoplasma gondii*, usually the encysted bradyzoites in immunosuppressed patients, such as cardiac transplant recipients or patients with AIDS or other forms of immunodeficiencies, either natural or iatrogenic.

GROSS FINDINGS: Usually nonspecific, although areas of necrosis may be seen in acute cases and fibrosis may be evident in chronic cases.

MICROSCOPIC FINDINGS: The microscopic hallmark is organisms in myocytes. These are usually bradyzoites in cysts, although tachyzoites have been seen. The associated myocarditis is usually lymphocytic and the cysts may not be associated with an inflammatory infiltrate. Chronically, fibrosis may develop.

REMARKS: If there are questions as to the identity of the intracellular organisms, a PAS stain, which is positive for *Toxoplasma,* and electron microscopy may be helpful.

DIFFERENTIAL DIAGNOSIS: Infections with other intracellular organisms such as *Trypanosoma cruzi* (see entry *Myocarditis, Chagas' disease*) and Sarcocystis, and acute mitochondrial calcification associated with ischemia may be confused with toxoplasmosis. Special stains, electron microscopy, and clinical correlation all may be helpful in differentiation.

KEY DIAGNOSTIC CRITERIA: Intracellular organisms and myocarditis.

POTENTIAL PITFALLS: The main pitfall is failure to examine noninflamed myocardium, because cysts may be present in normal appearing myocardium.

MYOCARDITIS, TRICHINOSIS-ASSOCIATED

Entry Author: H. Thomas Aretz

DEFINITION: Myocarditis caused by a hypersensitivity reaction to the parasite *Trichinella spiralis* resulting in an eosinophilic myocarditis or localized areas of necrosis in response to degenerating parasites.

GROSS FINDINGS: There may be areas of mottling, necrosis, and dilation. Foci of yellow necrosis may be present.

MICROSCOPIC FINDINGS: Trichinosis may cause necrosis in reaction to the larval forms, toxic changes, or a hypersensitivity reaction with prominent eosinophiles. There is therefore a mixture of findings which include localized areas of necrosis usually with a prominent eosinophilic response as well as a diffuse eosinophilic or lymphocytic myocarditis.

REMARKS: Clinical history and serology is helpful.

DIFFERENTIAL DIAGNOSIS: The localized areas of necrosis with associated eosinophilic myocarditis should raise one's suspicions about this entity. Clinical information is crucial, however, particularly in cases of pure hypersensitivity and/or toxic changes when organisms may not be present in the myocardium.

KEY DIAGNOSTIC CRITERIA: Clinicopathological correlation and careful examination of the myocardium for possible organisms.

POTENTIAL PITFALLS: The diagnosis may be missed because of insufficient history and the absence of organisms from the myocardium.

MYOCARDITIS, VIRAL

Entry Author: H. Thomas Aretz

DEFINITION: Myocarditis caused by a virus resulting in myocyte necrosis and myocardial inflammation. Many cases of idiopathic myocarditis are presumed to be viral in origin (see *Myocarditis, NOS*).

GROSS FINDINGS: The myocardium varies from unremarkable to flaccid, with or without mottling. Mural thrombi may be present, and the ventricles may be dilated.

MICROSCOPIC FINDINGS: Classically there is a lymphocytic myocarditis, but the infiltrate may be mixed and even giant cells may be seen. The vast majority of cases show the changes of myocarditis, NOS.

REMARKS: The most common cause of viral myocarditis is probably coxsackie virus B (see *Myocarditis, Coxsackie virus-associated*), but clinical cardiac abnormalities have been associated with many viral illnesses including mononucleosis and influenza. The diagnosis is usually made by circumstantial evidence. Molecular techniques have had varying successes in demonstrating viral genomes in myocarditis cases. Even if present, such genomic material may not indicate active infection. Serologic studies are usually only warranted during the course of a known epidemic and are otherwise a shot in the dark at best.

DIFFERENTIAL DIAGNOSIS: Because this is a diagnosis of exclusion, other causes of myocarditis have to be ruled out based on clinical history (e.g., drugs, collagen vascular disease). While molecular technique may be of only limited value, acute and chronic specific antibody titers may be the most supportive.

KEY DIAGNOSTIC CRITERIA: Lymphocytic or mixed inflammation with myocyte necrosis in a patient with rising antibody titers to a known virus. Myocarditis of this morphologic type occurring during the course of an epidemic is commonly accepted as due to the epidemic-causing virus.

POTENTIAL PITFALLS: Lack of clinical history or data to rule out other causes.

MYOCYTOLYSIS I

Entry Author: Robert J. Siegel

EDITORS NOTE—Because a significant difference of opinion has been expressed regarding this term, two separate entries have been used, each reflecting the views of a spokesman for a particular viewpoint.

SYNONYMS: Vacuolar degeneration, colliquative myocytolysis.

DEFINITION: Light microscopic appearance of vacuolated, cleared-out myocardial fibers.

GROSS FINDINGS: There is no specific gross appearance that correlates with this microscopic observation. The affected zone may display subendocardial pallor, yellow-tan discoloration, or no gross abnormality.

MICROSCOPIC FINDINGS: Cells exhibiting myocytolysis have a varying degree of cytoplasmic vacuolation. In its most pronounced form, the myocyte appears empty except for the nucleus and a peripheral rim of cytoplasm. Myocytolysis is detected in routine H&E-stained histologic sections. Special stains are not necessary in most cases; they may demonstrate glycogen but generally not lipid in the vacuolated fibers. Ultrastructurally, the cytoplasmic clearing corresponds to disorganization and loss of myofibrils, with accumulation of glycogen, cytoskeletal filaments, and mitochondria. Myocytolysis most frequently is seen in the subendocardial left ventricle and at the periphery of myocardial infarcts. Often it is perivascular. There is no associated inflammatory cellular reaction.

REMARKS: Myocytolysis most commonly is encountered in the setting of chronic ischemic heart disease but also may be seen in acute ischemia, in cardiomyopathies, myocarditis, and other miscellaneous disorders. Whether the change represents irreversible or reversible myocyte injury has been controversial. In previous usage, the term denoted *intracellular fluid uptake* (hydropic change), and although the definition given here is the most used, the true pathophysiology of the change described as "myocytolysis" is uncertain.

DIFFERENTIAL DIAGNOSIS: Myocardial fiber vacuolation also is seen in various storage diseases (glycogen, glycosaminoglycan, glycoprotein, etc.). The more diffuse nature of myocardial involvement, clinical presentation, and special techniques to detect the accumulated product aid in differentiating these disorders from myocytolysis.

KEY DIAGNOSTIC CRITERIA: The distinctive appearance of vacuolated myocyte cytoplasm allows for the recognition and diagnosis of myocytolysis.

POTENTIAL PITFALLS: Myocytolysis should be distinguished from tissue-sectioning artefact and from the other causes of myocardial fiber vacuolation, as just discussed.

References

1. Baroldi G, Falzi G, Mariani F. Sudden coronary death. A postmortem study in 208 selected cases compared to 97 "control" subjects. *Amer Heart J* 1979;98:20–31.
2. Greer JC, Crago CA, Little WC, Gardner LL, Bishop SP. Subendocardial ischemic myocardial lesions associated with severe coronary atherosclerosis. *Am J Pathol* 1980;98:663–680.
3. Flameng W, Suy R, Schwartz F et al. Ultrastructural correlates of left ventricular contraction abnormalities in patients with chronic ischemic heart disease: Determinants of reversible segmental asynergy postrevascularization surgery. *Am Heart J* 1981;102:846—857.
4. Edwards GM, Said JW, Block MI, Herscher LL, Siegel RJ, Fishbein MC. Myocytolysis (vacuolar degeneration) of myocardium: Immunohistochemical evidence of viability. *Hum Pathol* 1984:15:753–756.

MYOCYTOLYSIS II

Entry Author: Stephen M. Factor

EDITORS NOTE—Because a significant difference of opinion has been expressed regarding this term, two separate entries have been used, each reflecting the views of a spokesman for a particular viewpoint.

SYNONYMS: Microinfarction; coagulative myocytolysis; myofibrillar degeneration; organizing contraction band necrosis.

DEFINITION: Myofibrillar degeneration and/or dissolution that occurs in small groups of myocytes, often sharply delimited from the surrounding normal myocardium. Depending on the stage, myocytes may have recognizable structure (e.g., nucleus and myofibers) or they may appear as empty spaces surrounded by fine connective tissue and mononuclear inflammatory cells

GROSS FINDINGS: Foci of myocytolysis are usually not visible by gross examination, although minute (1-2 mm) areas of mottling may be seen on cut section. Larger areas of myocytolysis are dark red-brown or hemorrhagic when compared to surrounding myocardium. With organization, these foci develop a glassy, semi-translucent appearance.

MICROSCOPIC FINDINGS: Many stages of myocytolysis may be seen in the same heart. There may be minute foci (but usually no smaller than 200 μm in greatest dimension), and larger areas with myocellular dissolution, infiltration by mononuclear cells, and collapse of stroma. Initial lesion is contraction band necrosis, followed by progressive myofibrillar loss. Characteristically, lipofuscin pigment is maintained in the myocytolytic focus, often in histiocytes. These pigment-laden macrophages may persist for months until the lesion becomes a mature replacement scar.

REMARKS: This is the characteristic lesion of catecholamine-induced myocardial injury (see *Cardiomyopathy, catecholamine-associated*). Whether catecholamines or other agents damage myocytes directly by causing increased calcium flux or whether they act through the microvasculature by inducing microvascular spasm and reperfusion injury, is debatable. There is experimental evidence supporting both views. However, the grouping of affected myocytes, the visualization of experimental microvascular spasm leading to myocytolysis and the prevention of the lesions by agents that lead to vasodilation support a significant role for the microvasculature. Regardless of pathogenesis, however, it is important to recognize that myocytolysis is an irreversible form of myocardial injury, and that it is a major cause of microscopic fibrosis in the myocardium in many different types of heart disease.

DIFFERENTIAL DIAGNOSIS: Myocardial fiber vacuolization in various storage diseases (e.g., glycogen storage disease) and acquired myocardial injury (e.g., lipid in chronic anemia). Chronic ischemic damage produces vacuolization of myocytes that are viable. These changes have been correlated with the clinical condition of hibernating myocardium.

KEY DIAGNOSTIC CRITERIA: Grouped foci of damaged myocytes usually with residual myofibrils, and presence of lipofuscin-containing macrophages. Clinical states associated with high catecholamine levels (e.g., shock, stress, iatrogenic administration of adrenergically active drugs) are helpful in the diagnosis.

POTENTIAL PITFALLS: Important to differentiate from viable myocytes with vacuolation.

References

1. Todd GL, Baroldi G, Pieper GM, Clayton FC, Eliot RS. Experimental catecholamine-induced myocardial necrosis. I. morphology, quantification and regional distribution of acute contraction band lesions. *J Mol Cell Cardiol* 1985;17:317–338.
2. Baroldi G. Different types of myocardial necrosis in coronary heart disease: A pathophysiologic review of their functional significance. *Am Heart J* 1975;89:742–752.
3. Bloom S, Cancilla PA. Myocytolysis and mitochondrial calcification in rat myocardium after low doses of isoproterenol. *Am J Pathol* 1969:54:373–391.
4. Schlesinger MJ, Reiner L. Focal myocytolysis of the heart. *Am J Pathol* 1955;31:443–459.
5. Factor SM, Minase T, Cho S, Dominitz R, Sonnenblick EH. Microvascular spasm in the cardiomyopathic Syrian hamster: A preventable cause of focal myocardial necrosis. *Circulation* 1982;66:342-354.
6. Eng C, Cho S, Factor SM, Sonnenblick EH, Kirk ES. Myocardial micronecrosis produced by microsphere embolization. Role of an alpha adrenergic tonic influence on the coronary microcirculation. *Circ Res* 1984;54:74–82.
7. Ausma J, Schaart G, Thone F et al. Chronic ischemic viable myocardium in man: Aspects of dedifferentiation. *Cardiovasc Pathol* 1995;4:29–37.

PERIPARTUM CARDIOMYOPATHY

Entry Author: Sherman Bloom

SYNONYMS: Postpartum cardiomyopathy (PPCM), puerperal cardiomyopathy.

DEFINITION: Heart failure attributed to cardiomyopathy of unknown etiology and occurring in the last trimester of pregnancy or within 6 months of delivery. More common among persons of African ancestry than it is among Caucasians. It is morphologically indistinguishable from idiopathic dilated cardiomyopathy.

GROSS FINDINGS: Indistinguishable from idiopathic dilated cardiomyopathy. All chambers are dilated and the overall shape of the heart is globular. There is myocardial hypertrophy (increased weight), patchy myocardial and endocardial fibrosis, and, commonly, mural thrombi in the atria and ventricles.

MICROSCOPIC FINDINGS: Indistinguishable from idiopathic dilated cardiomyopathy. There may be myocyte hypertrophy, focal interstitial fibrosis, and scattered lymphocytes. The lymphocytic infiltrates may raise the question of myocarditis.

REMARKS: A variety of etiologies have been proposed for this condition. Whereas individuals with this clinical diagnosis have been found to have a variety of more specific conditions, no single etiology has emerged as especially important, and the majority of cases remain idiopathic. Sporadic reports of a similar condition in animals have appeared.

DIFFERENTIAL DIAGNOSIS: Because this is a form of idiopathic cardiomyopathy, all specific forms of cardiomyopathy must be considered and ruled out.

KEY DIAGNOSTIC CRITERIA: Idiopathic cardiomyopathy in the peripartum period.

POTENTIAL PITFALLS: Failure to recognize a specific etiology for heart failure, such as valvular disease or myocarditis.

References

1. Rizeg MN, Rickenbacher PR, Fowler MB, Billingham ME. Incidence of myocarditis in peripartum cardiomyopathy. *Am J Cardiol* 1994;74:474–477.
2. Desai D, Moodley J, Naidoo D. Peripartum cardiomyopathy experiences at King Edward VIII Hospital, Durban, South Africa and a review of the literature. *Trop Doct* 1995;25:118–123.

RIGHT VENTRICULAR DYSPLASIA

Entry Author: Renu Virmani

SYNONYMS: Right ventricular cardiomyopathy, arrhythmogenic right ventricle, arrhythmogenic right ventricular dysplasia.

DEFINITION: Dilation of the right ventricle with focal thinning and fat replacement. The histologic finding of focal loss of myocytes and partial or complete replacement of right ventricular muscle by fat and/or fibrous tissue with or without entrapped myocytes.

GROSS FINDINGS: There may not be cardiomegaly, but the right ventricle is dilated and thinned and focal fat and fibrosis may be visible. The left ventricle may also be involved and there is usually epicardial scarring with fat infiltration.

MICROSCOPIC FINDINGS: Right ventricle shows loss of myocytes with intermingling of fat, fibrous tissue, and myocytes. There may be associated myocarditis in the right or left ventricle (single cell necrosis with chronic inflammatory infiltrate). Similar findings may or may not be present in the left ventricle.

DIFFERENTIAL DIAGNOSIS: Usually patients present with sudden cardiac death or episodes of ventricular tachycardia. Death usually occurs with exercise in patients less than 30 years. Intermingling of fat, fibrous tissue, and myocytes in the right ventricular wall is characteristic. Ongoing myocarditis or healed myocarditis.

KEY DIAGNOSTIC CRITERIA: Right heart dilation with focal replacement of the myocardium by fat and fibrous tissue.

POTENTIAL PITFALLS: Normal fat infiltration of the right ventricle, especially in obese patients, may be difficult to distinguish from right ventricular dysplasia.

SPHINGOLIPIDOSIS, FABRY'S DISEASE

Entry Author: Renu Virmani

SYNONYM: Angiokeratoma corporis diffusum universale.

DEFINITION: Fabry's disease is caused by a deficiency of lysosomal galactosidase A (ceramide trihexosidase) and has an X-linked recessive mode of inheritance. Fabry's disease is manifested by skin lesions (angiokeratomas), pain, paresthesias in the extremities, and progressive renal and cardiovascular disease. Cardiovascular involvement occurs late with cardiomegaly, congestive heart failure, angina, and hypertension, all the result of deposits of ceramide trihexoside in lysosomes in the heart, blood vessels, and kidney. Cardiac valve lesions have been described and consist of mitral stenosis and regurgitation, aortic regurgitation, and pulmonary regurgitation. The disease is more severe in males. Heterozygous female will show some manifestations.

GROSS FINDINGS: Cardiac hypertrophy usually without dilation. This is often diagnosed clinically as hypertrophic cardiomyopathy. There may be focal areas of fibrosis or even myocardial infarction. The epicardial coronary vessels may show some thickening.

MICROSCOPIC FINDINGS: The myocytes show focal marked vacuolization that may also involve the specialized tissues of the atrioventricular conduction system. The vacuolar deposits occur in the central, perinuclear areas displacing the contractile elements toward the periphery. In frozen sections the vacuoles are sudanophilic, PAS-positive, and strongly birefringent. Vacuolar deposits are seen in endothelial cells, smooth muscle cells, and pericytes throughout the vascular system, especially in the intramyocardial and epicardial coronary arteries. Vacuolar deposits are also seen in valvular fibroblasts. Ultrastructural examination reveals that the ceramide trihexoside deposits form intralysosomal aggregates of concentric or parallel lamellae spaced 4 to 5 nm apart. The lamellae show a positive reaction with periodate-thiosemicarbazide-silver proteinate and periodate-thiosemicarbazide osmium tetroxide, which are both methods for demonstrating carbohydrate material ultrastructurally. The lamellar structures may also be demonstrated in freeze-fractured preparations.

SPECIAL PROCEDURES NEEDED FOR DIAGNOSIS: Demonstration of a deficiency of the galactosidase A lysosomal enzyme is diagnostic. Recently the gene rearrangement on X-chromosome (Xq22) has been identified and may become a useful diagnostic method.

DIFFERENTIAL DIAGNOSIS: Hypertrophic cardiomyopathy must be ruled out. The diagnosis of hypertrophic cardiomyopathy is made by showing myocyte hypertrophy with fibromuscular disarray without diffuse vacuolization. Dilated cardiomyopathy may show focal mild vacuolar degeneration but the lamellar deposits in cardiomyopathy lack birefringence in frozen sections and the highly organized substructure of lamellar deposits in Fabry's disease. Adriamycin-induced vacuolar degeneration on electron microscopy is distinct with massive sarcoplasmic reticular dilation.

KEY DIAGNOSTIC CRITERIA: Myocyte vacuoles on frozen sections are sudanophilic, PAS-positive, and strongly birefringent. Ultrastructural intralysosomal aggregates of concentric and parallel lamellae spaced 4 to 5 nm apart are not diagnostic. Clinical and morphologic findings together are fairly diagnostic but absolute certainty requires demonstration of ceramide trihexosidase deficiency.

POTENTIAL PITFALLS: Not all vacuolated cells indicate Fabry's disease and lamellar bodies can be seen in other storage diseases and cardiomyopathies.

SPHINGOLIPIDOSIS, GAUCHER'S DISEASE

Entry Author: Renu Virmani

DEFINITION: An uncommon inherited disorder (autosomal recessive) of glucosylceramide metabolism due to a deficiency of beta-glucosidase (glucocerebrosidase). This deficiency follows from mutations at the chromosome 1q21 locus and results in the accumulation of cerebrosides in spleen, liver, bone marrow, lymph nodes, brain, and myocardium. Clinically significant cardiac involvement is uncommon, but when present is characterized by left ventricular dysfunction, hemorrhagic pericardial effusion (related to bleeding diathesis that is frequent in Gaucher's disease), increased left ventricular wall mass, and calcification of left-sided valves. Adult patients develop pulmonary hypertension and cor pulmonale as a consequence of occlusion of alveolar capillaries by Gaucher cells derived from bone marrow.

GROSS FINDINGS: Constrictive calcific and hemorrhagic pericarditis have been reported. There is usually a lack of significant involvement of the heart in any of the types (infantile, juvenile, or adult) of Gaucher's disease.

MICROSCOPIC FINDINGS: Only a single adult with marked infiltration of the myocardial interstitium (not the conduction system) by Gaucher cells has been reported. Gaucher cells are large, and their cytoplasm shows a "wrinkled" appearance. Ultrastructural study demonstrates numerous elongated cytoplasmic inclusions that consist of membrane-bound accumulations of tubules that measure 20 nm in diameter.

SPECIAL PROCEDURES NEEDED FOR DIAGNOSIS: Presence of cellular accumulations of glucocerebroside and a deficiency in beta-glucosidase confirm the diagnosis. The gene locus has been identified on chromosome one (locus q21).

DIFFERENTIAL DIAGNOSIS: Chronic myeloid leukemia, acute leukemia, thalassemia, and dyserythropoietic anemia type II must be ruled out by clinical, morphologic, and biochemical assay. Pseudo-Gaucher cells show a strong birefringence which is not seen in Gaucher cells.

KEY DIAGNOSTIC CRITERIA: The ultrastructure of the Gaucher cell is fairly specific, and similar aspects are only found in the closely related galactosylceramidosis (Krabbe's disease). The lysosomes are enlarged, elongated, and fusiform, and contain tubular structures that are 20 nm in diameter. The walls of the lysosomes and tubules stain positive with phosphotungstic acid at low pH. Acid phosphatase in involved organs is increased.

POTENTIAL PITFALLS: Always interpret results with clinical findings because Gaucher-like cells may be seen in other conditions (see above).

Section 2

Acquired Diseases of the Valves and Endocardium

Section Editor: Malcolm D. Silver
Entry Authors: Francesca V. Lobo, Virginia M. Walley, and
Jagdish W. Butany

AORTIC ROOT DILATION, ANKYLOSING SPONDYLITIS OR RHEUMATOID DISEASE

Entry Author: Malcolm D. Silver

DEFINITION: Aortic root dilation in a patient who has ankylosing spondylitis or rheumatoid arthritis.

GROSS FINDINGS: See aortic root dilation. Findings in aortic root and ascending aorta may be those of syphilis with longitudinal wrinkling, but aortic changes usually confined to proximal 3–4 cm of aorta with thickening. Aortic valve may show changes associated with aortic incompetence.

MICROSCOPIC FINDINGS: Local destruction of elastic lamellae with replacement by scar. Excess glycosamine content seen in Marfan syndrome not a feature. Vasa vasorum may be thickened and show perivascular chronic inflammation but marked adventitial chronic inflammation of syphilis not obvious. Rheumatoid granulomata rare. Adventitial fibrosis prominent in ankylosing spondylitis.

REMARKS: Aortic root dilation is an uncommon complication of either of these "rheumatoid" diseases (and very rarely complicates Reiter's syndrome, Behçet's disease, and psoriasis). The age of the patient affected and their clinical history and findings including x-rays of joints and spine, should help differential diagnosis. Serologic tests for syphilis are negative.

DIFFERENTIAL DIAGNOSIS: Add that listed under previous entries for aortic root dilation.

AORTIC ROOT DILATION, EHLERS-DANLOS SYNDROME

Entry Author: Malcolm D. Silver

DEFINITION: Aortic root dilation in a patient with Ehlers-Danlos syndrome.

GROSS FINDINGS: Same as in aortic root dilation.

MICROSCOPIC FINDINGS: Nonspecific. Elastic tissue and collagen may be diminished with increased amounts of glycosaminoglycans in the sinus wall or that of the ascending aorta. "Cystic medionecrosis" is not a feature in the aortic wall.

REMARKS: Cardiovascular lesions are described in most forms of this syndrome which has a prevalence of 1/5000 to 1/10,000. Aortic root dilation is an uncommon complication of this heterogeneous group of inherited disorders of connective tissue (usually collagen) synthesis. It is often transmitted in an autosomal dominant manner but with some transmission through X-linked or autosomal recessive mechanisms. In some types, e.g., type 4, approximately half the cases are associated with new mutations. Types 1–3 account for 85% of diagnosed cases.

Family history, clinical, or autopsy findings may arouse suspicion of diagnosis. Fibroblast culture and analysis may help clinch it.

DIFFERENTIAL DIAGNOSIS: Ehlers-Danlos syndrome is best diagnosed, and the various forms distinguished from one another by biochemical analysis. Marfan syndrome should be suspected if the body habitus matches that phenotype. Aortic root dilation must be distinguished from fusiform or saccular aneurysms of the ascending aorta. These are generally located in the tubular portion of the vessel. An aortic dissecting aneurysm alone or complicated by aneurysm formation shows the dissecting hemorrhage in the sinus wall. Aneurysms of the sinuses of Valsalva usually cause a localized bulge beyond the confines of the sinus aorta. Dilation or aneurysm of ascending aorta caused by ankylosing spondylitis or rheumatoid disease may involve the aortic root. Inflammatory changes in these conditions extend into base of aortic cusps. In such cases, serological analyses and spinal x-rays may help differential diagnosis. Primary acute aortic sinus infections, although rare, can lead to aortic root dilation. These may be associated with surgical wounds or spread from aortic infective endocarditis.

Reference

1. Tilstra DJ, Byers PH. Molecular basis of hereditary disorders of connective tissue (Review). *Ann Rev Med* 1994;45:149–163.

AORTIC ROOT DILATION, MARFAN SYNDROME

Entry Author: Malcolm D. Silver

DEFINITION: Aortic root dilation in a patient with Marfan syndrome. May be an isolated condition or associated with aneurysm of tubular portion of ascending aorta.

GROSS FINDINGS: Same as aortic root dilation. Dissecting aortic aneurysms are a common complication. Aortic root dilation in this condition is prone to rupture.

MICROSCOPIC FINDINGS: Fragmentation atrophy, loss of elastic lamellae and accumulation of glycosamine glycans in the media forming pools in the sinus walls, adjacent aorta, and other blood vessels. No evidence of inflammation in aortic wall but increased medial vascularization possible. Medionecrosis not a feature. Monoclonal antibodies demonstrate fibrillin is absent in skin, blood vessels, and other tissues. The Movat pentachrome stain is useful to demonstrate mucopolysaccharide material.

REMARKS: This condition is caused by a mutation in the fibrillin gene on chromosome 15. It is inherited in an autosomal dominant manner. Eighty percent of cases have an affected parent, new mutations account for the remainder. Fibrillin is a major building block of microfibrils. More than 20 different mutations in the fibrillin gene are known to cause clinical manifestations. Aortic root dilation is most likely in affected individuals in their second to fifth decade. A family history or other physical findings suggestive of Marfan syndrome may help establish the diagnosis. Cultured fibroblasts can demonstrate the molecular defect.

In its florid form Marfan syndrome presents musculoskeletal, ocular and cardiovascular abnormalities. The latter develop in more than 95% of cases. Prolapse of the mitral valve and aortic valve cusps due to accumulation of mucopolysaccharide material with or without annular dilation may occur. Aortic valve cusps may be semitranslucent.

DIFFERENTIAL DIAGNOSIS: Ehlers-Danlos syndrome is best ruled in or out, and the various forms distinguished from one another, by biochemical analysis. Marfan syndrome should be suspected in any case in which the body habitus matches that phenotype. Aortic root dilation must also be distinguished from fusiform or saccular aneurysms of the ascending aorta. These are generally located in the tubular portion of the vessel. An aortic dissecting aneurysm alone or complicated by aneurysm formation shows the dissecting hemorrhage in the sinus wall. Aneurysms of the sinuses of Valsalva usually cause a localized bulge beyond the confines of the sinus aorta. Dilation or aneurysm of ascending aorta caused by ankylosing spondylitis or rheumatoid disease may involve the aortic root. Inflammatory changes in these conditions extend into base of aortic cusps. In such cases serological analyses and spinal x-rays may help differential diagnosis. Primary acute aortic sinus infections, although rare, can lead to aortic root dilation. These may be associated with surgical wounds or spread from aortic infective endocarditis.

AORTIC ROOT DILATION, NOS

Entry Author: Malcolm D. Silver

SYNONYMS: Sinus of Valsalva aneurysm; annulo-aortic aneurysm, ectasia or dilation.

DEFINITION: A generalized rather than a localized dilation of the proximal sinus portion of the aorta.
NOTE: This is a transitional zone between the left ventricle and the aortic wall and, functionally, is where aortic valve cusps are attached. Their attachments divide the sinus aorta into thirds forming the sinuses of Valsalva. The aortic diameter here is 1.5 times that of the tubular aorta, not well appreciated at autopsy but obvious in angiograms or casts. The cephalad margin of the sinuses are marked by a well-defined tissue ridge. The aortic "root" is the most caudal part of each sinus.

GROSS FINDINGS: The diameter of the sinus aorta exceeds 5 cm (normal 4.5 cm) but its conformation is preserved. Vessel wall may be semitranslucent and thinned. Mural thrombus in the affected segment is unlikely unless dilation is very marked (compare aneurysm).

MICROSCOPIC FINDINGS: Microscopic changes vary ·with etiology, which may be congenital (e.g., Ehlers-Danlos syndrome [rare], Marfan syndrome, [uncommon]) or acquired (inflammatory, e.g., syphilis [rare], rheumatoid arthritis [rare], or ankylosing spondylitis [rare] or noninflammatory, e.g., aortic arteriopathy or Takeyashus syndrome [not infrequent]). Dilation is caused by a weakening or destruction of support structures in the sinus wall. Thus, histology varies with cause but generally is not specific and involves some focal loss of elastic tissue, fibrosis, and/or increased glycosaminoglycan accumulation. Rheumatoid granulomas like those found in connective tissue elsewhere are rare in the sinus or aortic wall.

REMARKS: May be complicated by aortic valve regurgitation produced by alterations in the spatial relationships of the valve cusps. These are effectively shortened, which may interfere with coaption. Affected cusps have a thickened free margin (all or part of it) with the margin rolled toward the ventricular lumen. Dilated aortic root can rupture into pericardium producing cardiac tamponade or into adjacent tissue leading to sinuses passing into the aorta or any of the four heart chambers.

DIFFERENTIAL DIAGNOSIS: Ehlers-Danlos syndrome is best diagnosed, and the various forms distinguished from one another, by biochemical analysis. Marfan syndrome should be suspected if the body habitus matches that phenotype. Aortic root dilation must be distinguished from fusiform or saccular aneurysms of the ascending aorta. These are generally located in the tubular portion of the vessel. An aortic dissecting aneurysm alone or complicated by aneurysm formation shows the dissecting hemorrhage in the sinus wall. Aneurysms of the sinuses of Valsalva usually cause a localized bulge beyond the confines of the sinus aorta. Dilation or aneurysm of ascending aorta caused by ankylosing spondylitis or rheumatoid disease may involve the aortic root. Inflammatory changes in these conditions extend into base of aortic cusps. In such cases, serological analyses and spinal x-rays may help differential diagnosis. Primary acute aortic sinus infections, although rare, can lead to aortic root dilation. These may be associated with surgical wounds or spread from aortic infective endocarditis.

KEY DIAGNOSTIC CRITERIA: Generalized dilation of the proximal sinus portion of the aorta.

AORTIC ROOT DILATION, OSTEOGENESIS IMPERFECTA

Entry Author: Malcolm D. Silver

DEFINITION: Aortic root dilation in a patient with osteogenesis imperfecta (uncommon complication).

GROSS FINDINGS: See aortic root dilation. Aortic cusps may be elongated and semitranslucent. Mitral insufficiency may complicate the condition. Likely to be evidence of fractured bones and their sequelae.

MICROSCOPIC FINDINGS: Changes in sinus wall not specific.

REMARKS: Osteogenesis imperfecta is a rare congenital defect in collagen (type 1) synthesis. Family history, clinical, or autopsy findings help arouse suspicion of diagnosis.

DIFFERENTIAL DIAGNOSIS: Ehlers-Danlos syndrome is best ruled in or out and the various forms distinguished from one another by biochemical analysis. Marfan syndrome should be suspected in any case in which the body habitus matches that phenotype. Aortic root dilation must also be distinguished from fusiform or saccular aneurysms of the ascending aorta. These are generally located in the tubular portion of the vessel. An aortic dissecting aneurysm alone or complicated by aneurysm formation shows the dissecting hemorrhage in the sinus wall. Aneurysms of the sinuses of Valsalva usually cause a localized bulge beyond the confines of the sinus aorta. Dilation or aneurysm of ascending aorta caused by ankylosing spondylitis or rheumatoid disease may involve the aortic root. Inflammatory changes in these conditions extend into base of aortic cusps. In such cases, serological analyses and spinal x-rays may help differential diagnosis. Primary acute aortic sinus infections, although rare, can lead to aortic root dilation. These may be associated with surgical wounds or spread from aortic infective endocarditis.

AORTIC ROOT DILATION, SYPHILITIC

Entry Author: Malcolm D. Silver

DEFINITION: Aortic root dilation in a patient with tertiary syphilis.

GROSS FINDINGS: See aortic root dilation. The sinus wall may show marked secondary atherosclerosis and/or calcification. A fine, longitudinal wrinkling of the aortic intima may be apparent but more often is obscured by severe atherosclerosis of the dilated or aneurysmal vessel wall. Thrombus may fill the lumen. Commissures of aortic valves appear separated. Valve cusps may show secondary changes because of associated aortic incompetence (QV).

MICROSCOPIC FINDINGS: Histological changes are those found in the aortic wall in syphilis with patchy elastic tissue destruction and fibrosis and increased medial vascularization. Chronic adventitial inflammation with prominent plasma cells, increased medial vascularization, and thickening of vasa vasorum. Changes are often obscured by severe atherosclerosis. They do not extend into the base of the aortic cusps. Treponema are not demonstrable in the tissue.

REMARKS: This is an uncommon complication of the tertiary stage of infection with *Treponema pallidum*. Rarely seen nowadays because the infection can be treated. Usually associated with syphilitic aneurysm of ascending aorta. In the past, observed most often in fifth to seventh decades.

Clinical history and serological tests help diagnosis. Rarely, a syphilitic gumma in the annular area produces aortic insufficiency.

DIFFERENTIAL DIAGNOSIS: Dilation or aneurysm of ascending aorta caused by ankylosing spondylitis or rheumatoid disease may involve aortic root. Atherosclerotic changes usually affect intima, but, if severe, extend into media destroying it as process advances, not in piecemeal fashion. Adventitial mononuclear cell reaction occurs in atherosclerosis but plasma cells not a feature nor are vasa vasorum thickened.

AORTIC VALVE INCOMPETENCE

Entry Author: Malcolm D. Silver

SYNONYMS: Aortic valve incompetence, aortic valve regurgitations.

DEFINITION: Incompetence (QV) of a native or prosthetic aortic valve. The former is caused by a congenital anomaly or acquired pathology that affects, singly or in combination, components of the aortic valve complex so that the valve does not close normally, permitting blood to regurgitate into the left ventricle.

An aortic valve prosthesis becomes incompetent when the cusps of a tissue valve separate from their attachments, ulcerate or perforate, or cannot coapt properly. If the occluder of a mechanical valve becomes fixed or cannot seat properly (thrombus or vegetations usually, rarely a foreign body) or fractures or escapes its cage or diminishes in size because of structural wear or degeneration, that valve becomes incompetent.

GROSS FINDINGS: Varies with underlying pathology. May be associated with an anomaly like a congenitally bicuspid valve where a cusp's height is shortened or anatomic arrangement or tethering near a raphe shortens the conjoined cusp or allows prolapse. The latter occurs too when a raphe is represented by a fibrous cord extending from the sinus wall to attach near the conjoined cusp's free margin, and it ruptures. This is uncommon. Rarely, too, a jet lesion from a membranous subaortic stenosis can damage normal aortic valve cusps producing incompetence.

Typically, the cusps of the free margins of incompetent aortic valves are thickened (by fibrous tissue) and appear rolled toward the ventricular lumen. A regurgitant blood jet may strike the endocardial surface in the distal outflow tract of the left ventricle (often the septal wall or the ventricular surface of the anterior mitral valve leaflet) producing gray-white patches of endocardial thickening or small valve-like structures (jet lesions), both composed of fibroelastic tissue. The ostia of such "valves" usually open toward the aortic valve and may give clue as to direction of the jet and the site of incompetence.

Volume overload is the physiological consequence of aortic incompetence. The result is a left ventricle that is dilated and hypertrophied. The heart appears globular and the left ventricular wall may not be markedly thickened. Other signs of left ventricular or generalized heart failure may be observed.

MICROSCOPIC FINDINGS: Varies with cause and may be specific or nonspecific.

REMARKS: Aortic insufficiency can develop at any age and may be of acute onset or chronic in nature. Incompetent valves are prone to infection. In this setting, the areas of endocardial thickening produced by jet lesions can be secondarily infected. Rarely, they are the site of a primary infection.

Valvular lesions are the most frequent cause of aortic insufficiency with supravalvular lesion less frequent and subvalvular causes infrequent.

Of acquired lesions affecting native valves, common ones include active or healed endocarditis (QV) with cusp ulceration or perforation; healed rheumatic valvulitis (QV) which shortens cusps; myxomatous degeneration (QV) or Marfan syndrome which allows cusp prolapse, perforation or shredding and trauma (QV). Dilation of the aortic root (QV) or proximal ascending aorta can change spatial relationships, effectively shortening cusps allowing prolapse or inhibiting proper coaption. If cusps are markedly stiffened by processes that cause aortic stenosis (QV) the patient may have associated aortic incompetence. Rarely material in the valve lumen (e.g., thrombus, infected vegetations, foreign body, or tumor) prohibit valve closure. Deposits in annular tissue can also interfere with valve closure. Rheumatoid nodules may act in this manner—see *Myocarditis, rheumatoid.*

Detailed gross findings and microscopic examination of excised tissue in surgical pathology will usually define an underlying cause. If cusps are normal, suspect a supravalvular cause. History and clinical findings may help differentiation. At autopsy supra- and subvalvular areas must be examined carefully.

DIFFERENTIAL DIAGNOSIS: See above under gross findings.

A paravalvular leak caused by a dehisced heart valve prosthesis or a fistula resulting from rupture of an aortic annular abscess or sinus of valsalva aneurysm induces clinical symptoms identical to those caused by insufficiency.

CARCINOID VALVULAR DISEASE (INCLUDING COMMENT ON METHYSERGIDE- AND ERGOTAMINE-INDUCED DISEASE)

Entry Authors: Jagdish W. Butany and Malcolm D. Silver

DEFINITION: Valve incompetence or stenosis that develops in approximately 50% of patients with a functional carcinoid syndrome. Most often, develops with a primary intestinal carcinoid tumor, usually of the small bowel, that has metastasized to lymph nodes and liver. Much less commonly, carcinoid tumors of lung or ovary, where venous return bypasses the liver, may be associated with carcinoid valvular disease.

GROSS FINDINGS: Right-sided heart valves are affected most frequently, but overall this is not a common cause of valvular heart disease. Left-sided valves may be involved too, especially if there is a right to left shunt at atrial level or if venous return from tumor bypasses the liver.

Diffuse, plaque-like endocardial thickening affects the right heart chambers and associated valves. The plaques are a pale gray-white and predominate on the sinus side of pulmonary valve cusps and the ventricular aspect of posterior and septal leaflets of the tricuspid valve. Both surfaces of the anterior tricuspid valve leaflet may show them. Plaques may extend onto commissural areas; chordae and leaflet tissue can become tethered to the ventricular endocardium. They usually induce an incompetent tricuspid valve and stenosis of the pulmonary valve.

MICROSCOPIC FINDINGS: The microscopic architecture of the valve is largely preserved with plaques deposited on them. In this location and elsewhere on the endocardium, they are composed of myxoid tissue containing stellate cells and abundant interstitial matrix. Elastic fibers are not a feature.

REMARKS: Substances (likely serotonin and bradykin) secreted by functionally active tumors (primary or secondary) induce both clinical symptoms (flushing, diarrhea, and wheezing being the main ones) and endothelial plaques.

Similar lesions that encase mitral valve leaflets, chordae tendineae causing their fusion, and the apices of the left ventricular papillary muscles as well as the aortic valve cusps, are described in a few patients treated with methysergide and rarely in those receiving ergotamine tartrate therapy. The predominant involvement of left-sided heart valves in the cases associated with these therapies differs from mainly right-sided valvular disease in carcinoid valvular disease. Histologically, elastin fibers may be prominent in methysergide/ergotamine-induced plaques or absent from them. Endocardial fibrosis is also present in this condition.

DIFFERENTIAL DIAGNOSIS: The gross findings and histologic features of this condition are virtually diagnostic, especially if there is a carcinoid tumor with liver metastases—see above.

ENDOCARDITIS, INFECTIVE

Entry Authors: Francesca V. Lobo and Malcolm D. Silver

SYNONYMS: Valvulitis, infective; endocarditis, infectious.

DEFINITION: Presence of infected thrombotic vegetations attached to the endocardium of native or bioprosthetic heart valves or to mechanical heart valve prostheses. (NOTE: this term is also used to describe infection occurring in a mural thrombus, a much less frequent occurrence).

GROSS FINDINGS: Left-sided native valves are infected more often than right-sided ones. An affected valve may have been normal or show congenital anomaly or pre-existing disease. Usually, this induces valve incompetence but stenosed valves can be infected. The condition predominates in middle-aged males, but with intravenous drug abuse the incidence of right-sided infection is high and young males are affected. Prosthetic valves in the left heart are more often infected, with mitral and aortic prostheses affected equally.

On native valves, infected vegetations usually occur at the line of closure but may involve adjoining cusps/leaflets or contiguous structures. They are commonly attached to the atrial aspect of atrioventricular valves and the ventricular aspect of semilunar valves. They rarely arise away from the line of closure. If so, a reason is usually obvious. The size of vegetations can vary from 0.5 cm to 4.0 cm in diameter, or be larger. They may be smooth surfaced or irregular, single or multiple (on the same or different/opposing cusps), gray-pink, soft and friable, or gray, yellow-brown and firm.

On bioprosthetic valves vegetations occur on valve cusps and may spread to their sewing ring/annulus whereas infections on mechanical prostheses start on the sewing ring.

An excised infected valve at surgical pathology or examined at autopsy may reveal local complications. They include cusp/leaflet ulceration or perforation (common) or aneurysm formation, chordal rupture or annular abscesses (less common). These lesions can present acute features or evidence of healing. The latter process can induce fusion of adjacent sides of semilunar valves at commissural areas. Generalized complications are caused by bland or infected emboli or immune-mediated phenomena. Infected emboli may be excised surgically.

MICROSCOPIC FINDINGS: Freshly formed vegetations consist of platelet-fibrin thrombi containing neutrophils and lesser number of other white blood cells. Later, neutrophils are also present in subjacent valve tissue. Colonies of microorganisms may be demonstrated at the edge or within the thrombus and also in the valve substance. Organisms may be present within macrophages in rickettsial endocarditis, for example. In longstanding or indolent infections, vegetations show varying degrees of organization, with or without calcification or the presence of chronic inflammatory cells, and occasional giant cells (the latter are particularly noticeable in Q fever endocarditis). Findings in the cusp/leaflet and subjacent tissue may include preexisting changes (if any), varying degrees of edema, inflammation, necrosis, and later, reparative changes. At autopsy secondary changes related to complication may be present. After effective treatment, thrombotic vegetations stop growing, organize from their base and bacterial colonies calcify. This may leave a thickened deformed valve like that resulting from rheumatic disease.

REMARKS: An infecting microorganism may damage the valve substance directly or localize on previously sterile vegetations occurring at sites of endothelial trauma, turbulence, or scarring. Thus, infective endocarditis has an increased frequency in hearts with valves affected by congenital anomalies or acquired valvular lesions. Mural endocarditis is frequently associated with high pressure shunts, e.g., VSD or perforated aortic valve cusp developing where the blood jet impinges on the endocardium. Seeding of a valve with microorganisms occurs during infection and is associated with a variety of diagnostic or therapeutic procedures. Alcoholism and various forms of immunosuppression are also predisposing factors. Any microorganism may cause infective endocarditis, but bacterial infections, especially those caused by gram-positive cocci, are most common, with fungal infection much less frequent. Viral and parasite infection are rare. There may be mixed infection and superinfection. Infective endocarditis should be suspected clinically when a heart murmur and unexplained fever are present for 1 week, or in febrile intravenous drug abusers even without a heart murmur. Diagnosis requires confirmation by blood culture. Symptoms and signs are related to the location of the infection and its local and general complications.

Echocardiography, especially by the transesophageal mode, detects vegetations greater than 3 mm in diameter on a native valve. Serial phonocardiography and cine radiography are useful to diagnose prosthetic valve infections. Blood cultures (x3) assist in identifying an infecting organism in over 95% of cases. Samples of vegetations, emboli, or tissue obtained at surgery may be cultured or subject to smears and staining if the diagnosis is suspected.

DIFFERENTIAL DIAGNOSIS: Demonstrable microorganisms in thrombi attached to heart valves establish the diagnosis for a pathologist. That material may derive directly from a heart valve, an embolus, or be obtained during cardiac catheterization. A combination of Gram and GMS stains is most useful to demonstrate microorganism but histology or clinical suspicion may demand others or molecular diagnostic techniques. If a pathologist is the first to encounter the infection, material must be submitted for culture.

A previous infective endocarditis may be inferred by observing healed lesions and/or complications. The diagnosis may be suspected if thrombotic vegetations and adjacent valve show a marked acute inflammatory/destructive/reparative response in the absence of demonstrable microorganisms.

ENDOCARDITIS, INFECTIVE,
ANNULAR INFECTION/ABSCESS

Entry Author: Francesca V. Lobo

SYNONYMS: Annular abscess of heart valve; valve ring infection or abscess.

DEFINITION: Infection involving the valve ring (annulus) of either a native or a prosthetic heart valve almost invariably associated with infective endocarditis.

GROSS FINDINGS: Native valve annular infections are most frequently associated with aortic valve infections and, in descending order of frequency, those on mitral and tricuspid valves. Right-sided heart valves are rarely affected. May be associated with infection of a calcified mitral annulus. In prosthetic heart valves, ring abscesses are more often associated with mechanical prostheses, particularly those in the aortic position, where infection usually begins on the sewing ring and spreads to the annulus. It may occur, though less often, as a complication of an infected bioprosthetic valve where infections start on the cusps subsequently spreading to the sewing ring. An annular abscess can cause dehiscence of a prosthetic valve.

In the acute phase a lesion presents as pus in the valve annulus, involving varying arcs of its circumference. Subsequently, burrowing abscesses develop presenting pus with surrounding acute inflammation or sinuses or fistulous tracts that in healing are defined by scar tissue. Such lesions may not be obvious on initial examination and require detailed dissection. Thus, at autopsy an infected heart valve prosthesis must always be removed to examine the annulus. A pathologist encounters these lesions both in surgical pathology and post mortem. One must be aware of the anatomy of the annular region to understand pathways taken by these burrowing abscess sinuses or fistulae. For example, one extending distally from the aortic annulus may rupture onto the adventitial surface or into the aortic lumen producing a paravalvular leak; extending proximally they pass into (a) the interventricular septum and can rupture into either ventricle or destroy the membranous interventricular septum inducing a ventricular septal defect or the adjacent conducting system causing arrhythmias or complete heart block; (b) the anterior leaflet of the mitral valve (which shares a common relationship with the aortic annulus) rupturing at its base or extending further toward its free margin before rupturing toward left atrium or ventricle. Lateral extension depends on the site of infection. It can be toward the pericardium, causing pericarditis or a hemopericardium with cardiac tamponade or an endocardial bulge or fistula that impinges on the right atrial wall proximal or at the region of the membranous interventricular septum, the outflow tract of the right ventricle, or proximal pulmonary artery, or into the left atrium. Thus, fistulae from annular abscesses may pass to any heart chamber.

An annular abscess of the mitral valve most frequently extends laterally to the epicardial surface, causing pericarditis or a hemopericardium. It may compress the right coronary artery with subsequent thrombotic occlusion and myocardial infarction or rupture into the left atrial or ventricular lumen. Again, sinuses or fistulae result.

MICROSCOPIC FINDINGS: Presence of microorganisms, pus, and inflammatory exudate in annulus or burrowing abscess, with neutrophilic infiltration in surrounding tissues. Sinuses or fistulous tracts are lined by thrombus and defined by scar tissue. At this stage, microorganisms may not be demonstrable on special stains. Heavy calcification in area if associated with mitral annular calcification. Demonstrable by x-ray postmortem.

KEY DIAGNOSTIC CRITERIA: A valve ring abscess should be suspected in a patient with infective endocarditis and evidence of accelerated valve dysfunction, pericarditis, cardiac tamponade, an acquired ventricular septal defect, or complete heart block. The key pathological criterion is the presence of a loculated collection of pus at a valve ring in a patient with infective endocarditis or residua subsequent to extension of a burrowing abscess in its perforation.

REMARKS: Sinus of Valsalva aneurysms (QV) may extend like burrowing annular abscesses and produce intracardial sinuses or, on rupture, fistulae. In early stages, presence of pus and microorganisms in annular abscess allows differentiation. Later, sinus aneurysm or healed annular abscess could have comparable gross and microscopic morphology. In those circumstances, patient's history or finding other stigmata of healed endocarditis may help differentiation.

ENDOCARDITIS, INFECTIVE, BACTERIAL

Entry Author: Francesca V. Lobo

SYNONYMS: Infectious endocarditis, bacterial; bacterial endocarditis (acute or subacute); valvulitis, bacterial.

DEFINITION: A subset of infective endocarditis produced by bacterial infection.

REMARKS: Bacterial endocarditis with a rapidly progressive course and much tissue destruction often occurs on a normal valve and is caused by *Staphylococcus aureus* or *Enterococcus*. A more indolent clinical course may be seen with *Streptococcus viridans* infection occurring on a previously damaged native valve. In indolent infections vegetations may be tiny.

"Early onset prosthetic valve endocarditis," which occurs within 60 days of surgery, is usually fulminant. Fifty percent of cases are caused by staphylococcal infections (particularly *Staphylococcus epidermidis*). "Late onset prosthetic valve endocarditis" may be fulminant or indolent.

SPECIAL PROCEDURES NEEDED FOR DIAGNOSIS: Clinically, blood cultures (x3) assist identification of the infecting organism in over 95% of cases. The most common are gram-positive cocci, staphylococci and streptococci which account for 90–95% of cases. Gram-negative bacilli, while a less common cause of infection, are not infrequent in intravenous drug abusers, those with diabetes mellitus or who have a calcified posterior mitral annulus complicated by endocarditis. Infection by almost all species in addition to mycoplasma, rickettsiae (*Coxiella burnetii*), spirochetes, chlamydia, and organisms not normally pathogenic, is possible. One notes that the staining characteristics of bacteria in Gram stains may be changed after antibiotic therapy; also, that dead organisms frequently calcify.

ENDOCARDITIS, INFECTIVE, FUNGAL

Entry Author: Francesca V. Lobo

SYNONYMS: Infectious endocarditis, fungal; valvulitis, fungal; mycotic endocarditis.

DEFINITION: A subset of infective endocarditis produced by fungal infection.

GROSS FINDINGS: Thrombotic vegetations are often large, friable, and prone to produce embolic phenomena, which may be the presenting symptom (this possibility must be considered in examining any embolus in surgical pathology). For example, pulmonary embolism/abscess is prevalent when these infections affect the tricuspid valve.

MICROSCOPIC FINDINGS: Fungal vegetations most often consist of fungal elements with platelet aggregates and relatively little fibrin. The organisms penetrate the underlying valve substance with variable degrees of destruction associated with acute, mixed, or granulomatous inflammation.

REMARKS: Fungal endocarditis rarely involves native valves of healthy people but may do so in patients with debilitating or lymphoreticular diseases, in intravenous drug abusers, or in association with IV catheters. Steroid, broad spectrum antibiotic, cytotoxic drug, and radiotherapy increase risk as do prosthetic heart valves.

The most frequent infecting organism is *Candida* followed by *Aspergillus* and *Histoplasma*. *Candida* accounts for 10% of early onset prosthetic valve endocarditis with a lessened frequency in late onset cases. The prognosis is usually grave owing to relatively poor activity of antifungal agents. Surgical removal of infected tissue is an important form of treatment.

ENDOCARDITIS, INFECTIVE, OF AORTIC VALVE

Entry Author: Francesca V. Lobo

DEFINITION: Infected thrombotic vegetations attached to endocardium of the aortic valve or to a heart valve prosthesis in that area.

GROSS FINDINGS: Findings vary with the virulence of the causative microorganism and duration of infection. Late complications, whether acute or healed, may be observed. See *Endocarditis, NOS.*

REMARKS: Infective endocarditis of the aortic valve is common, being second in frequency to mitral endocarditis on native valves. Infection of mitral and aortic heart valve prostheses occur with equal frequency.

Affected aortic valve may be normal and have three cusps or show congenital anomaly (especially bicuspid valve) or acquired pathology of which rheumatic valvular disease (QV), degenerative calcification (QV), or myxomatous change are common. Incompetent valves are particularly affected but stenosed valves are also infected. An aortic valve distal to a congenital membranous subaortic stenosis is prone to infection.

Of local complications cusp ulceration and perforation are common. The resultant valve incompetence may produce mural endocarditis on the left ventricular septal wall or the ventricular aspect of the anterior mitral leaflet (and chordae). Infective aortic intimitis is a rare complication of an infected and stenosed aortic valve. Nowadays, acute lesions and excised annular abscesses are encountered in surgical pathology; also, healed lesions that cause aortic incompetence.

Considering infective organisms, comments made under endocarditis of the mitral valve (QV) also apply to aortic valve infections.

KEY DIAGNOSTIC CRITERIA: See *Endocarditis, infective, NOS.*

ENDOCARDITIS, INFECTIVE, OF MITRAL VALVE

Entry Author: Malcolm D. Silver

DEFINITION: Infected thrombotic vegetations attached to endocardium of the mitral valve or to a heart valve prosthesis in that area.

GROSS FINDINGS: Findings vary with the virulence of the causative microorganism and duration of infection. Local complications, whether acute or healed, may be observed. See *Endocarditis, infective NOS.*

REMARKS: Infective endocarditis of the mitral valve is common. The valve often shows underlying pathology, most often rheumatic valvular disease (QV). But infective endocarditis is also associated with prolapsed mitral valve (QV) calcification of mitral annulus (QV), and other congenital anomalies or acquired disease.

An unusual location of infected vegetations may give clues to underlying pathology. Thus, those at the base of the anterior mitral leaflet are associated with a burrowing abscess extending from an aortic annular infection; those at the base of the posterior leaflet with mitral annular calcification; those on the ventricular aspect of the anterior leaflet with muscular subaortic stenosis in hypertrophic cardiomyopathy or an infected jet lesion associated with an infected, incompetent, aortic valve. A mural left atrial jet lesion produced by an incompetent mitral valve may be secondarily infected.

Of local complications, leaflet ulceration and perforation are common. Chordal rupture and leaflet aneurysm formation are uncommon. These are seen in surgical pathology as acute or healed lesions. Annular infection (QV) is also uncommon, if more frequent, with mechanical heart valves.

Gram-positive cocci are the most frequent cause of mitral valve endocarditis. Staphylococci and streptococci infect native valves about equally whether they are normal or abnormal. Streptococcal infections are still commonly associated with damage caused by rheumatic disease. These organisms are also a frequent cause of mitral prosthetic valve endocarditis. Fungal infections are not rare in these latter circumstances.

KEY DIAGNOSTIC CRITERIA: See *Endocarditis, infective NOS.*

ENDOCARDITIS, INFECTIVE, PULMONARY VALVE

Entry Author: Jagdish W. Butany

DEFINITION: Infected thrombotic vegetations attached to the endocardium of the pulmonary valve or to a heart valve prosthesis located in that area.

GROSS AND MICROSCOPIC FINDINGS: Findings vary with the virulence of the causative organism and duration of infection. See *Endocarditis, infective NOS.*

REMARKS: Infective endocarditis of the pulmonary valve is rare. It may be an isolated lesion on a normal valve but usually is associated with a congenital anomaly, acquired disease, or following surgical repair in the area. Usually associated with infective endocarditis on other heart valves. In fact, fungal infection in IV drug abusers associated with tricuspid valve endocarditis (QV) is frequent. Local complications occur but are infrequent. Recurrent pulmonary infarctions and abscesses result from emboli to lungs.

KEY DIAGNOSTIC CRITERIA: Demonstration of microorganisms in thrombotic vegetations—see *Endocarditis, infective NOS.*

ENDOCARDITIS, INFECTIVE, TRICUSPID VALVE

Entry Author: Jagdish W. Butany

DEFINITION: Infected thrombotic vegetations attached to the endocardium of the tricuspid valve or a heart valve prosthesis located in that area.

GROSS AND MICROSCOPIC FINDINGS: Findings vary with the virulence of the causative organism and duration of infection. See *Endocarditis, infective NOS.*

REMARKS: Infective endocarditis of the tricuspid valve is not common. Approximately 50% of cases develop on previously damaged valves. Can be associated, if not commonly, with indwelling catheter/pacemaker leads. Occurs most often in intravenous drug abusers. Nonetheless, left-sided endocarditis is still more common in this population. In these cases, fungal infections are not uncommon. Blood and infected thrombi impact on the lungs producing recurrent pulmonary infarcts or abscesses. Chordae may rupture and leaflets ulcerate or perforate. Associated annular abscesses are rare.

KEY DIAGNOSTIC CRITERIA: Demonstration of microorganisms in thrombotic vegetations with acute inflammatory cells and with or without destruction of leaflet tissue. See *Endocarditis, infective NOS.*

ENDOCARDITIS, INFECTIVE, VIRAL

Entry Author: Francesca V. Lobo

SYNONYMS: Infectious endocarditis viral, nonrheumatic; valvular disease; postinflammatory valvulitis.

DEFINITION: A subset of infective endocarditis is thought produced by viral infection.

REMARKS: The possibility of viral endocarditis has been suggested by demonstrating viral antigens (Coxsackie B, polio, and echovirus 16) in surgically excised mitral and aortic valves, and the observation that cytomegalovirus and other human viruses may be associated with an endomyocarditis in immunosuppressed patients.

An acute and chronic valvulitis can be produced in mice and monkeys with coxsackie B and adenovirus infections. The tricuspid valve is affected most frequently followed by mitral, aortic, and pulmonary valves in descending frequency. Viral valvulitis/endocarditis may or may not occur together with viral myocarditis or pericarditis.

In mice, the acute valvulitis consists of localized areas of marked edema, necrosis of individual endothelial and stromal cells, and slight round cell infiltration. From the 7th to the 14th day of infection there is proliferation of endothelial cells and stromal fibroblasts and an obvious mononuclear infiltrate. After the 3rd to 5th week, changes of chronic valvulitis appear, with irregular thickening by fibroblasts and occasional fibrotic verrucal nodules on the surface. Mononuclear inflammatory cells decrease after three months. Subsequently (chronic stage), there is thickening and deformity of valves with extensive fibrosis with or without myxomatous degeneration, slight round cell infiltration, occasional cartilaginous metaplasia at the root of the valve and, in some, chordal shortening (which may occur quite early in the inflammation).

Viral culture and serology could become part of the routine investigation in patients with acquired valvular heart disease, otherwise viruses go undetected. May occur alone or as mixed viral and bacterial infection. Viral antigen may be localized by immunofluorescent technique on damaged valve tissue, or amplified using molecular diagnostic techniques.

ENDOCARDITIS, INFECTIVE, WHIPPLE'S DISEASE

Entry Author: Francesca V. Lobo

DEFINITION: A rare subset of infective endocarditis caused by a bacterial organism, the so-called "Whipple bacillus." The organism has been detected on ultrastructural examination or molecular diagnostic techniques. The latter suggest the possibility of a gram-positive aerobic actinomycete not closely related to any other known genus.

GROSS FINDINGS: Produces vegetations resembling those of nonbacterial thrombotic endocarditis. Fine vegetations with erosion of the surface of valve leaflets have been described. In addition to endocarditis, there may be myocarditis and, more frequently, pericarditis. However, cardiac lesions may be clinically insignificant in patients with systemic involvement by Whipple's disease (intestinal lipodystrophy).

May produce valvular deformities. The mitral valve is most commonly involved followed by tricuspid and aortic valves. Involvement of a porcine bioprosthesis by Whipple's disease has been reported. Resembles chronic rheumatic heart disease with diffuse thickening and fibrosis of valve leaflets, rolling of free edges, and chordal fibrosis that may be associated with shortening and fusion.

MICROSCOPIC FINDINGS: Affected valves and vegetations contain large macrophages full of PAS-positive granular material (similar to that found in small intestinal mucosa) at the base of the vegetation and in the valve substance. There is associated proliferation of fibrous tissue and presence of chronic inflammatory cells. Intracellular and extracellular rod-shaped PAS-positive bodies 1.5 to 2 microns long and 0.2 to 0.4 microns in diameter are found on ultrastructural examination in affected valves and also in the myocardium. These, as well as membrane-bound masses of fibrillar material within the macrophages are of bacterial origin.

SPECIAL PROCEDURES NEEDED FOR DIAGNOSIS: Diagnosis of Whipple's disease by jejunal biopsy in patients with malabsorption. PAS stain on such biopsies is of assistance.

DIFFERENTIAL DIAGNOSIS: With vegetations exclude nonbacterial thrombotic endocarditis with valvular deformity. Exclude chronic rheumatic valvular disease (see below).

KEY DIAGNOSTIC CRITERIA: Presence of the Whipple bacillus in vegetations or valve substance. The presence of PAS-positive granules in macrophages in the valvular lesions as well as elsewhere is characteristic. But electron microscopic examination may be needed to exclude some congenital enzyme deficiencies whose products thicken valve cusps/leaflets.

ENDOCARDITIS, NONBACTERIAL THROMBOTIC

Entry Authors: Francesca V. Lobo and Jagdish W. Butany

SYNONYMS: NBTE; nonbacterial endocarditis; noninfective endocarditis; marantic endocarditis; terminal endocarditis; valvular vegetation, thrombotic; verrucal endocardiosis; verrucal endocarditis.

DEFINITION: Presence of sterile, thrombotic vegetation(s) on heart valves associated with terminal (e.g., malignancy) and debilitating (e.g., TB) diseases, as well as sporadically in other conditions (e.g., blood dyscrasias). Presumably related to endocardial injury though the precise pathogenesis is not known. NOTE: The thrombotic vegetation found in acute rheumatic fever and systemic lupus endocarditis (Libman-Sacks endocarditis) may be considered examples of NBTE, albeit of small size.

GROSS FINDINGS: Pink to grayish vegetations usually occur on valve cusps/leaflets most frequently along the line of closure. They vary in size but are usually 1.0 mm to 1.0 cm in maximum diameter. May be smooth surfaced and firmly attached, or bulky, nodular, friable, and spread over the adjacent surface of a cusp. "Kissing lesions" can affect adjacent sides of cusps. In the aortic and pulmonary valves, vegetations usually start at the noduli Arantii and spread to adjacent closure lines.

MICROSCOPIC FINDINGS: Fresh vegetation composed of platelets admixed with fibrin and red blood cells. Special stains do not reveal microorganisms. Underlying valve usually shows little host response or edema, fibrin, and a few white blood cells related to the vegetation. Fragmented elastic and collagen may be found in some instances, evidence of underlying pathology, e.g., rheumatic or degenerative valve disease. Later, vegetations may lyse, endothelialize, organize, fibrose, or calcify.

DIFFERENTIAL DIAGNOSIS: Must be differentiated from infective endocarditis. Diagnose by exclusion—no microorganisms demonstrable histologically.

REMARKS: These vegetations are present in 1–2% of autopsy cases, more often in males than females, and more common in the 4th to 8th decades. Likely, but not exclusively, occur in those with malignancy, terminal, and wasting diseases. The mitral valve is most frequently affected, followed by the aortic or combined left-sided lesions. Right-sided valves may be affected, particularly in patients with indwelling cardiac lines. NTBE lesions produce emboli.

Blood and verrucal cultures are negative. Circulating phospholipid antibodies may be detected. These could promote valve thrombosis by a "procoagulant" effect. If of adequate size, vegetations can be detected by echocardiography. NBTE is the most common cause of endocarditis. It may be asymptomatic and found incidentally at autopsy or present with heart murmurs in life or sequelae including embolization. NOTE: On rare occasions tumor cells are found in thrombotic vegetations in patients with metastatic malignancy.

ENDOCARDITIS, NONBACTERIAL THROMBOTIC IN ACUTE RHEUMATIC FEVER

Entry Author: Francesca V. Lobo

SYNONYM: Rheumatic endocarditis.

DEFINITION: Nonbacterial thrombotic endocarditis associated with inflammation of heart valves occurring in episodes of acute rheumatic fever.

GROSS FINDINGS: Mitral, aortic, tricuspid, and pulmonary valves involved in descending order of frequency. Wart-like vegetations or verrucae 1.0 to 2.0 mm in diameter are present on the contact margins of the valve cusps/leaflets. Vegetations are initially translucent, later opaque gray or brown. They occur singly or in clusters, are firmly attached, and rarely embolize. May also occur on chordae tendineae or mural endocardium, particularly of the left atrium and sometimes the left ventricle. In healing, help to contribute to valvular deformity found in rheumatic valvular disease (QV).

MICROSCOPIC FINDINGS: Vegetations consist of fibrin-platelet thrombi that overlie areas of edema, fibrinoid necrosis, and a polymorphic inflammatory cell infiltrate in the valve substance. At a later stage there is vascularization of the leaflet and organization of vegetations with scarification. Aschoff bodies are rare in valves, except in severe cases (they are better seen in the mural endocardium or myocardium). The extent of subsequent damage to a cusp/leaflet varies with duration, severity, and presence or absence of recurrent episodes.

DIFFERENTIAL DIAGNOSIS: See nonbacterial thrombotic endocarditis. Clinical history is important in establishing diagnosis. Inflammatory lesions in cusp/leaflet are prominent. Patients rarely die in acute phase. At autopsy Aschoff nodules may be seen in myocardium as described.

KEY DIAGNOSTIC CRITERIA: Rheumatic fever most often affects children and young adults 10 days to 6 weeks following a throat infection by B-hemolytic group A streptococci. In the acute phase, cardiac manifestations may include mitral or aortic regurgitation and, less commonly, tricuspid valve dysfunction.

ENDOCARDITIS, NONBACTERIAL THROMBOTIC IN SYSTEMIC LUPUS ERYTHEMATOSUS (SLE)

Entry Author: Francesca V. Lobo

SYNONYMS: Atypical verrucous endocarditis; Libman-Sacks endocarditis.

DEFINITION: Nonbacterial thrombotic endocarditis occurring in patients with SLE.

GROSS FINDINGS: The thrombotic vegetations are often found on heart valves at lines of closure but are scattered elsewhere, e.g., on valvular endocardium, chordae tendineae, or mural endocardium of atria or ventricles (i.e., in atypical locations). May affect any valve but mitral and tricuspid valves more often affected. These lesions are predominantly located on the ventricular surface of leaflets. Observed in 25–60% of autopsy cases of SLE, though only 6–20% are clinically symptomatic.

Vegetations usually between 0.1–0.4 cm in diameter, rarely up to 0.8–1.0 cm), dry, granular, pink, or tan-yellow, relatively flat and adherent. May be single, multiple, or aggregated. May cover both surfaces of a leaflet, extend onto atrial and ventricular endocardium, and occupy angles between leaflet and ventricular endocardium. Can predominate along the line of closure. Leaflet perforation (usually related to steroid therapy) or chordal rupture are complications. Rarely a source of emboli.

Healed chronic lesions are morphologically indistinguishable from rheumatic disease of mitral or aortic valve. May cause adhesion of the posterior mitral valve leaflet to the posterior ventricular wall producing valvular insufficiency.

MICROSCOPIC FINDINGS: Acute lesions show fibrinoid necrosis of valve substance that may erode the endothelium with superimposed thrombus formation. These verrucae contain finely granular fibrinous material. Varying degrees of exudative and proliferative cellular reaction associated with inflammatory cells, histiocytes and, on occasion, "hematoxyphilic bodies" not only within the valve substance but also in the valve ring, sinuses, and mural endocardium. Palisading granulomatous inflammation is noted occasionally.

Healing is by granulation tissue and may produce focal fibrous thickenings of the valve or mural endocardium. Chronic lesions resemble rheumatic valvular disease grossly. Microscopically, there is continuing fibrinoid necrosis and quite heavy inflammatory infiltration.

DIFFERENTIAL DIAGNOSIS: Distinguished from NTBE by patients' clinical history, younger age, and female predominance. In acute stage, verrucae have a distinctive distribution on valves, mural endocardium, and angles between leaflets and ventricular endocardium. Hematoxyphilic bodies may be present within verrucae and in valve substance. Circulating phospholipid antibodies (lupus anticoagulant) can be detected.

ENDOCARDITIS, NOS

Entry Author: Francesca V. Lobo

SYNONYMS: Infective endocarditis or nonbacterial thrombotic endocarditis.

DEFINITION: Presence of thrombi on heart valves or, less frequently, on mural endocardium. Thrombi may or may not be infected.

GROSS FINDINGS: Thrombotic vegetations on the contact margins of cusps/leaflets, with gross and histologic features varying according to etiology, the specific microorganism involved and host response.

MICROSCOPIC FINDINGS: Vegetations composed of fibrin platelet thrombus—variable numbers of inflammatory cells and/or microorganisms. Heart valve may exhibit underlying pathology with tissue disruption, necrosis, inflammatory infiltration or microorganisms, or show very little damage. See *Endocarditis, infective* and *Endocarditis, nonbacterial thrombotic*.

REMARKS: Thrombotic vegetations forwarded for study in surgical pathology may be artifactually colonized by microorganisms if not soon covered with fixative solution. Artifactual colonization can also occur post mortem. In these instances, microorganisms are confined to the immediate surface of vegetations and are not intimately mixed within the thrombus. Also, the vegetation does not contain many acute inflammatory cells and no inflammatory/reparative reaction is present in the valve cusp/leaflet.

ENDOCARDITIS, PARASITIC

Entry Author: Malcolm D. Silver

REMARKS: Extremely rarely parasitic organisms are found in thrombotic vegetations attached to a heart valve showing an inflammatory reaction, with or without an associated reparative response. For example, *Entameba histolytica* has produced tricuspid valve and right ventricular mural endocarditis with nodular vegetations.

KEY DIAGNOSTIC CRITERIA: Likely hematogenous spread from another site of infestation. Geographic location of patient or clinical history may arouse suspicion. Parasites may be demonstrable by PAS stain.

Reference

1. Trinz P. A case of tricuspid valvular and right parietal endocarditis due to *E. histolytica* in the course of fatal systemic amebiasis. *Bull Soc Pathol Exot* 1974;67:359.

HEART VALVE, ACUTE RHEUMATIC DISEASE

Entry Author: Francesca V. Lobo

See *Endocarditis, nonbacterial, thrombotic, in acute rheumatic fever.*

HEART VALVE, AGE CHANGES

Entry Author: Malcolm D. Silver

SYNONYMS: Heart valve sclerosis, senile valve changes, degenerative valve changes, atherosclerosis of mitral valve, lipid deposits in heart valves, calcification of heart valves.

DEFINITION: A galaxy of minor, usually nonpathogenic changes, found affecting heart valves with increasing age.

GROSS FINDINGS: 1. Heart Valve Fibrosis—Most heart valves thicken with age, the change though due to mechanical factors. It is recognized by increased opacity and is most noticeable on left-sided valves. Produces firm, nodular, thickenings along line of closure (on corpus Arantius of semilunar valves) and in "rough" zone, i.e., area of contact during closure of atrioventricular valves, whole cusp/leaflet may thicken slightly. Chordae tendineae, too, may thicken.

2. Lipid Deposits—They can develop on any heart valve with increasing age but are most obvious at the base of the anterior mitral leaflet or on its ventricular aspect and in aortic valve cusps (and sinuses of Valsalva). They appear as opaque yellowish plaques, 5 mm in diameter or larger, if they coalesce. Occasionally they calcify, rarely ulcerate. Lipid deposits also develop in the cusps of tissue heart valve prostheses with time.

3. Fenestrations—These small, oval, single or multiple, 1–2 mm diameter defects in cusp substance are located above the line of closure of semilunar valves usually near commissures. They do not have thickened edges. Children often have very thin, delicate membranous tissue in these areas. They can have fenestrations but their number increase with age. (NOTE: in rare instances, a fenestration may extend beyond the line of closure and induce aortic incompetence).

4. Isolated Amyloid Deposits—Isolated amyloid deposits occur in heart valves (both native or those of tissue prosthetic valves). Usually a microscopic diagnosis but can cause nodular deposits 2.5 mm in diameter.

5. Calcification—A fine calcification, often associated with lipid deposits, may be noticed as a grittiness when cutting left-sided heart valve leaflets/cusps in surgical pathology. Deposits can coalesce to produce nodules, especially in the distal two thirds of semilunar valves. (NOTE: when these changes are marked and stiffen aortic valve cusps, they induce clinical stenosis—see *Aortic valve stenosis, calcification.*

6. Lambl's Excrescences—These 1–4 mm long whisker-like lesions may be single or, if multiple, produce a filiform appearance. They are common especially on left-sided heart valves and at a cusp's/leaflet's free margin or along the line of closure including corpora Arantii. They are also found, occasionally, on chordae. They become more obvious when a valve is placed under water.

7. Myxomatous Change—A microscopic diagnosis—see below.

8. Isolated Tricuspid Valve Ulceration—Pomerance described single or multiple ulcerations on the atrial aspect of tricuspid valve leaflets, appearing as 0.5–1 cm diameter erosions or punched-out craters at the contact margins. They are yellowish and have hemorrhagic margins. Pomerance noted these lesions more frequently in the English winter.

MICROSCOPIC FINDINGS: 1. Heart Valve Fibrosis—Fibroelastic tissue thickening (that may incorporate Lambl's excrescences) deposited on surface of cusp/leaflet/chordae. Elastic lamellae in new tissue are usually fine. Original elastic lamellae deep to plaque can be fragmented.

2. Lipid Deposits—Have microscopic morphology comparable in some ways to atherosclerotic plaque. Early deposits of sudanophilic droplets or produce a foamy appearance in fibrosa. Later macrophages and crystalline material seen often accompanied by a fine stippling of calcium but other complications of atherosclerotic plaque (e.g., hemorrhage) not seen. NOTE: Such lipid deposits, often associated with calcification, develop in cusps of tissue heart valve prostheses.

3. Fenestrations—May or may not show fibroelastic tissue thickening of their edges.

4. Isolated Amyloid Deposits—Usually ATTR amyloid is derived from transthyretin. They have the histologic, special stain, and electron microscopic morphology of amyloid deposits elsewhere—see *Amyloidosis.*

5. Calcification—The histology is that of calcium deposits elsewhere. See *Mitral valve annulus calcification.* However, putaceous deposits do not occur.

6. Lambl's Excrescence—Contain fibrin progressing to endothelialized fibrous tissue, little glycosamine glycan content. In elastic tissue, stains often demonstrate concentric rings of granular tissue that stains for elastin.

7. Myxomatous Change—Normally glycosamine glycan material is confined to the loosely arranged spongiosa of a valve leaflet/cusp. With increasing age, this material is observed in small quantities in the valve fibrosa. Such deposits are never as widespread or florid as those found in a myxomatous valve nor does the affected leaflet prolapse.

8. Isolated Tricuspid Valve Ulceration—The affected leaflet has an ulceration in its surface with dense linear aggregates of granular elastic-staining material at its margin and fibrin on the ulcer floor. No inflammatory reaction is seen.

DIFFERENTIAL DIAGNOSIS: 1. Heart Valve Fibrosis—The thickening associated with age is never as marked as that caused by rheumatic valvular disease or deposits associated with methysergide therapy nor found in places where thrombi commonly deposit and become organized.

2. Lipid Deposits—Any heart valve may be affected, but the deposits are never as severe nor do they develop as early in life as those associated with hyperlipidemia. The role of these deposits in subsequent valve calcification is controversial.

3. Fenestrations—Very rarely a fenestration may extend beyond the line of closure and be associated with aortic valve incompetence. Congenitally double orifice tricuspid and mitral valves have chordae distributed to the perimeter of the second orifice. A healed perforation associated with infective endocarditis is usually larger and has thickened edges.

4. Calcification—Normally, calcium deposits occurring with age are not marked. Deposits at the base of the posterior mitral leaflet can be associated with calcification of the mitral annulus.

5. Lambl's Excrescences—Lambl's excrescences are distinguishable from papillary fibroelastomas on histological grounds—see Section 5, *Tumors of Pericardium, Myocardium,* and *Blood vessels.*

Reference

1. Pomerance A. Isolated ulceration of the tricuspid valve. *J Pathol* 1970:102:171.

HEART VALVE INCOMPETENCE, MITRAL VALVE

Entry Author: Virginia M. Walley

SYNONYMS: Mitral valve insufficiency, mitral valve regurgitation.

DEFINITION: Incompetence (QV) of this valve caused by congenital anomaly or acquired pathology. See remarks below on "functional" mitral insufficiency.

GROSS FINDINGS: Varies with underlying valve pathology. May be associated with congenital anomaly like corrected transposition of great vessels with ventricular discordance in adult life; double mitral valve orifice; congenital cleft in anterior mitral leaflet associated with endocardial cushion defect, each of which presents easily definable gross morphology.

Of acquired lesions infective endocarditis of a mitral valve or transferred to that valve from an aortic valve infection may ulcerate or perforate a leaflet and healed rheumatic valvulitis shorten one. Trauma can also perforate a leaflet. Each of these presents specific gross morphology. Leaflets may have appearance of prolapsed mitral valve (QV).

See specific entries under: *Heart valve myxomatous degeneration; Heart valve mitral prolapse; Mitral valve annular calcification; Heart valve incompetence, mitral, associated with ischemic heart disease.*

An atrial myxoma or thrombus may project into the valve lumen and interfere with its closure.

Sequelae depend on the chronicity as well as severity of the insufficiency. Acute severe insufficiency may be evidenced only by severe lethal pulmonary congestion and edema, whereas chronic mild insufficiency causes left atrial dilation and hypertrophy accompanied by atrial fibrillation. Occasional cases show a left atrial jet lesion consisting of an endocardial plaque of fibrous thickening and roughening of the surface. A mural thrombus may form at this site.

MICROSCOPIC FINDINGS: Varies with underlying pathology.

REMARKS: "Functional" mitral insufficiency occurs but is less frequent than functional tricuspid valve insufficiency (QV). Mitral insufficiency is most likely to have a pathological basis. Once established, mitral incompetence seems to become self-perpetuating. The enlarging left atrium alters spatial relationships in the annular region, effectively rolling the posterior leaflet more and more toward the left atrium, with effective shortening so that coaption with the anterior leaflet worsens.

DIFFERENTIAL DIAGNOSIS: Between conditions listed, usually not difficult.

HEART VALVE INCOMPETENCE, NOS

Entry Author: Malcolm D. Silver

DEFINITION: Incompetence of a native heart valve caused by a congenital anomaly or pathology that interferes with the function of one or more components of a valve's "complex" or the anatomic structures involved in valve closure. Incompetence of a prosthetic heart valve is produced by changes within a valve or in its paravalvular region that interfere with cusp or occluder function or permit valve dehiscence.

REMARKS: Valvular insufficiency may develop acutely over a long period or acutely aggravating pre-existing insufficiency.

The valvular pathology varies with the cause of incompetence.

Structures important in atrioventricular valve closure include the valve annulus, leaflets, chordae, and left ventricular myocardium including the papillary muscles. Thus, dilation of a valve annulus and its heavy calcification or deposits in its fibrous tissue cause valve incompetence as do anomalies or pathology that (a) interfere with leaflet coaption, e.g., vegetations or tumor; (b) effectively lengthen them allowing "overshooting" of their free margins, e.g., myxomatous change or other causes of leaflet prolapse; (c) effectively shorten them, e.g., ulceration or scarring; or (d) perforate them, e.g., trauma or infective endocarditis. Chordal rupture or avulsion and papillary muscle rupture or dysfunction, the latter often associated with ischemic heart disease and having several mechanisms also cause atrioventricular valve incompetence. Structures important in closing semilunar valves include the valve annulus, cusps, the ventricular myocardium, and the integrity of the sinus and tubular portions of the ascending aorta and corresponding regions of the main pulmonary trunk. The observed pathology of annulus, cusps, and ventricle are like those just described. Aortic and pulmonary root dilation from whatever cause must also be considered.

At autopsy heart chambers proximal and distal to the incompetent valve are hypertrophied and/or dilated. Jet lesions, on the left side particularly, may cause endocardial thickening or valve-like structures on septal wall or ventricular aspect of the anterior mitral leaflet or on the endocardium of the left atrium. Secondary changes, caused by heart failure, develop rapidly within proximal organs and incompetence of sudden onset. They may be lethal.

Pathological changes that destroy annular tissue allow a prosthetic valve dehiscence. Interference with closure of a mechanical valve occluder and changes to the cusps of biological valves like those just described are observed. Degenerative changes may affect any valve component with time, including mechanical wearing or metal fatigue allowing structure fracture. These must be considered if a prosthetic valve is incompetent.

Further details are found under causative diseases or the heading "insufficiency" related to a particular valve.

HEART VALVE INCOMPETENCE OR STENOSIS ASSOCIATED WITH METABOLIC OR ENZYME-DEFICIENCY DISEASES

Entry Author: Malcolm D. Silver

GROSS FINDINGS: Cusp/leaflets or annular tissue thickened with or without secondary calcification and changes found in valvular stenosis or incompetence.

MICROSCOPIC FINDINGS/DIFFERENTIAL DIAGNOSIS: Conditions distinguished by light or electron microscopic morphology.

REMARKS: Very rarely abnormal deposits or materials occur in heart valve cusps/leaflets or annular tissue in metabolic or enzyme-deficiency diseases and induce valvular incompetence or stenosis. See *Myocardium—Glycogen storage diseases; Mucopolysaccharidosis; Sphingolipidosis; Gout and oxalosis.*

HEART VALVE INCOMPETENCE, TRICUSPID VALVE

Entry Author: Jagdish W. Butany

SYNONYMS: Tricuspid valve insufficiency, tricuspid valve regurgitation.

DEFINITION: Incompetence (QV) of this valve caused by congenital anomaly or acquired pathology. See remarks below on functional tricuspid incompetence.

GROSS FINDINGS: Varies with underlying valve pathology. May be associated with congenital anomaly like Ebstein's anomaly or double tricuspid valve orifice, each of which presents easily definable gross morphology.

Of acquired lesions, infective endocarditis can ulcerate or perforate a leaflet and healed rheumatic valvulitis shorten one. Endocardial plaques in carcinoid heart disease induce incompetence as does the valve's complete surgical excision to treat infective endocarditis or its traumatic perforation during passage of catheter, pacemaker wire, or instrument. Myxomatous change in the leaflets or chordae may allow incompetence. Tumor or thrombus may project into the valve lumen and interfere with its closure.

Regardless of the cause, chronic tricuspid insufficiency is associated with dilation and hypertrophy of the right atrium. The liver is enlarged and congested initially and may subsequently develop "cardiac" cirrhosis associated with ascites.

MICROSCOPIC FINDINGS: Varies with underlying pathology.

REMARKS: Tricuspid incompetence due to pathological changes is not particularly frequent. Much more often it is "functional." In those circumstances, leaflets and chordae show no pathology, but heart failure causes annular dilation, effectively shortening the leaflets. Functional incompetence resolves when right heart failure is controlled.

DIFFERENTIAL DIAGNOSIS: Between conditions listed, usually not difficult.

HEART VALVE, MYXOMATOUS DEGENERATION

Entry Author: Malcolm D. Silver

SYNONYMS: Myxomatous valve, floppy valve, mucoid degeneration.

DEFINITION: Congenital or acquired marked accumulation of sulfated glycosamine glycans, especially in lamina spongiosa, with associated degeneration of collagen and elastic tissue. Changes may also affect valve annulus and chordae tendineae.

GROSS FINDINGS: Left-sided valves affected more often than right-sided ones. Cusp/leaflet tissue more voluminous than usual. May be semitranslucent or opaque due to fibroelastic tissue deposition. Cut edge has a grayish, gelatinous appearance. Changes cause weakening of integrity of cusp/leaflet tissues so chordae can elongate and have a reduced diameter and valve prolapse Alternatively, chordae are thickened, especially near insertion. Chordal or commissural fusion not a feature. Tiny thrombi found on valve surface with linear ones at base of prolapsed posterior mitral leaflet (QV).

Look for complications including perforation or spontaneous rupture of aortic valve cusps (rare); valve prolapse (common) with or without signs of valvular insufficiency; rupture of chordae (uncommon); calcification of leaflet base and annulus (rare); infective endocarditis (rare); and evidence of TIAs or stroke (uncommon).

MICROSCOPIC FINDINGS: Lamina fibrosa widened through most of cusp's/leaflet's length by glycosamine accumulation, with loss of collagen and elastic tissue disruption. Changes also present in chordae and annulus. They are well demonstrated by Movat's stain. Fibroelastic thickening of leaflets/chordae often present and marked if mitral valve prolapsed. Look on valve surface and at base of posterior mitral valve for fresh or organized thrombi and dystrophic calcification.

REMARKS: May affect any age, but symptoms associated with Marfan syndrome common in 3rd to 5th decade.

Idiopathic form may induce midsystolic click syndrome in teenagers and young adults, especially women. A small percentage of these cases subsequently develop complications.

DIFFERENTIAL DIAGNOSIS: Minor and focal accumulations or glycosamine glycans not uncommon in valve cusps/leaflets with age or as reactive change associated with other disease processes (e.g., rheumatic disease). Deposits not as marked as in myxomatous degeneration and affected valves do not prolapse.

Glycosamine glycans deposited in Marfan syndrome. Patient has family history and other stigmata/complications of this condition. In this congenital condition, all four heart valves may be affected.

Chordae may be thickened in this condition but no commissural or chordal thickening as in rheumatic disease of atrioventricular valves. History should help distinguish methysergide-related thickening. Myxomatous change not a feature in that condition.

Myxomatous change in right-sided valves may accompany pulmonary hypertension.

Idiopathic myxomatous degeneration usually affects mitral valve (see *Myxomatous degeneration, mitral valve*) with some involvement of aortic valve.

HEART VALVE, RHEUMATIC VALVULITIS, HEALED

Entry Author: Malcolm D. Silver

DEFINITION: Valvular pathology induced by repeated attacks of acute rheumatic fever (see *Endocarditis, nonbacterial, thrombotic in acute rheumatic fever*).

MICROSCOPIC FINDINGS: Cusps/leaflets and chordae show nonspecific fibrous thickening with mild degrees of elastosis. The usual arrangement of layers in cusps/leaflets is lost. Vascularization and a few collections of mononuclear inflammatory cells may be present in the basal third of a leaflet. Specific histological features of rheumatic fever (e.g., Aschoff nodules) are seldom seen in valves at this stage.

REMARKS: The healing of the nonbacterial thrombotic vegetations and valve damage induced by the cross-immune reaction to heart tissue following streptococcal throat infection in susceptible individuals leads to valve stenosis (QV), incompetence (QV), or a combination of these changes.

These valvular changes develop rapidly in childhood and early adulthood in tropical countries or take many years to become manifest after the last attack of acute rheumatic fever in Western countries, appearing in adults in their 4th decade or later. In the latter instance, organization of minute mural thrombi deposited as a result of turbulent blood flow may aid progression. Secondary calcification is more prominent in westerners too. Affected valves are prone to infective endocarditis (QV).

For further details see discussion of valve incompetence/stenosis under specific valves.

HEART VALVE STENOSIS, AORTIC

Entry Author: Malcolm D. Silver

DEFINITION: Stenosis (QV) affecting the aortic valve orifice. In adults, occurs when valvular outflow area is reduced below 0.75 cm^2.

Because of their design, prosthetic valves, both tissue and mechanical, induce minor stenosis when inserted. They may become further stenosed subsequently.

GROSS FINDINGS: See separate entries for specific forms of aortic valve stenosis.

The jet of blood leaving a stenosed valve generates turbulence in the aortic lumen. This leads to a variety of forces acting on the aortic wall that can induce post-stenotic dilation, a localized aneurysm or a patch of intimal thickening, usually in the mid-third of the ascending aorta. A jet lesion may become infected. Mural thrombus is likely in an aneurysm but not in a dilation.

Due to pressure overload the left ventricle is hypertrophied with marked thickening of its wall. There may be signs of left or generalized heart failure. A stenosed aortic valve can develop infective endocarditis, may induce red cell hemolysis, and be associated with calcium or thrombotic emboli. The former occurs when calcium masses ulcerate. Such ulcerated lesions may damage nearby cusps, where they come in contact, and ulcerate or perforate them. When cusps are completely immobilized, some degree of aortic incompetence accompanies valve stenosis.

MICROSCOPIC FINDINGS: Varies with underlying pathology and presents specific or nonspecific changes. Generally, the latter are seen histologically with a combination of cusp sclerosis caused by fibrous or fibroelastic tissue and variable calcification. Cartilaginous or bony metaplasia is possible in calcium deposits and both lipid and amyloid deposits can be found in cusps. If calcium deposition predominates the descriptive term "calcific aortic stenosis" is applied.

Various specific deposits associated with inborn errors of metabolism may, through their bulk, cause cusp stiffening. The deposits may be recognizable by light or electron microscopy or by appropriate immunohistochemical analysis.

The aortic wall in areas of post-stenotic dilation often shows focal elastic tissue destruction with replacement by fibrous tissue. Glycosaminoglycans are often increased in the area and may form pools in the media.

DIFFERENTIAL DIAGNOSIS: Signs and symptoms caused by subvalvular (uncommon) or supravalvular (rare) stenosis may mimic those of valvular stenosis. These areas should be examined carefully to exclude nonvalvular causes of left ventricular outflow tract obstruction.

Aortic stenosis may present at any age, with a causative pathology varying in particular decades. It is the most common cause of left ventricular outflow tract obstruction.

REMARKS: In surgical pathology, provided that a native stenosed aortic valve is not severely fragmented during excision, the underlying pathology can be defined in the majority of cases (>95%). It is important to know the history, the number of cusps received, their size, whether or not raphes are present, the form of the valve orifice if cusps are excised in toto, and the presence and extent of commissural fusion. Even with the most careful examination, if a valve is severely stenosed and heavily calcified it may be impossible to establish underlying pathology.

HEART VALVE STENOSIS, AORTIC, ASSOCIATED WITH TYPE 2 HYPERLIPIDEMIA

Entry Author: Malcolm D. Silver

DEFINITION: Aortic stenosis caused by cusp stiffening produced by marked lipid deposits and accompanying calcification in this congenital hyperlipoproteinemia.

GROSS FINDINGS: Cusps are thickened and yellow because of lipid deposits. Secondary calcification may add to these changes. All may affect sinus region and ascending aorta.

MICROSCOPIC FINDINGS: Marked lipid deposition within aortic /valve cusps is a major finding together with associated calcification. Extensive amorphous lipid deposition including crystalline material as found in an extensive atheromatous atherosclerotic plaque. Marked associated fibroelastic thickening and calcium deposits that may be finely granular or large and modular.

REMARKS: Rare form of aortic valve stenosis seen in homozygous type 2 hyperlipidemia. Patients usually in their third to fourth decade. Family and clinical history with histological findings aid diagnosis.

NOTE: Small quantities of lipid may be demonstrated in calcified heart valves and may form part of that process. However, deposits never as marked as in this rare form of aortic valve stenosis.

HEART VALVE STENOSIS, AORTIC, CONGENITAL ANOMALY, INCLUDING ACOMMISSURAL, UNICOMMISSURAL, AND BICUSPID VALVES

Entry Author: Malcolm D. Silver

SYNONYMS: Congenital aortic stenosis, calcific aortic stenosis with unicommissural or bicuspid valves.

DEFINITION: Aortic stenosis associated with acommissural, unicuspid, or bicuspid valves.

GROSS FINDINGS: An acommissural aortic valve is dome or frustum shaped. Its small lumen appears central and the diaphragm-like valve has no well-defined commissures. Ridges of tissue marking their aborted formation may or may not be seen on the sinus side of the cusp.

A unicommissural valve presents with one well-defined commissure. Its orifice is shaped like an exclamation mark. Usually one or more raphes are apparent on its sinus side.

A congenitally bicuspid valve occurs in about 2% of the adult population but is more frequent when associated with coarctation of the aorta (10%). At autopsy, the commissures may be located anywhere around the circumference of the sinus aorta but most often are medial and lateral, less often anterior and posterior. In the former instance, one coronary artery arises from each sinus, in the latter both take origin from the anterior sinus.

MICROSCOPIC FINDINGS: Nonspecific. Histological examination of commissural areas do not help diagnosis.

REMARKS: Both unicommissural and bicuspid aortic valves are more frequent in males than females.

DIFFERENTIAL DIAGNOSIS: In surgical pathology acommissural, unicommissural, and aortic valves are often received, excised in toto, allowing examination of both their shape and orifice. A bicuspid valve may be excised with cusps joined at a commissural area but more often appears as two separate cusps.

Using the following points of differentiation the underlying congenital cause of the aortic stenosis can be established by gross examination in the majority of cases.

Accommissural valve—This valve is stenosed from birth and usually produces clinical symptoms then or within the first year of life. Its dome shape and central valve orifice are characteristic. It may not be calcified in children but can calcify subsequently, especially if a commissurotomy is done and the valve excised in teen-age. At this stage, gross differentiation from a unicommissural valve may be difficult and clinical history becomes important.

Unicommissural valve—This too is stenosed from birth but to a lesser degree than an acommissural valve. It may not be calcified when examined but usually calcifies with time. The resultant cusp stiffening worsens stenosis and prompts excision in second through fourth decade. From the side, the excised tissue mass is frustrum shaped. If the orifice is open at one end where excised from the single commissure, it is "U" shaped. If intact, it has the shape of an exclamation mark.

Bicuspid valve—If both cusps are of equal size this valve may not sclerose or calcify in life. More often, however, one cusp is larger than the other and with time both sclerose and calcify becoming stiff and causing valve stenosis usually in the fifth to eighth decade. Fusion of adjacent sides of the cusps produces commissural fusion, explaining why both cusps may be joined on receipt, but this change is usually not marked. If the valve is in toto the orifice may be semilunar. A raphe marking the aborted third commissure is found as a ridge of tissue on the sinus side of the larger on conjoined cusps in most cases (60–95%) but is not always present. A raphe's morphology varies in height (extension from base of sinus toward a cusp's free margin), length (extension from sinus wall toward cusp), and degree of separation at its upper or free margin. It is often heavily calcified. A congenitally bicuspid valve produces isolated aortic stenosis. Differentiation from acquired bicuspidization resulting from fusion at one commissure may be difficult. Here a history, especially of rheumatic disease, an involvement of other valves, especially the mitral valve, may be helpful. However, a few patients with a congenitally bicuspid aortic undoubtedly acquire rheumatic disease.

Healed rheumatic valvulitis—Here a valve has 3 cusps with stenosis caused in the main by commissural fusion, producing a triangular orifice. Acquired bicuspidization is uncommon. Secondary calcification may worsen stenosis and is particularly prominent at commissural areas. In the tropics, aortic stenosis caused by repeated attacks of acute rheumatic fever may develop rapidly, producing clinical symptoms in first to third decades. Such valves may not be calcified. In Western countries calcification and continuing stenosis likely caused by organization of minute thrombi induce valve stenosis in the fourth through sixth decade. Again, minor rheumatic valvular disease is a frequent accompanying lesion.

Mönckeberg's calcification—Here the "D"-shaped excised cusps show the calcification that stiffened them mainly in their distal two-thirds. They may be sclerosed. Commissural fusion is not usually a feature. This form of aortic stenosis usually affects older patients (with males predominating) in their seventh through ninth decades.

The cuspal free margin(s) in all of these forms of aortic stenosis is usually normal. If thickened or rolled toward the ventricular aspect in any area, a modicum of concomitant aortic incompetence must be suspected. These points also help differentiation at autopsy.

The rare quadricuspid aortic valve may calcify causing stenosis.

NOTE: Patients with the Singleton-Merten syndrome may develop severe calcification of both aortic valve cusps and ascending aorta with associated aortic valve stenosis.

HEART VALVE STENOSIS, AORTIC, HEALED RHEUMATIC VALVULITIS

Entry Author: Malcolm D. Silver

SYNONYMS: Chronic rheumatic aortic valve disease with stenosis; calcific aortic stenosis.

DEFINITION: Aortic stenosis resulting from repeated attacks of acute rheumatic fever.

GROSS FINDINGS AND DIFFERENTIAL DIAGNOSIS: See under *Heart valve stenosis, aortic, congenital anomaly.*

MICROSCOPIC FINDINGS: Nonspecific. Aschoff nodules usually not found within the cusps. Cusps show varying degree of thickening caused by fibrous or fibroelastic tissue. Fusion of adjacent sides of cusps in commissural area (commissural fusion) is common. Cusps and commissural areas may be heavily calcified. Increased vascularization is usual at the base of cusps together with some mononuclear inflammatory cell infiltrate. Foci of myxomatous change may be apparent but are not usually marked.

REMARKS: Providing valve not heavily calcified, diagnosis in autopsy suite or surgical pathology usually not a problem. Usually associated with mitral valvular disease caused by healed rheumatic valvulitis.

HEART VALVE STENOSIS, AORTIC, MÖNCKEBERG'S CALCIFICATION

Entry Author: Malcolm D. Silver

SYNONYMS: Degenerative aortic stenosis; aortic stenosis in the elderly; calcific aortic stenosis; calcific degenerative aortic stenosis.

DEFINITION: Aortic stenosis caused by calcium deposits within cusps. Etiology ascribed to degenerative processes within cusps.

GROSS FINDINGS: Yellowish calcium deposits found mainly in the basal two thirds of the cusps and most noticeable on their sinus sides. Initially, deposits are separate and 2 to 3 mm in diameter but become confluent and multinodular with increasing size. They thicken cusps up to 1 cm and can ulcerate the endocardial surface. Peripheral emboli (calcium or thrombi) may arise from the ulcerated calcium deposits. Resultant cusp stiffening is the main cause of valve stenosis. The free margins are normal. Commissural fusion is not a feature of this form of aortic stenosis.

MICROSCOPIC FINDINGS: Calcium (mainly) and fibrous tissue thicken the cusp. Cartilaginous and bony metaplasia found rarely. Some lipid deposits usual in the cusp substance. Focal amyloid deposits possible.

REMARKS: The term *calcific aortic stenosis* is used both in a generic sense, where it describes aortic stenosis caused by any mechanism and associated with marked cusp calcification and specifically, where it refers to this form which occurs in older individuals. I prefer the term Mönckeberg's calcification to distinguish this form of calcific aortic stenosis.

If calcification is severe (irrespective of the underlying cause of aortic stenosis) a bar of calcium can extend from the base of the posterior aortic cusp into the base of the anterior mitral valve leaflet. In rare instances, this involves the conducting system and by damaging it induces cardiac arrhythmias or complete heart block. Also, calcification of the posterior mitral valve annulus occurs.

Mönckeberg's calcification usually occurs as an isolated aortic valve disease. Affects valves with 3 cusps. Seen in older patients in their seventh to ninth decades; more frequent in males than females.

DIFFERENTIAL DIAGNOSIS: See under *Heart valve stenosis, aortic, congenital anomaly.*

HEART VALVE STENOSIS, MITRAL

Entry Author: Virginia M. Walley

SYNONYMS: Rheumatic valvular disease, healed rheumatic valvulitis, chronic rheumatic disease—all of the mitral valve.

DEFINITION: Stenosis (QV) of the mitral valve orifice may be caused by a congenital anomaly producing encroachment of adjacent tissues but is usually acquired and due almost invariably to healed rheumatic valvulitis (QV).

GROSS FINDINGS: Changes caused by healed rheumatic valvulitis may affect leaflets only with chordae showing no change or slight thickening without fusion. In that case, valve orifice appears reduced when viewed from the atrial aspect because fusion of adjacent sides of anterior and posterior leaflets at commissural areas (commissural fusion) extends toward center of valve lumen. This may affect only one commissure or both. At autopsy, secondary atrial dilation may give a clue to the condition. Leaflets are usually thickened, especially in their distal two-thirds, and the anatomic clefts in the posterior leaflet that define its scallops are obliterated. Secondary calcification with or without overlying endocardial ulceration and thrombosis is often present in patients from Western countries and is most marked near commissural areas. If chordae are affected they are usually shortened, thickened, and may be fused together. Secondary calcification develops. If these changes are marked, fused chordae produce a subvalvular obstruction.

At autopsy, changes in the right atrium, lungs, other chambers and organs, due to heart valve stenosis and its complications, must be sought.

MICROSCOPIC FINDINGS: Usually not specific—see *Rheumatic valvulitis, healed.*

REMARKS: Females develop mitral stenosis more often than males. It may be an isolated condition following repeated attacks of recognized rheumatic fever but can develop without a clear-cut history of acute rheumatic fever. Often associated with healed rheumatic valvulitis affecting in decreasing order of frequency—aortic, combined aortic and tricuspid valves, or other valves. The distribution of associated valvular disease can vary with geographic location. Mitral stenosis can develop rapidly in tropical countries. Elsewhere 10–25 years may elapse between last attack of rheumatic fever and its valvular heart disease.

DIFFERENTIAL DIAGNOSIS: Approximately 99% of cases of mitral stenosis are caused by healed rheumatic valvulitis. However, left-sided carcinoid heart disease and methysergide/ergotamine treatment (QV) are rare causes with distinction based on history and histological findings. The role of viruses and rheumatic fever in producing these changes is controversial—see *Endocarditis, infective, viral.* Antiphospholipid antibodies have been demonstrated in patients with mitral stenosis. Exact relationship to valve stenosis is subject to further investigation.

Acquired mitral stenosis caused by thrombus or tumor, e.g., atrial myxoma impinging on the valve lumen is usually differentiated with ease.

HEART VALVE STENOSIS, NOS

Entry Author: Malcolm D. Silver

DEFINITION: Narrowing of native valve orifice (reduction of luminal area) caused by congenital anomaly or acquired pathology that (a) thickens and/or stiffens cusps/leaflets inhibiting their free movement; (b) induces fusion of adjacent sides of cusps/leaflets at commissural areas (commissural fusion); or (c) produces a combination of these changes. Rarely, a native valve is stenosed by encroachment on its lumen by intraluminal processes, e.g., vegetation or tumor or by extraneous pathology compressing the orifice, e.g., pericardial calcification.

Biological and mechanical heart valve prostheses are stenosed by similar acquired changes affecting their particular morphology.

REMARKS: Left-sided heart valves stenose more frequently than those in right-sided chambers.

Changes observed in valve cusps/leaflets vary with the underlying pathology. Thus, a valve may be congenitally domed or have frustrum shape, whereas congenital anomalies of leaflets, chordae, endocardium, or myocardium, including papillary muscles, can encroach on its valve lumen. Cusp/leaflets thicken/stiffen when fibrous tissue thickens their surface or materials, e.g., calcium especially or products resulting from enzyme deficiencies are deposited in their substance. Where commissural fusion is a major cause it is fibrous initially. This can cause a diaphragm-like appearance of the tricuspid valve, a "fish-mouth" narrowing of mitral valve or the particular gross morphology found in stenosed aortic valves (QV). With time, fibrous commissural fusion becomes calcified, especially in Western countries. Indeed, irrespective of the process that initiates valve stenosis secondary changes, particularly further commissural fusion and calcification, gradually worsen it. Stenosed valves are prone to infection. Severe stenosis of left-sided heart valves can cause hemolysis. Large calcium deposits ulcerate. Such lesions and small thrombi deposited in these areas are a source of peripheral emboli.

At autopsy the heart chamber proximal to the stenosis is hypertrophied and/or dilated, and free-floating or mural thrombi develop in atria. Their endocardium may thicken or calcify. The resultant localized cardiomegaly can compress surrounding organs. Back pressure effects on proximal organs, e.g., lungs or liver, develop if heart failure ensues. Poststenotic dilation is possible.

Further details are found under causative diseases or the heading "stenosis" related to a particular valve.

HEART VALVE STENOSIS, PULMONARY

Entry Authors: Jagdish W. Butany and Malcolm D. Silver

DEFINITION: Stenosis (QV) affecting pulmonary valve orifice.

GROSS FINDINGS: Isolated pulmonary stenosis is usually congenital rather than acquired and may present as an isolated finding at autopsy. Here, the annular circumference is in the 4–5 cm range. A quadricuspid pulmonary valve can calcify or fibrose.

Pulmonary valvular stenosis may be a congenital anomaly and part of Fallot's tetralogy, Noonan syndrome or LEOPARD syndrome, with the patient manifesting associated findings of those conditions. The affected pulmonary valve may have a reduced annular circumference, be dome-shaped, or have dysplastic valve cusps.

Acquired pulmonary stenosis is not common. When it occurs it is usually associated with diseases affecting other heart valves of which rheumatic valvular disease (QV) or carcinoid valvular disease (QV) are the most frequent. Rheumatic pulmonary stenosis occurs with greater frequency where patients with rheumatic fever live at high altitudes.

MICROSCOPIC FINDINGS: Dysplastic valve cusps show a disorganization of the usual layered architecture. See also under *Rheumatic* and *Carcinoid valvular disease.*

DIFFERENTIAL DIAGNOSIS: Usually not a problem. Possibility of an isolated congenital stenosis must be considered if annular circumference much reduced.

HEART VALVE STENOSIS, TRICUSPID

Entry Authors: Francesca V. Lobo, Jagdish W. Butany, and Malcolm D. Silver

SYNONYMS: Rheumatic valve disease, healed rheumatic valvulitis, chronic rheumatic disease—all of the tricuspid valve.

DEFINITION: Stenosis (QV) affecting tricuspid valve orifice, and most commonly caused by healed rheumatic valvulitis (QV). Females are affected more often than males.

GROSS FINDINGS: Rheumatic tricuspid valve stenosis is almost invariably associated with healed rheumatic valvulitis of mitral and aortic valves. Combined pulmonary and tricuspid valve stenosis are more common at higher altitudes with frequency of tricuspid valve involvement increasing in tropical countries. In severe cases, the tricuspid valve orifice area is less than 1 cm^2 (annular circumference <8 cm). Commissural fusion is most often seen at anteroseptal commissure. If all commissures are affected, a diaphragm or funnel-like stenosed orifice is produced. Leaflets are thickened and shortened. Chordae tendineae show only slight thickening and shortening. Chordal fusion is not common or severe calcification.

At autopsy, right atrium is dilated and may contain thrombi. Liver congestion occurs and may be associated with portal fibrosis.

MICROSCOPIC FINDINGS: See *Rheumatic valvulitis, healed.*

REMARKS: Rheumatic tricuspid valve stenosis is often accompanied by some degree of valve incompetence (QV) with resultant right ventricular hypertrophy.

DIFFERENTIAL DIAGNOSIS: Other unusual causes of tricuspid valve stenosis include carcinoid heart disease (QV), Whipple's disease (QV), prolonged methysergide treatment (QV), endocarditis (QV), right atrial myxoma, or other tumor or thrombus. An aneurysm of the sinus of Valsalva or aortic valve annular abscess can impinge on the orifice of this valve. Morphological differentiation between these conditions is not likely to be a problem.

KEY DIAGNOSTIC CRITERIA: Past history of acute rheumatic fever-associated involvement or left-sided heart valves by healed rheumatic endocarditis with valve stenosis and/or incompetence.

HEART VALVE, TRAUMA

Entry Author: Jagdish W. Butany

DEFINITION: Penetrating, hydrostatic, rotational, or iatrogenic injury to components of a valve "complex." May produce valve incompetence or have no functional significance.

GROSS FINDINGS: Varies with type of trauma. Thus, gunshot or stabbing wounds can destroy a valve or perforate or sever parts of its complex. Raised hydrostatic pressure caused by marked abdominal or chest compression can tear cusps of semilunar valves or rupture them at their bases. Rotational injuries produce tears at points where cardiovascular structures are "fixed," or relatively immobile. They can extend into valvular tissues. Most of these injuries are associated with severe trauma and may contribute to a fatal outcome.

In the hospital setting, passage of catheters, insertion of pacemaker leads, and other instrumentation (e.g., endomyocardial biopsy) offer potential trauma. Severe forms are rare, the majority have no functional significance. Thus, indwelling catheters/leads damage the endocardium and become encased in thrombus or fibrous tissue. Pacemaker wires are often incorporated with tricuspid valve tissue by fibrous tissue. Attempted removal may tear leaflets or chordae. A common autopsy finding are right-sided leaflet/cusp injuries associated with the use of Swan-Ganz catheters. Fresh ones present as small areas (up to 5 mm in diameter) of congestion, ulceration, or thrombus deposition either on the posterior tricuspid leaflet (with corresponding "kissing" lesions on the anterior leaflet) or on the posterior pulmonary valve cusp. They may be a source of emboli and very rarely become infected.

MICROSCOPIC FINDINGS: Varies with type of trauma—when fresh catheter/lead-associated injuries present fresh hemorrhage in endocardial tissue.

If ulcerated, a minimal acute inflammatory reaction is found and overlying thrombus in healing patchy endocardial fibrosis may mark the course of a catheter/lead, with many becoming partly or completely encased in a fibrous tissue tunnel. Cusp/leaflet lesion scar producing small fibrous tissue plaques.

DIFFERENTIAL DIAGNOSIS: Generally not a problem. The history of an endomyocardial biopsy, the presence of a pacemaker lead or Swan-Ganz catheter help clinch the diagnosis.

HEART VALVE, TUMOR

Entry Author: Malcolm D. Silver

DEFINITION: Primary or secondary tumor involving the heart valve.

GROSS FINDINGS: Appearance varies. Tumor may be smooth or nodular with shiny gelatinous surface (myxoma); papillary (fibroelastoma) thicken cusp/leaflet tissue, or the valve tissues may be incorporated in a tumor mass.

MICROSCOPIC FINDINGS: Papillary fibroelastomas (QV) usually arise from the mid-region of a valve and in aortic valves can originate from either surface. Usually consists of multiple papillary fronds arranged on a stalk projecting from the valve's surface. Have a central core of dense connective tissue surrounded by fine meshwork of elastic fibers but core may be wholly elastic tissue. Fronds mainly endocardium-coated connective tissue containing delicate elastic lamellae.

Myxomatous and other primary or secondary tumors involving heart valves have the histology of those tumors.

Rarely, vegetations or nonbacterial thrombotic endocarditis contain tumor cell emboli.

REMARKS: Primary or secondary tumors involving heart valves are very rare, with secondary involvement more frequent.

DIFFERENTIAL DIAGNOSIS: Papillary fibroelastoma can be distinguished histologically from Lambl's excrescences by location on valve and different histology. This tumor does not contain fibrin, has a prominent glycosamine glycan content, and contains smooth muscle.

Differentiation of other tumors usually not a problem.

MITRAL INCOMPETENCE, IN ISCHEMIC HEART DISEASE

Entry Author: Malcolm D. Silver

DEFINITION: Mitral incompetence developed during episodes of ischemic heart disease or during course of, or subsequent to, an acute myocardial infarction.

GROSS FINDINGS: The mitral incompetence may be functional and transient appearing during acute ischemic episodes or occur during the acute phase of a myocardial infarction. In these cases, the mitral valve complex may show no abnormality but the annulus is dilated. Mitral incompetence initiated suddenly during the course of a myocardial infarction is usually caused by avulsion of chordae from a papillary muscle (rare) or by papillary muscle rupture. The latter occurs in approximately 3% of acute myocardial infarcts, affects anterior and posterior papillary muscles with equal frequency and develops most frequently within the first week of infarction. The severity of resultant valve incompetence depends on the number of chordae set free. In avulsion of chordae they have a tiny fragment of connective tissue or myocardium attached to their distal end. A varying length of myocardium is attached to chordae when a papillary muscle ruptures. Its free margin is usually jagged and may have tiny thrombi attached to it. The released chordae may twist upon themselves in the axis of the ruptured papillary muscle. The healing of a myocardial infarction leads to fibrosis. If this causes atrophy of a papillary muscle (flattening of its normally rounded contour) and fibrosis in the adjacent left ventricular wall, mitral incompetence can result. An aneurysm developing in an acute myocardial infarction or subsequently on healing can, in expansion, change the spatial relationships of the papillary muscles and cause the same valvular dysfunction. These forms of mitral insufficiency may develop with the acute infarction or months or years afterward.

Rarely the dysynchronous arrival at papillary muscles of the impulse to contract produces mitral valve incompetence. In this instance the valve may be normal.

MICROSCOPIC FINDINGS: See under *Myocardial infarction.*

REMARKS: Right-sided myocardial infarctions may be complicated by papillary muscle rupture with tricuspid valve incompetence. However, this is a very rare occurrence.

See *Myocardial infarct with rupture.*

DIFFERENTIAL DIAGNOSIS: See *Heart valve, incompetence.*

MITRAL INSUFFICIENCY DUE TO LEFT VENTRICULAR ENDOCARDIAL DISEASE

Entry Author: Malcolm D. Silver

DEFINITION: Mitral insufficiency resulting from tethering of chordae or posterior mitral leaflet to the endocardium of posterior left ventricle.

GROSS FINDINGS: Varies with underlying pathology (see *Myocarditis eosinophilic, hypereosinophilia syndrome*) and endomyocardial fibrosis, tropical.

Essential pathology involves a thickening of left ventricular endocardium with direct incorporation of posterior leaflet/chordae into the thickening endocardial process, with their tethering.

REMARKS: These are rare cases of mitral insufficiency.

DIFFERENTIAL DIAGNOSIS: 1. Small linear streaks of endocardial thickening in the base/apex direction (friction lesions) are produced if chordae rub against the endocardium in hypertrophied hearts. Chordae may become incorporated in them, but this does not often cause valvular insufficiency.

2. In calcification of the mitral annulus large calcium deposits may effectively rotate annular tissue toward the left atrium allowing posterior mitral leaflet/chordae to come into contact with the left ventricle that may or may not overlie a calcium mass. Tissue then incorporated into friction lesions or directly attached.

3. Nonbacterial thrombotic endocarditis associated with systemic lupus erythematous may heal and atypically located vegetations on organization tether chordae/leaflets.

MITRAL VALVE ANNULUS, CALCIFICATION

Entry Author: Virginia M. Walley

SYNONYMS: Age-related calcification of mitral valve; mitral ring calcification; mitral annular calcification.

DEFINITION: Age-related or degenerative calcification of the mitral annulus. May be seen in younger age groups when there are disorders of calcium metabolism or renal failure.

GROSS FINDINGS: Calcification of the part of the mitral annulus that supports the posterior leaflet, where the muscular left ventricular free wall joins the left atrium at the A-V groove. Earliest deposits affect annular connective tissue deep to the middle scallop of the posterior leaflet. Calcification may then become more widespread. Large nodules of calcium may form and erode endocardium and the base of the posterior mitral leaflet, which is draped over the deposits and elevated into the left atrium. Both changes can induce mitral insufficiency. Areas of leaflet ulceration are occasionally complicated by infection. Fragments of calcium may embolize. Sometimes the center of the deposits soften, become grumous, and contain much lipid. Calcium deposits associated with surrounding chronic inflammation and reactive fibrosis replace annular tissue. Giant cell inflammatory reaction in approximately 10% of cases.

MICROSCOPIC FINDINGS: Generally, large deposits may show central necrosis and be very rich in lipids on special stain.

SPECIAL PROCEDURES NEEDED FOR DIAGNOSIS: Specimen radiography at autopsy will demonstrate a C-shaped ring of calcification of the posterior leaflet annulus.

REMARKS: Process affects approximately 10% of the elderly population, with complications (e.g., mitral insufficiency or infective endocarditis)—rare. May be combined with calcification of aortic annulus.

POTENTIAL PITFALLS: Large grumous deposits may be mistaken for granulomas, especially TB. Ziehl-Nielsen stains negative. Misinterpretation as atherosclerosis a possibility.

MITRAL VALVE CHORD RUPTURE

Entry Author: Virginia M. Walley

SYNONYMS: Chordal rupture, mitral valve prolapse with chord rupture, ruptured chordae tendineae.

DEFINITION: Rupture of a single chord or of chordae tendineae passing to the mitral valve leaflets.

GROSS FINDINGS: Discontinuity of one or more of the chords which normally join the left ventricular wall or papillary muscles to a mitral valve leaflet. If associated with myxomatous mitral valve disease, chords may be elongated and thinned, and ruptured ends will be tapered or whisker-like. If the rupture is secondary to infective endocarditis, then infected thrombi may be evident on chords or other portions of the valve. If the rupture is related to trauma, chords may appear torn with jagged free ends. If much time has passed since rupture, the ends of torn chords become "rounded" and nodular as a result of reactive fibrosis. Rarely the ruptured ends of chords recurve and reattach through inflammation and repair to the ventricular aspect of a leaflet, presenting a looped appearance.

Associated manifestations vary. If rupture is acute, and chords provide major structural leaflet support, sequelae of severe mitral valve incompetence will occur. If chord is less structurally important, there may be fewer sequelae and chronic mitral insufficiency develop. In this instance, gross features of a chronic prolapsed mitral leaflet are evident.

MICROSCOPIC FINDINGS: If myxomatous degeneration is the underlying process, then myxomatous degeneration is found in the chord. With infective endocarditis, infected thrombotic vegetations and/or inflammation are present. Ruptured end appears frayed. Acutely, focal necrosis and neutrophils will be seen along with small deposits of thrombus and tissue necrosis. Eventually, there is healing with fibrosis, thickening a chord.

SPECIAL PROCEDURES NEEDED FOR DIAGNOSIS: Connective tissue stains aid diagnosis with myxomatous mitral valve; special stains identify microorganisms.

REMARKS: Cords cut by a surgeon have square cut or angled ends. If chordal rupture is suspected on gross examination, embed and cut it at several depths through block. That will increase yield of positive diagnoses. Movat's stain useful in this instance.

Most cases associated with myxomatous degeneration of mitral valve. Many cases classified as idiopathic in the past have this cause. Other causes are infrequent. Rarely, rough deposits of calcium in the posterior mitral annulus can fray chorda to posterior leaflet.

NOTE: Artificial cords of thread are constructed by surgeons and inserted. With time they may rupture, presenting frayed cloth edges.

DIFFERENTIAL DIAGNOSIS: Clinical history may help differential diagnosis. Must be distinguished from chordae avulsion from tip of papillary muscle. Look for a fragment of connective tissue or tag or myocardium (from tip of papillary muscle) at distal attachment. This condition is associated with acute myocardial infarcts.

MITRAL VALVE PROLAPSE

Entry Author: Virginia M. Walley

SYNONYM: Floppy mitral valve.

DEFINITION: A genetic term describing the abnormal excursion of mitral valve leaflets into the left atrium during mitral valve closure.

GROSS FINDINGS: Overall findings vary with the underlying pathology that allows real or effective lengthening of a leaflet or chordae permitting leaflet "overshooting." As a result, normal leaflet coaption and valve closure does not occur. Thus, the condition may be associated with signs of mitral insufficiency (QV). It is caused by congenital or acquired conditions. See *myxomatous degeneration of heart valve and mitral valve, ruptured chordae tendineae or mitral insufficiency associated with ischemic heart disease.*

In the acute phase, and if the cause is extravalvular, leaflets may be normal. If the condition is prolonged, the affected part or whole leaflet appears redundant, thickened, and deformed by a dome-like protrusion toward the left atrium. The leaflet tissue may bear tiny thrombi or they are found sometimes as a linear deposit at the base of the prolapsed leaflet in the angle produced by its base and the adjacent atrial wall. These thrombi may produce emboli and, if organized, a linear scar in this area.

MICROSCOPIC FINDINGS: Varies with underlying cause. Healed leaflet thickened by fibroelastic tissue and may show mural thrombi.

MYXOMATOUS DEGENERATION, MITRAL VALVE

Entry Author: Virginia M. Walley

SYNONYMS: Myxomatous mitral valve; floppy mitral valve, Barlow's disease; ballooned mitral valve; mitral valve insufficiency.

DEFINITION: Myxomatous degeneration (QV) affecting mitral valve leaflets, chordae, and annulus.

GROSS FINDINGS: Depends on severity. An affected leaflet may be semi-translucent but more often is opaque, thickened, and on cut section, grayish and gelatinous in texture. It is redundant in width and length with eventual hooding and prolapse into the left atrium. The chordae elongate and become thinned or are thickened, especially near their insertion into leaflets. Thickened chordae do not fuse. Condition tends to involve the posterior leaflet preferentially and in its earliest form the middle scallop. Part, or all, of the anterior leaflet, or all leaflet tissue may be affected.

Eventually leaflets are thickened by overlaid reactive fibrosis. Thrombi may form on leaflet/chordal surface or in the angle produced by the redundant posterior leaflet and the left atrium. They can embolize. Dystrophic calcification can develop in leaflets or mitral annulus. Occasional cases are complicated by infection or chord rupture. Chords may rub on left ventricular endocardium and cause small plaques of reactive fibrosis there or become adherent.

MICROSCOPIC FINDINGS: Lamina spongiosa of valve usually shows mucopolysaccharide material. In this condition widened with glycosamine glycan deposits, which are also prominent in the lamina fibrosa, with eventual distortion and weakening of valve elements. Collagen loss and elastic fiber destruction are usual. If chronic overlying fibrosis is seen, thrombi and dystrophic calcification may also be demonstrated. Annulus and chordae also show increased glycosamine glycan content.

SPECIAL PROCEDURES NEEDED FOR DIAGNOSIS: Special stains (e.g., Movat's) will accentuate any changes in lamina spongiosa.

DIFFERENTIAL DIAGNOSIS: See *Heart valve, myxomatous degeneration.* NOTE: *Parachute mitral valve* describes a unique congenital anomaly where all chordae arise from a single papillary muscle.

KEY DIAGNOSTIC CRITERIA: Marked glycosamine glycan deposits in lamina spongiosa of the valve, with resultant weakening and distortion of valve elements.

RHEUMATIC VALVULITIS, AORTIC, HEALED

Entry Author: Francesca V. Lobo

SYNONYMS: Healed rheumatic valvulitis, aortic valve; chronic rheumatic aortic valve disease; rheumatic valvulitis, healed, aortic.

DEFINITION: Deformity and functional abnormality (stenosis, insufficiency, or both) occurring in the aortic valve usually years (10 to 20) after episodes of acute rheumatic fever. In developing countries, the process may be accelerated owing to frequent recurrence of rheumatic fever, and present at a younger age (children or teenagers), at times in conjunction with verrucal endocarditis (acute rheumatic valvulitis).

GROSS FINDINGS: Fibrosis causes shortening of cusps and valvular insufficiency. Alternatively, fusion of adjacent cusps at their commissures leads to valvular stenosis. Combined stenosis and incompetence possible. Commissural fusion often results in a small triangular orifice or, less frequently, an acquired bicuspidization. Dystrophic calcification is present more frequently and to a greater degree in stenosed valves. However, in developing countries sclerosis may be the dominant feature with little or no calcification.

MICROSCOPIC FINDINGS: Thickened valve cusps show fibrosis, collections of chronic inflammatory cells (especially at their base), foci of myxomatous change, increased vascularity with thick-walled small blood vessels, and calcification of varying degree affecting the cusps and commissural areas. Foci of surface erosion and small deposits of thrombus may occur over calcified areas. Infected thrombotic vegetations are occasionally found, particularly in conjunction with an insufficient valve. Aschoff nodules are rarely seen in the valve.

REMARKS: Healed rheumatic valvulitis of the aortic valve usually presents in conjunction with mitral valve disease. It is the most frequent cause of combined aortic stenosis and insufficiency and the second most frequent cause of isolated aortic stenosis (after calcific degenerative aortic stenosis).

DIFFERENTIAL DIAGNOSIS: Other causes of valve stenosis: Congenital (supravalvular, valvular, or subvalvular) aortic stenosis, calcific bicuspid aortic valve, Mönckeberg's calcification, and other causes of post-inflammatory valvulitis.

Other causes of valve insufficiency:

Any lesion causing distortion, destruction, or perforation of the cusps, including congenitally bicuspid aortic valve, traumatic or iatrogenic lesions, infective endocarditis, and rheumatoid disease.

KEY DIAGNOSTIC CRITERIA: Past history of rheumatic fever. Long-standing heart murmurs.

RHEUMATIC VALVULITIS, MITRAL, HEALED

Entry Authors: Francesca V. Lobo and Virginia M. Walley

SYNONYMS: Healed rheumatic valvulitis, mitral valve; chronic rheumatic mitral valve disease; rheumatic heart disease.

DEFINITION: Deformity and functional abnormality (stenosis, insufficiency, or both) of the mitral valve, usually years (10 to 20) after episodes of acute rheumatic fever. In developed countries, this lesion is rarely seen in patients less than 20 years old. In developing countries, the process may be accelerated owing to frequent recurrence of acute rheumatic fever and be present at a younger age (children or teenagers), at times in conjunction with evidence of acute rheumatic valvulitis.

GROSS FINDINGS: Fibrous thickening and rigidity of leaflets with obliteration of clefts and effacement of the posterior leaflet scallops, as well as shortening and puckering of leaflets. There is fusion of adjacent sides of leaflets at commissural areas, particularly in stenosed valves. There is shortening, thickening, and fusion of chordae tendineae. These changes result in an oval, slit-like (fish-mouthed), or buttonhole orifice. Dystrophic calcification is frequent within leaflets but sometimes also occurs in the annulus, chordae, or papillary muscles. In some instances, subvalvular fusion is marked. Lambl's excrescences are frequent.

Effective shortening of leaflets or their tethering produces valve insufficiency.

MICROSCOPIC FINDINGS: There is thickening of valve leaflets with fibroelastic connective tissue. Musculoelastic blood vessels and a variable number of chronic inflammatory cells, with an occasional Anitschkow cell, are observed particularly at the leaflet base, around blood vessels, and around calcium deposits. Foci of surface erosion can occur particularly overtraumatized areas and calcific nodules and may have small thrombi associated with them. The thrombus is usually sterile in cases with pure mitral stenosis. Infected thrombi may occur in conjunction with an insufficient valve. The chordae show variable fibrosis with or without foci of calcification. Papillary muscles exhibit fibrosis, the presence of thick-walled small vessels and an occasional Aschoff body.

REMARKS: Healed rheumatic valvulitis is the most common cause of pure mitral stenosis. It is more frequent in women. However, some patients may have combined mitral stenosis and insufficiency. Alternatively, mitral insufficiency may be the dominant functional abnormality.

In cases with an incompetent valve, there may be a patch of endocardial thickening on the posterior left atrial wall.

DIFFERENTIAL DIAGNOSIS: Pathological—Other causes of mitral stenosis (rare): Atrial myxoma or other mass lesion obstructing orifice. Other causes of postinflammatory valvulitis. Large vegetations of infective endocarditis. Mitral annular calcification ± infective endocarditis.

Congenital malformations (rare) including congenital mitral stenosis, parachute mitral valve, cor triatriatum, anomalous fibromuscular bands, or stenosing supravalvular fibrous rings.

Miscellaneous—carcinoid syndrome (in presence of intra-atrial communication or lung involvement), methysergide therapy, storage diseases, e.g., Fabry's and Hurler's syndromes, pseudoxanthoma elasticum, Whipple's disease, etc.

Other causes of mitral insufficiency: Affecting annulus—senile mitral annular calcification and other hypercalcemias, left ventricular cavity dilation, and Marfan's syndrome.

Affecting leaflets ± chordae (a) Prolapse: floppy valve, Marfan's syndrome. (b) Infection, destruction, perforation; infective endocarditis and other causes of post-inflammatory valvulitis. (c) Deficiency: congenital clefts ± endocardial cushion defects. Affecting chordae ± papillary muscles—trauma, ischemia (acute or chronic), cardiomyopathy (congestive or hypertrophic).

Clinical—In addition to the above listed, conditions to exclude are: Coexistent stenosis or insufficiency of other heart valves.

Chronic lung disease, primary pulmonary hypertension, atrial septal defect (mimicking mitral stenosis). Other congenital anomalies (endocardial cushion defect, corrected transposition); endocardial fibroelastosis; prolapsing mitral valve syndrome, etc. (mimicking mitral regurgitation).

KEY DIAGNOSTIC CRITERIA: A scarred deformed valve, often with a funnel-shaped, fishmouth, or buttonhole orifice in a patient with prior rheumatic disease evidenced either clinically by the Jones' criteria or pathologically by the presence of Aschoff nodules in the atrial or ventricular myocardium.

RHEUMATIC VALVULITIS, PULMONARY, HEALED

Entry Author: Francesca V. Lobo

SYNONYMS: Healed rheumatic valvulitis, pulmonary valve; chronic rheumatic pulmonary valve disease.

DEFINITION: The changes in a pulmonary valve caused by healing subsequent to repeated episodes of acute rheumatic pulmonary valvulitis. In North America, the pulmonary valve is least frequently involved in this process. When it is, it is almost always in conjunction with all three other valves being affected.

GROSS FINDINGS: Usually mild cusp thickening and slight commissural fusion. Changes may be more severe in certain geographic regions where it is associated with longstanding pulmonary hypertension (as in areas of high altitude, such as Mexico City). The hypertension possibly increases stress and makes the valve more prone to damage.

MICROSCOPIC FINDINGS: The thickened valve cusps show features similar to healed rheumatic valvulitis in the other heart valves but to a lesser degree. Calcification has not been described.

REMARKS: Rheumatic pulmonary involvement occurs so rarely in North America it is of little practical significance. Should be thought of where the valve is primed by pre-existing pulmonary hypertension and other heart valves are involved.

DIFFERENTIAL DIAGNOSIS: Other causes of pulmonary obstruction. Among subvalvular lesions these include congenital subvalvular isolated infundibular stenosis (fibrous or muscular), tetralogy of Fallot, and aneurysm of the membranous septum. Among subvalvular acquired lesions are marked septal hypertrophy (rarely in hypertrophic obstructive cardiomyopathy). Valvular obstructive lesions to be ruled out are congenital isolated pulmonary valve stenosis, pulmonary valve stenosis associated with other defects (Noonan syndrome, tetralogy of Fallot, LEOPARD syndrome), and quadricuspid pulmonary valve with secondary fibrosis and calcification. Among acquired valvular lesions of concern are changes due to carcinoid tumor and cardiac tumor. Supravalvular pulmonary obstruction occurs in congenital pulmonary arterial stenosis, and (rarely) is caused by a fibrous membranous ring in the pulmonary artery distal to the pulmonary valve.

Pulmonary insufficiency may be secondary to dilation of the pulmonary ring as a consequence of severe pulmonary hypertension of any cause.

KEY DIAGNOSTIC CRITERIA: Thickened, scarified pulmonic valve in a patient with clinical or pathologic evidence of prior rheumatic disease. Rheumatic pulmonary valve involvement, when present, invariably is a component of multivalvular disease.

TRICUSPID VALVE, BLOOD CYSTS

Entry Author: Jagdish W. Butany

DEFINITION: Small (3–5 mm diameter) brownish cystic lesion on the endocardial surface of valve leaflets, usually in infants. Have no functional significance.

Their etiology is uncertain but they are most commonly seen along the line of valve closure in the newborn. It is possible that they are related to trauma to the small blood vessels in the leaflet tissue.

GROSS FINDINGS: Elevated solitary or multiple hemispherical brownish cysts along the line of closure of the valve leaflets.

MICROSCOPIC FINDINGS: Small collection of blood deep to the endocardium.

REMARKS: The cause of these lesions is uncertain. Possibly secondary to trauma of small blood vessels in the leaflets.

DIFFERENTIAL DIAGNOSIS: Traumatic lesions (usually show superficial ulceration with deposition of thrombus).

Section 3

Diseases of the Blood Vessels

Section Editor: J. T. Lie
Entry Authors: Avrum I. Gotlieb, J. T. Lie, and Alan G. Rose

ADVENTITIAL CYSTIC DISEASE (ACD)

Entry Author: J. T. Lie

SYNONYM: Cystic adventitial disease or "degeneration" ("CAD" may be confused with coronary artery disease).

DEFINITION: A dysplastic lesion of vascular wall, of unknown cause, characterized by the formation of a mucoid cystic mass, with or without a true cellular lining, in or around the adventitia of an otherwise normal blood vessel (artery or vein).

GROSS FINDINGS: ACD occurs near a joint, 10 to 15 times more commonly in the wall of medium or small arteries (especially the popliteal artery behind the knee joint) than comparable-sized veins, as a firm localized swelling that may compress the affected blood vessel. Rarely, the cyst circumferentially envelopes the affected blood vessel.

MICROSCOPIC FINDINGS: An encapsulated cystic cavity with a gel-like content that histochemically stains like glycoproteins and acid mucopolysaccharides and contains collagen fragments with minimal or no inflammatory reaction around the vessel wall. The cystic mass may be unilocular or multilocular and its inner surface is rarely lined with a flattened cell layer of undetermined origin.

REMARKS: ACD occurs in about one in 1200 cases of limb claudication; 5 to 8 times more often in men than in women, usually manual laborers, with a mean age of 40 (range 10–70) years; the total number of popliteal and non-popliteal ACD reported in the literature up to 1990s is about 250. ACD appears angiographically as a smooth-walled fluted stenosis or, rarely, occlusion of the affected artery which may be displaced laterally or in an anteroposterior direction; it may recur after incomplete excision.

DIFFERENTIAL DIAGNOSIS: Ectopic ganglion; popliteal artery entrapment syndrome; arteriosclerosis obliterans or thrombosis; fibromuscular dysplasia; vasculitis.

References

1. Flanigan DP et al. Summary of cases of adventitial cystic disease of the popliteal artery. *Ann Surg* 1979;189:165–175.
2. Ishikawa K. Cystic adventitial disease of the popliteal artery and of other stem vessels in the extremities *Jap J Surg* 1987;17:221–229.
3. Lie JT, Jensen PL, Smith RE. Adventitial cystic disease of the lesser saphenous vein (Review). *Arch Pathol Lab Med* 1991;115:946–948.

ALLOGRAFT TRANSPLANT ARTERIOPATHY

Entry Author: J. T. Lie

DEFINITION: Arterial and arteriolar occlusive disease of chronic allograft rejection, developed usually several months posttransplant.

GROSS FINDINGS: Clear evidence of arterial occlusive disease without distinctive features in naked-eye appearance.

MICROSCOPIC FINDINGS: Progressive myointimal proliferation leading to the development of accelerated atherosclerosis or intimal foam cell accumulation and, in severe cases, a necrotizing vasculitis of small arteries and arterioles.

REMARKS: The lesions in any given instance may be quite variable, depending on donor organs (heart, kidney, liver, lung), the posttransplant period, anti-rejection and other drug treatment, size of the blood vessels in question and, possibly, the recipient's underlying disease, such as hyperlipidemia.

DIFFERENTIAL DIAGNOSIS: None really except, perhaps, undetected or unsuspected existing lesions of the donor organ or a primary vasculitis of undetermined cause.

Reference

1. Hammond EH (ed). *Solid organ transplantation pathology*. Philadelphia, WB Saunders; 1994:285.

ANEURYSM, FALSE

Entry Author: Alan G. Rose

SYNONYM: Pseudoaneurysm.

DEFINITION: An arterial or venous aneurysm that is not delimited by all the original elements of the vessel wall (intima, media, and adventitia), usually only the adventitia remains.

GROSS FINDINGS: The aneurysm is saccular in appearance and communicates with the artery via an ostium, the incomplete rupture site.

MICROSCOPIC FINDINGS: There is an abrupt interruption in the continuity of the wall of the artery at the ostium of the aneurysm and externally the aneurysm is bound by the tunica adventitia only. Presence of hemosiderin and granulation tissue with inflammatory infiltrate may be observed within the fibrous tissue layer of the aneurysm.

SPECIAL PROCEDURES NEEDED FOR DIAGNOSIS: Doppler ultrasound, computed tomography, and/or angiography clinically; histologic sections of the circumference of the aneurysm, as well as of the vessel-aneurysm junction.

DIFFERENTIAL DIAGNOSIS: True aneurysm, pulsating vascular tumor.

KEY DIAGNOSTIC CRITERIA: History of trauma or interventional procedures; absence of systemic arteritis, aneurysm wall lacking all normal components.

POTENTIAL PITFALLS: A longstanding true aneurysm may have eroded normal vessel wall components.

ANEURYSM OF THE ABDOMINAL AORTA

Entry Author: Alan G. Rose

SYNONYMS: Atherosclerotic aortic aneurysm; inflammatory aneurysm of the aorta. [The term *aneurysm of the abdominal aorta* is nonspecific and an aneurysm may have more than one cause, but because atherosclerosis is the commonest cause of such aneurysms, the term has become synonymous with atherosclerotic aneurysms of the abdominal aorta; inflammatory aneurysm is a subset.]

DEFINITION: An aneurysm situated somewhere along the course of the aorta after it has passed through the diaphragm and before it bifurcates into the common iliac arteries.

GROSS FINDINGS: A segment of the abdominal aorta (commonly infrarenal) forms a fusiform-shaped and rarely saccular dilation due to uniform or asymmetric circumferential weakening of the wall by atherosclerosis which is usually also severe in the adjacent, nonaneurysmal aorta. The aneurysm wall is usually thin, but a thick layer of laminated thrombus, which seldom undergoes complete organization even after months and years, may reduce the lumen to a similar diameter to that of the nonaneurysmal aorta and be misleading angiographically.

MICROSCOPIC FINDINGS: Features are nonspecific: fibrous aneurysm wall with or without calcification, cholesterol crystals, lipid-laden macrophages, and (organizing) thrombus covered by a thick layer of unorganized thrombus on the luminal aspect. Remnants of the aortic wall will be detectable at the margins of the aneurysm.

SPECIAL PROCEDURES NEEDED FOR DIAGNOSIS: Elastic van Gieson stain is essential for detecting atrophic medial remnants within aneurysm wall.

DIFFERENTIAL DIAGNOSIS: Clinically a large retroperitoneal tumor (e.g., pancreatic carcinoma or lymphoma) may transmit the aortic pulsation to the epigastric area on palpation and an aortic dissection may extend down the abdominal aorta. The usual atherosclerotic abdominal aortic aneurysm differs from the so-called "inflammatory aneurysm" or "periaortitis" which is a variant of the former and is characterized by an atrophic media and marked fibrosis with perivascular/perineural lymphoplasmacytic infiltrate and rare giant cells, obliteration of venules and incorporation of lymph nodes in the fibrous response. The histologic appearance of the latter is reminiscent of retroperitoneal fibrosis. In non-Westernized societies, atherosclerosis is still rare, and other aortic diseases, e.g., Takayasu's arteritis may assume greater importance as a cause of aortic aneurysms.

KEY DIAGNOSTIC CRITERIA: A fusiform aneurysm of the abdominal aorta, with weakened wall, arising in association with severe atherosclerosis in an elderly patients. Normally, a nonspecific chronic inflammatory change may be noted in the periaortic tissues but without the thick rind of fibrosis of the inflammatory aneurysm. There may be a familial incidence of this condition.

POTENTIAL PITFALLS: Current surgical practice is to leave the aneurysm *in situ* and to place the prosthetic graft within the aneurysm's lumen. Samples of tissue, if taken at all, will more likely come from the central portion of the aneurysm, i.e., the site least likely to yield evidence of its previous aortic structure. Inflammatory variant should not be mistaken for arteritis.

ANEURYSM OF THE THORACIC AORTA

Entry Author: Alan G. Rose

SYNONYMS: Aneurysm of the ascending aorta, aneurysm of the aortic arch, aneurysm of the descending thoracic aorta.

DEFINITION: An aneurysm of the aorta situated anywhere from the aortic root to the level of the diaphragm.

GROSS FINDINGS: The gross appearance will vary according to the underlying cause. An aortic dissection associated with hypertension or medionecrosis may have the appearance of an aneurysm; syphilitic aortitis is characterized by tree bark wrinkling of the intima plus saccular aneurysm(s) situated in the proximal aorta. Atherosclerotic aneurysms are more often fusiform than saccular in appearance and these aneurysms are now more common than syphilitic aneurysms. A saccular aneurysm may also result from focal weakening of the aortic media due to an incomplete tear associated with medionecrosis. False aneurysms of the thoracic aorta due to trauma usually occur just distal to the site of the ligamentum arteriosum and the origin of the left subclavian artery, i.e., at the junction of the fixed and mobile portions of the aorta. Up to 30% of Takayasu aortitis may present as thoracic aneurysms often with aortic insufficiency.

MICROSCOPIC FINDINGS: The microscopic features will vary according to the etiology of the underlying condition [see individual entities].

SPECIAL PROCEDURES NEEDED FOR DIAGNOSIS: Elastic and alcian blue-PAS stains are not only useful but essential for demonstrating a possible intrinsic defect of the arterial wall, such as Erdheim's cystic medionecrosis.

DIFFERENTIAL DIAGNOSIS: Aneurysm of the thoracic aorta is a term that may be applied to a number of conditions producing aneurysms and just discussed.

KEY DIAGNOSTIC CRITERIA: Evidence of active or healed aortitis may be in keeping with syphilitic or Takayasu aortitis and obliteration of the vasa vasorum is observed in both conditions. The two conditions may be difficult to separate on histologic grounds alone. Serology for syphilis is useful. Medionecrosis is characterized by focal loss of medial myocytes, disruption of the elastica, and collagen with replacement by pools of acid mucopolysaccharides. False aneurysm has no aortic medial or intimal components in its wall. Aortic dissections show separation of the intima and inner half to two thirds of the media from the outer one third of the media and the adventitia by an intramural hematoma which has originated from a tear of the inner aortic wall. The pattern of elastic fiber fragmentation is more generalized in medionecrosis of Marfan's syndrome as opposed to that in the more commonly seen *forme fruste* variety or aging-related changes.

POTENTIAL PITFALLS: Aneurysm of the thoracic aorta is a descriptive rather than a diagnostic term.

ANEURYSM, TRUE

Entry Author: Alan G. Rose

SYNONYMS: Arterial ectasia; focal dilation of arterial lumen; arteriomegaly.

DEFINITION: An aneurysm is a focal dilation of the lumen of a vessel (usually an artery) or of the heart. A true aneurysm will have remnants of the original parent structure (i.e., arterial intima, media, or myocardium) in the wall of the aneurysm.

GROSS FINDINGS: The gross appearance of the aneurysm will vary according to the etiology. Thus, circumferential weakening of the arterial wall (e.g., due to atherosclerosis) will produce a fusiform aneurysm, whereas focal weakening of the wall (e.g., due to syphilis or a tear in medionecrosis) may produce a saccular aneurysm that communicates via an ostium with the parent artery. Berry aneurysm arises at the site of a medial defect at branch points of the circle of Willis.

MICROSCOPIC FINDINGS: The aneurysm will show remnants of the original arterial wall or myocardium in the wall of a ventricular aneurysm.

SPECIAL PROCEDURES NEEDED FOR DIAGNOSIS: Elastic stains are invaluable in detecting remnants of elastic laminae in the arterial aneurysm wall.

DIFFERENTIAL DIAGNOSIS: False aneurysm, dissecting aneurysm, kinking of a vessel, aging-related ectasia of arteries.

KEY DIAGNOSTIC CRITERIA: Remnants of the parent structure (artery or heart) are present in the aneurysm wall.

POTENTIAL PITFALLS: A true aneurysm of long duration may have few, if any, persisting remnants of the parent structure in the aneurysm wall. Rupture of the aorta which interrupts the intima and media but is contained by an intact adventitia, is termed a false aneurysm because the adventitia is poorly demarcated from the surrounding connective tissue.

ANGIODYSPLASIA

Entry Author: J. T. Lie

SYNONYMS: Arteriovenous malformation; nontraumatic arteriovenous fistula; congenital hemangiomas; angiohamartomas.

DEFINITION: The traditional term *arteriovenous malformation* (AVM) refers to a heterogenous group of vascular anomalies for which the current preferred term is *angiodysplasia*. According to the Hamburg Classification there are four morphologic types:
1. Predominantly arterial defects
2. Predominantly venous defects
3. Predominantly AV shunting defects
4. Combined vascular defects (including the lymphatics)

Angiodysplasia may occur anywhere in the body: the skin, soft tissue, viscera, and the central nervous system. Some vascular lesions commonly diagnosed as AVM are various types of hemangiomas or lymphangiomas and not AVM.

GROSS FINDINGS: Angiodysplasia occurs as a solitary mass or multiple space occupying lesions as delineated by angiography, ultrasound, computed tomography, or magnetic resonance imaging techniques, and a tangled mass of vascular tissue to the naked eye.

MICROSCOPIC FINDINGS: The unifying features are an entanglement of thick- and thin-walled vascular channels, which, morphologically may be arteries, veins, lymphatics, or hybrids (non-artery non-vein vascular channels). Arteriovenous communications are seldom demonstrable histologically.

References

1. Malan E. *Vascular malformations (angiodysplasia)*. Milan: Carlo Erba Foundation; 1974.
2. Special Symposium Issue. *Int Angiol* 1990;9:133–227.
3. Leu HG, Lie JT. In: Stehbens WE, Lie JT, eds. *Vascular Pathology*. London, Chapman & Hall; 1995: 489–516.

ANGIOLYMPHOID HYPERPLASIA WITH EOSINOPHILIA (ALHE)

Entry Author: J. T. Lie

SYNONYM: Kimura's disease (see REMARKS).

DEFINITION: An unusual type of dermal and subcutaneous inflammatory vascular and lymphofollicular proliferation, occurring predominantly in the head and neck areas, with about equal gender ratio, most commonly Caucasians between the age of 20 and 50 years.

GROSS FINDINGS: The cutaneous lesions are characterized by single or multiple smooth-top papules or plaques of varying color, with palpable indurations.

MICROSCOPIC FINDINGS: Historically, ALHE consists of atypical vascular proliferation with nodular and diffuse lymphoid infiltrates and prominent eosinophils in the dermis and subcutaneous tissue. In about 50% of cases, an arterial/arteriolar structure (confirmed by elastic stains) can be observed in close association with or is the site of the histiocytoid endothelial cell proliferation. Involvement of a major named artery has been identified only rarely.

REMARKS: Although once considered as synonymous with Kimura's disease, ALHE and Kimura's disease are currently accepted by most investigators as two distinct and separate entities in the family of histiocytoid hemangiomas or epithelioid hemangioendotheliomas.

References

1. Rosai J et al. The histiocytoid hemangiomas. A unifying concept embracing several previously described entities of skin, soft tissue, large vessels, bone, and heart. *Human Pathol* 1979;10:707–730.
2. Rosai J. Angiolymphoid hyperplasia with eosinophilia of the skin. Its nosological position in the spectrum of histiocytoid hemangioma. *Am J Dermatopathol* 1982;4:175–184.
3. Weiss SW et al. Epithelioid hemangioendothelioma and related lesions. (Review). *Semin Diag Pathol* 1986;3:259–287.

ANTERIOR TIBIAL COMPARTMENT SYNDROME

Entry Author: J. T. Lie

DEFINITION: Ischemic necrosis of the anterior tibial compartment (ATC) muscles. ATC is a closed anatomic compartment, bound by bone, interosseous membrane and fascia, and contains the anterior tibial muscle and the long extensor muscles of the toes, with blood supply from the anterior tibial artery. Expansion within the compartment is greatly limited and the syndrome occurs typically in otherwise fit young men in the following manner: unaccustomed exertion, trauma to the muscles resulting in swelling with increase in pressure within the compartment and compression of the anterior tibial artery and its branches.

GROSS FINDINGS: Mostly clinical, with pain/tenderness, swelling, and induration over the anterior tibial compartment associated with footdrop and inability to dorsiflex the toes.

MICROSCOPIC FINDINGS: Where applicable, may show thromboembolic occlusion of the otherwise normal anterior tibial artery or its parent trunk and, later, edema, congestion, and ischemic necrosis of the muscles in ATC.

REMARKS: The diagnosis of ATC is clinical and seldom requires biopsy except for confirmation of tissue necrosis.

ANTIPHOSPHOLIPID SYNDROME

Entry Author: J. T. Lie

SYNONYMS: Anticardiolipin syndrome; anti-phospholipid antibody syndrome.

DEFINITION: An autoimmune disease characterized by the presence of autoantibodies against the negatively charged phospholipids, the three major components are cardiolipin, lupus anticoagulant, and reagin, with the clinical manifestations of recurrent, large and small vessel arterial and venous thrombosis/embolism as systemic, pulmonary, and cerebral vaso-occlusive disease; thrombocytopenia; recurrent miscarriages; vegetative, noninfective thrombotic endocarditis and intracardiac mural thrombosis. The syndrome may occur unassociated with an underlying connective tissue disease (primary) or in association with systemic lupus erythematosus or a lupus-like disorder (secondary).

GROSS FINDINGS: Changes are those of recurrent, arterial and/or venous large and small vessel and intracardiac thromboses and their sequelae and complications, e.g., tissue necrosis, ulceration, infarction, and noninfective thrombotic endocarditis.

MICROSCOPIC FINDINGS: Noninflammatory thromboses of different histologic ages and any of the sequelae that may be present in the target organs.

DIFFERENTIAL DIAGNOSIS: Inflammatory vaso-occlusive disease, such as true vasculitis.

Reference

1. Lie JT. In: Asherson RA, Cervera R, Piette JC, Shoenfeld Y (eds). *The antiphospholipid syndrome.* Boca Raton, FL: CRC Press; 1996:89–104.

AORTIC DISSECTION

Entry Author: Alan G. Rose

SYNONYMS: Dissecting aneurysm of the aorta; intramural or dissecting hematoma of the aorta.

DEFINITION: A partial tear of the inner aortic wall that leads to separation of the medial layers by aortic blood flow with variable extension of the travelling intramural hematoma.

GROSS FINDINGS: The commonest site of the initial aortic wall defect is a transverse tear, seldom more than a few centimeters above the aortic valve. The aortic outline is widened by the contained intramural hematoma. Cases associated with medionecrosis may exhibit a very dilated, thin-walled aorta. The dissection may extend from the aorta into the visceral or peripheral arteries. Organization of the intramural hematoma, which is the most advantageous outcome, may take place over a period of time. A reentry tear may lead to the false channel supplying blood flow to the distal tissues/organs. External rupture usually occurs close to the site of the entrance intimal tear, with hemorrhage into the pericardial sac to produce cardiac tamponade and death.

MICROSCOPIC FINDINGS: There is separation of the intima and inner half to two thirds of the media from the remainder of the outer media plus the adventitia by the passage of blood via a focal tear through the inner aortic wall. Severe medionecrotic changes in a normotensive patient may implicate such changes as a possible cause of aortic weakening.

SPECIAL PROCEDURES NEEDED FOR DIAGNOSIS: Elastic van Gieson or Movat's pentachrome, and colloidal-iron or alcian blue-PAS stains are absolutely essential.

DIFFERENTIAL DIAGNOSIS: Other causes of aortic aneurysm only come into the differential diagnosis on chest radiography and grossly prior to cutting across the aorta. On transection of the aorta the diagnosis is easily made.

KEY DIAGNOSTIC CRITERIA: Longitudinal splitting of the aortic media by blood which communicates with the lumen.

POTENTIAL PITFALLS: Aging aorta develops medionecrotic-like changes, seen in the majority of hypertension-related aortic dissection, may be confused with the true idiopathic or primary medionecrosis associated with Erdheim, Marfan, and Ehlers-Danlos syndromes.

ARTERIAL CALCIFICATION
OF INFANCY (ACI)

Entry Author: J. T. Lie

DEFINITION: A rare and often fatal, probably autosomal recessive arterial dysplasia of infancy, characterized by abnormal and excessive calcification of the arterial wall, with little more than 100 cases reported in the literature, to date. Death from myocardial infarction usually results within the first 6 months of life. ACI is unrelated to and should not be confused with idiopathic hyperparathyroidism or other secondary causes of hypercalcemia.

GROSS FINDINGS: ACI occurs most commonly in the coronary arteries and it may also affect the aorta, visceral and peripheral systemic arteries, pulmonary arteries and possibly the central nervous system, with the gross appearance of a vaso-occlusive disease, and the arterial calcification may be detected radiologically.

MICROSCOPIC FINDINGS: Unexplained (idiopathic) and usually extensive arterial calcification at the intima-media junction or in the media, associated with occlusive intimal proliferation and occasionally an inflammatory reaction around the calcification.

REMARKS: ACI has been observed in stillborn and newborn infants and among the siblings with no apparent gender predilection. Very few affected infants survived past the first decade of life and there is only one known reported case of survival to adulthood.

References

1. Moran JJ. Idiopathic arterial calcification of infancy: A clinicopathologic study. *Pathol Annual* 1975; 10:393–417.
2. Chen H et al. Generalized arterial calcification of infancy in twins. *Birth defects: Original article series* 1982;18:67–80.
3. Juul S et al. New insights into idiopathic infantile arterial calcinosis. Three patient reports. *Am J Dis Child* 1990;144:229–233.

ARTERIAL EMBOLUS

Entry Author: Alan G. Rose

SYNONYM: Arterial thromboembolus.

DEFINITION: Solid matter traveling within the arterial circulation. Note that gas bubbles may have the properties of solid particles.

GROSS FINDINGS: The commonest type of embolus is a thromboembolus (composed from elements of the blood). The head/initial portion of the thrombus has a dry, greyish-white appearance due to its constituent platelets and fibrin. Lines of Zahn may be seen. A detached portion of propagated thrombus that has embolized will have a red color due to its greater erythrocyte component. An embolus will lodge in the appropriate-sized arterial segment.

Other types of emboli will have a different appearance, e.g., foreign body (bullet, gelfoam); or amniotic fluid, bone marrow, or atheroembolism, which is not apparent to the naked eye.

MICROSCOPIC FINDINGS: Alternate layers of platelets and fibrin with a variable erythrocyte component as described under thromboembolus. Gelfoam will be birefringent. Amniotic fluid embolism will appear as vacuoles within the plasma in association with desquamated squames and lanugo hairs. Bone marrow emboli consist of adipocytes plus variable numbers of hemopoietic cells. Atheroemboli should be self-evident histologically.

SPECIAL PROCEDURES NEEDED FOR DIAGNOSIS: Martius scarlet-blue stain for fibrin. Differential staining may give some indication of the age of the fibrin but not of the thromboembolus. Polarized light shows refractivity of the Gelfoam.

DIFFERENTIAL DIAGNOSIS: The term *thromboembolus* is often used because it is not always possible to distinguish a traveling thrombus (embolus) from *in situ* thrombosis. An "embolus" is thrombotic in origin unless otherwise specified, e.g., atheroembolus or bone marrow embolus.

KEY DIAGNOSTIC CRITERIA: History of sudden, acute arterial occlusion in a patient with possible sources of arterial embolism; hypercoagulable state.

POTENTIAL PITFALLS: Local *in situ* thrombosis may be difficult to distinguish and a thromboembolus may be infected.

ARTERIAL HYPOPLASIA

Entry Author: Alan G. Rose

SYNONYMS: Underdevelopment of an artery, embryological underdevelopment of an artery.

DEFINITION: The term *hypoplasia* means incomplete or under development of an organ or part. Here it applies to an artery.

GROSS FINDINGS: According to the above definition a hypoplastic artery should appear smaller and narrower than a fully formed one. The concept is fraught with difficulties since normal arteries show a wide anatomical variation and the condition is probably greatly over diagnosed. Quantitative studies of suspected hypoplastic arteries usually show that the area of supply is adequately supplied by arterial branches.

In the coronary circulation one coronary artery may be larger than the other (nondominant) vessel. Hypoplastic cardiac ventricles will of necessity have smaller coronary arteries supplying them—these arteries are in fact "normal" for the size of the ventricle which they are supplying.

Short left coronary artery occurs when the vessel bifurcates into its two branches shortly after its origin.

MICROSCOPIC FINDINGS: Normal histological appearance apart from the small arterial diameter.

DIFFERENTIAL DIAGNOSIS: Most of the arteries suspected of being hypoplastic are probably normal; it is a subjective evaluation. Chronic or healed abdominal Takayasu aortitis with a long-segment stenosis.

POTENTIAL PITFALLS: There is a tendency to overdiagnose arterial hypoplasia without reference to the ethnic group, body size, age, and gender-matched controls.

ARTERIAL THROMBOSIS

Entry Author: Alan G. Rose

SYNONYMS: Primary and secondary arterial thrombosis.

DEFINITION: Arterial thrombosis is defined as coagulated blood formed during life and within the lumen of an artery.

GROSS FINDINGS: The artery is distended by an intraluminal fibrin-platelet thrombus that has a firm, dry, white appearance. The degree of adherence to the vessel wall on gross inspection is not always useful in separating the thrombus from a postmortem clot. A large mural thrombus may have visible lines of Zahn. Underlying ulcerated atherosclerosis may be evident in mural thrombosis.

MICROSCOPIC FINDINGS: The microscopic appearance will depend on the age of the thrombus (varying stages of organization), whether one is examining the white (fibrin-platelet) head or the propagated (erythrocyte-rich) portion of the thrombus.

SPECIAL PROCEDURES NEEDED FOR DIAGNOSIS: Martius scarlet-blue or phosphotungstic acid hematoxylin stain may assist in identifying and highlighting a thrombus.

DIFFERENTIAL DIAGNOSIS: Thrombosis is difficult to distinguish from thromboembolism. A source for the embolus such as a myocardial infarction with mural thrombus, infective endocarditis, or dilated cardiomyopathy may provide a clue, because *in situ* thrombosis may closely resemble a thromboembolus. Indeed, the very term thromboembolus was coined for that very same reason.

KEY DIAGNOSTIC CRITERIA: Fibrin-platelet coagulum lies within the lumen of an artery. Variable entrapment of erythrocytes within the thrombus.

POTENTIAL PITFALLS: See differential diagnosis above regarding thromboembolus.

ARTERIAL TRAUMA

Entry Author: Alan G. Rose

SYNONYM: Physical damage to an artery.

DEFINITION: Damage to an artery usually by physical agents but occasionally due to ionizing radiation. Trauma is sometimes used in a wider sense to include any noxious influence on the artery.

GROSS FINDINGS: The traumatized artery may appear bruised, disrupted, show an aneurysmal bulging or an intramural hematoma. Hyperflexion injury of the aorta may lead to multiple transverse tears of the inner portion of the vessel or complete avulsion/transection.

MICROSCOPIC FINDINGS: The damaged portion of the arterial wall may appear hypereosinophilic with a smudged eosinophilic appearance within which nuclear detail is scanty or nonexistent. Ionizing radiation may lead to foam cell transformation of the intima and fibrinoid necrosis of the media. Intimal fibroplasia may also occur.

SPECIAL PROCEDURES NEEDED FOR DIAGNOSIS: Injection of dye or contrast material may show a leak in the arterial wall within a specimen. Elastic van Gieson stain is essential in tracing the original arterial wall into the traumatized portion.

DIFFERENTIAL DIAGNOSIS: Damage to an artery may elicit an inflammatory response that can mimic a primary arteritis. Chronic or repeated cannulation injury to an artery may produce changes histologically identical to endarteritis obliterans; also possibly chronic ergotism.

KEY DIAGNOSTIC CRITERIA: History of trauma, physical disruption of the artery, loss of cellular detail. Radiation damage may lead to foam cell transformation of the artery.

POTENTIAL PITFALLS: Changes in the artery may develop decades after the original radiation damage occurred (see *Irradiation arteriopathy*).

ARTERIOLAR HYALINIZATION

Entry Author: Avrum I. Gotlieb

SYNONYM: Arteriolar hyalinosis.

DEFINITION: Deposition of homogenous, strongly eosinophilic PAS-positive material, called *hyalin*, in the extracellular matrix of the vessel wall, commonly observed in otherwise normal splenic arterioles and also elsewhere in the body.

GROSS FINDINGS: Not visible.

MICROSCOPIC FINDINGS: The presence of homogenous eosinophilic material in the subintima and media. The material is PAS-positive and remains extracellular in location. The hyalin deposition results in a thickening of the vessel wall, a reduction in the size of the lumen, and atrophy of the medial smooth muscle cells.

SPECIAL PROCEDURES NEEDED FOR DIAGNOSIS: For research purposes, electron microscopy shows finely granular osmiophilic material and, occasionally, immunofluorescence may reveal the presence of C3 and IgM.

DIFFERENTIAL DIAGNOSIS: None.

KEY DIAGNOSTIC CRITERIA: Amorphous, eosinophilic mass in the arteriolar walls.

ARTERIOLOSCLEROSIS

Entry Author: Avrum I. Gotlieb

SYNONYM: Arteriolar sclerosis.

DEFINITION:A general term referring to fibrosis or sclerosis of an arteriole.

GROSS FINDINGS: Not visible.

MICROSCOPIC FINDINGS: In general, the medial tissue is partially or completely replaced by fibrous tissue. The nature of the other changes in the media and changes in the intima will provide a more precise diagnosis. For example, in hypertension there is prominent hyalin deposition in the lumen with lumenal narrowing and thickening of the wall.

DIFFERENTIAL DIAGNOSIS: Clinical information should also be considered in establishing a definitive diagnosis, such as the presence of hypertension, diabetes mellitus.

ARTERIOSCLEROSIS

Entry Author: Avrum I. Gotlieb

DEFINITION: A general term that refers to sclerosis or fibrosis of an artery and, therefore, is inclusive of physiological arteriosclerosis of aging, hypertensive arteriopathy, atherosclerosis, and medial calcification (Mönckeberg sclerosis). The common usage of the term *arteriosclerosis* excludes atherosclerosis and Mönckeberg sclerosis.

GROSS FINDINGS: Usually uniformly thick-walled arteries which may show calcification.

MICROSCOPIC FINDINGS: In general, there is replacement of medial muscle with fibrous tissue. The nature of the replacement and the changes in the intima will provide a more precise diagnosis. For example, in hypertension there is hyalinization of the media. There is intimal thickening due to smooth muscle cell proliferation and some increase in elastic tissue in the intima in the early stages. In severe hypertension, fibrinoid necrosis is present.

ATHEROSCLEROTIC PLAQUE

Entry Author: Avrum I. Gotlieb

SYNONYMS: Fibrofatty plaque.

DEFINITION: Predominantly an intimal disease characterized by fibrocellular proliferation, sometimes with calcification, foam cells, and fatty acid deposits in its central core. The composite plaque may be necrotic, often vascularized, and with plaque hemorrhage.

GROSS FINDINGS: An elevated focal lesion, pearly white to yellow in color, with a surface that is smooth and/or focal erosions with or without adherent mural thrombi. May be brittle and hemorrhagic.

MICROSCOPIC FINDINGS: A lesion with fibrocellular cap with a central necrotic core of debris. Cells include smooth muscle cells, foam cells, macrophages, lymphocytes, and occasionally foreign body giant cells; the latter are often associated with cholesterol clefts. The matrix contains fibrous tissue and proteoglycans and shows both punctate calcification and more diffuse calcification. On occasion, this dystrophic calcification leads to bone formation. Neovascularization is prominent, especially toward the base of lesion. Some lesions will not show fatty acid deposits and central necrotic core, and are known as fibrous plaques.

Complicated or complex lesions are defined as those with plaque hemorrhage, surface erosions, mural thrombi, prominent varying thickness calcification, and/or aneurysmal formation. The atherosclerotic vessel may show mild to prominent inflammatory cell infiltrate, mainly in the plaque but sometimes in the adventitia. The latter condition is usually associated with prominent thinning of the media with aneurysm formation. Some refer to this as an *inflammatory plaque*, however, it is more likely that the inflammation is secondary to the presence of inflammatory mediators released in the plaque.

SPECIAL PROCEDURES NEEDED FOR DIAGNOSIS: Elastic stain is essential to identify and separate the intima from the media.

ATYPICAL COARCTATION OF THE AORTA

Entry Author: Alan G. Rose

SYNONYMS: Acquired coarctation; abdominal coarctation; stenosis due to healed Takayasu arteritis; vasculopathy of neurofibromatosis (type 1) [see separate individual listings].

DEFINITION: A constriction of the aorta at a site other than that which occurs developmentally opposite the insertion of the ductus arteriosus, most commonly involving the abdominal aorta.

GROSS FINDINGS: The aorta is affected by dysplastic fibromuscular proliferation or healed aortitis with stricture formation. The thickened intima has a wrinkled appearance, the media appears dysplastic and adventitia appear sclerotic.

MICROSCOPIC FINDINGS: Healed mesaortitis is the characteristic feature together with intimal and adventitial fibrosis. Contraction of the fibrous tissue leads to stenosis (coarctation) of the aorta. Intimal thickening also reduces the lumen. Inflammatory cells are scanty or absent. In neurofibromatosis, there is proliferative fibromuscular dysplasia of the intima and/or media.

SPECIAL PROCEDURES NEEDED FOR DIAGNOSIS: Elastic and trichrome, or combined elastic-trichrome, or Movat's pentachrome stain.

DIFFERENTIAL DIAGNOSIS: Congenital (classic) coarctation is distinguished by its developmental nature and specific site of occurrence.

KEY DIAGNOSTIC CRITERIA: Young adults with acquired stenosis of the abdominal aorta or clinicopathologic stigmata of neurofibromatosis. Histology of healed mesaortitis.

POTENTIAL PITFALLS: The term *coarctation of the aorta* refers to the congenital narrowing of the aorta whereas the term *atypical coarctation* creates confusion and should not be used. It is preferable to speak of acquired stenosis of the aorta due, e.g., to Takayasu aortitis or vasculopathy of neurofibromatosis.

BEHÇET'S DISEASE

Entry Author: J. T. Lie

SYNONYM: Behçet syndrome.

DEFINITION: Originally described in 1937 as a clinical triad of recurrent oral and genital ulceration and relapsing iridocyclitis, it is now universally accepted as a systemic disease that may affect virtually any and multiple organ systems of the body with vascular disease as the common pathologic basis of its various clinical manifestations.

GROSS FINDINGS: Vascular involvement in Behçet's disease affects arteries and veins and blood vessels of all sizes (from aorta to arterioles, venules, and capillaries). Arterial involvement comprises aneurysms, thrombosis, and angiitis of systemic and pulmonary arteries, large and small. Venous involvement consists of recurrent thrombosis, thrombophlebitis, and veno-occlusive disease, as well as pulmonary thromboembolism and pulmonary hypertension.

MICROSCOPIC FINDINGS: The small vessel disease is a necrotizing angiitis; pulmonary involvement is typically a form of thromboangiitis with aneurysm formation; and the large artery involvement is usually thrombosis or aneurysmal disease and, more frequently, a lymphoplasmacytic systemic and pulmonary arteritis.

References

1. Lakhanpal S, Tani K, Lie JT. Pathologic features of Behçet's syndrome: A review of Japanese autopsy registry data. *Human Pathol* 1985;16:790–795.
2. Lakhanpal S, O'Duffy JD, Lie JT. In: Plotkin GR, Calabro JJ, O'Duffy JD, eds *Behçet's disease.* Mount Kisco, NY, Futura; 1988:101–142.
3. Lie JT. Vascular involvement in Behçet's disease: Arterial and venous and vessels of all sizes. *J Rheumatol* 1992;19:341–343.

BERRY ANEURYSM

Entry Authors: Alan G. Rose and J. T. Lie

SYNONYM: Congenital intracranial aneurysm. The term *congenital* may be misleading because it is the underlying medial defect at arterial branching, and not the aneurysm, which is congenital. Some have even suggested that the medial defect may be acquired.

DEFINITION: A saccular aneurysm, sometimes multiple, arising at branching points of the circle of Willis at the base of the brain on the basis of defects in the medial muscle. On the basis of autopsy and angiographic series, the frequency of intracranial berry aneurysms is estimated to be 1–8% in the general population, of these about 90% develop subarachnoid hemorrhage.

GROSS FINDINGS: A small saccular aneurysm at a branching point of the circle of Willis. Usually the aneurysm lies within the subarachnoid space, but occasionally it may burrow into the cerebral cortex. Initial hemorrhage into the wall of the aneurysm may be followed by external rupture of the aneurysm yielding a subarachnoid hemorrhage.

MICROSCOPIC FINDINGS: The saccular aneurysm arises on the basis of a congenital (often familial) defect in the medial muscle layer at a branching point of the circle of Willis. At this site of medial deficiency, the intima and adventitia are in direct contact, and the aneurysm arises due to ballooning outward of these two layers.

SPECIAL PROCEDURES NEEDED FOR DIAGNOSIS: Radiopaque contrast material may be injected into the cerebral vessels to demonstrate the (multiple) aneurysms. The entire circle of Willis may be dissected off the brain to better demonstrate the aneurysm(s) at autopsy.

REMARKS: Most berry aneurysms are idiopathic and isolated. However, polycystic kidney disease, fibromuscular dysplasia, coarctation of aorta, connective tissue diseases, arteriovenous malformations, moyamoya disease, and unilateral carotid arterial or vertebral occlusion or agenesis have all been known to be associated with intracranial berry aneurysms. These disease-associated aneurysms are at sites similar to those of idiopathic aneurysms.

DIFFERENTIAL DIAGNOSIS: The site of a berry aneurysm is fairly specific. Atherosclerosis seldom produces a saccular aneurysm; usually a fusiform aneurysmal bulging of the basilar artery is the change noted in this vicinity. Mycotic aneurysms come into the differential. Rarely, other forms of arteritis may affect the vessels of the circle of Willis, e.g., giant cell arteritis. Berry aneurysm is a common cause of subarachnoid hemorrhage; other causes include hematological abnormalities, trauma, or hypoxia in neonates.

KEY DIAGNOSTIC CRITERIA: Saccular aneurysm arising at or close to a branching point of the circle of Willis. Increased incidence of the condition in patients with systemic hypertension or coarctation of the aorta.

POTENTIAL PITFALLS: Rupture of the aneurysm may lead to the wall of the aneurysm being destroyed. Massive subarachnoid hemorrhage may also obscure the ruptured aneurysm.

BLACKFOOT DISEASE

Entry Author: J. T. Lie

SYNONYM: Environmental chronic arsenism.

DEFINITION: Blackfoot disease is the clinical description of an endemic occlusive peripheral vascular disease found among the inhabitants of selected geographical regions (e.g., southwest Taiwan and north-central Chile) where artesian water with a high concentration of arsenic (up to 1.8 ppm) has been the drinking water supply for several generations. Lower limb involvement occurs in 98% with an annual rate for major amputation of 3.8 per 100 patient-years. The name "blackfoot disease" is a folk term used to indicate the discoloration of the affected limbs which, when ischemic and gangrenous, become black and well demarcated from the adjacent unaffected tissues.

MICROSCOPIC FINDINGS: There are two types of histopathologic findings: the majority (70%) of cases are indistinguishable from premature, severe arteriosclerosis obliterans and the remainder (30%) resembles thromboangiitis obliterans (Buerger's disease). The possible causal role of tobacco use in the latter group has not been independently evaluated.

Reference

1. Tseng WP. Blackfoot disease in Taiwan: A 30-year follow-up study. *Angiology* 1989;40:547–557.

BUDD-CHIARI SYNDROME

Entry Author: J. T. Lie

DEFINITION: An uncommon clinical disorder produced by obstruction to hepatic venous outflow. The first clinical observation of this disorder was attributed to George Budd in 1845; Hans Chiari, in 1898, added the first pathologic description of a liver with "obliterating endophlebitis of the hepatic vein." Clinically, the syndrome is characterized by ascites, hepatomegaly, and abdominal pain. Jaundice is usually mild or absent.

GROSS FINDINGS: The gross features are usually those of the underlying disease, if one exists, and of thrombosis in hepatic veins and their tributaries.

MICROSCOPIC FINDINGS: Hepatic congestion and the incriminating thrombosis of the hepatic veins and their tributaries may be detectable by MRI, ultrasound, or computed tomography. Needle biopsies of the liver may show only variable degrees of (usually marked) centrilobular congestion and, fortuitously, recent or organized thrombi in the tributaries of hepatic veins. Hepatic infarction may be observed occasionally.

DIFFERENTIAL DIAGNOSIS: Portal vein thrombosis; hepatic veno-occlusive disease. Hepatic vein thrombosis may be associated with myeloproliferative disorders, malignancy, nocturnal hemoglobinuria, pregnancy, and the use of oral contraceptives, or the cause may be undetermined (idiopathic).

References

1. Parker RGF. Occlusion of the hepatic veins in man. *Medicine* 1959;38:369–402.
2. Gibson JB. Chiari's disease and the Budd-Chiari syndrome. *J Pathol Bacteriol* 1969;79:381–401.
3. Sons HU, Borchard F. Budd-Chiari syndrome: Some pathologic-anatomic aspects. *Angiology* 1985;36: 603–607.

BUERGER'S DISEASE

Entry Author: J. T. Lie

SYNONYM: von Winiwarter-Buerger's disease (in European literature); thromboangiitis obliterans.

DEFINITION: Buerger's disease is a nonarteriosclerotic, segmental, inflammatory occlusive disease of medium-sized and small arteries and veins of the upper and lower limbs, and it only rarely affects visceral blood vessels. Involvement of central nervous system is questionable, and of the aorta has never been proven. The etiology is unknown but the disease has a strong causal association with tobacco use (smoking and nonsmoking). It occurs predominantly in young men (M/F = 9/1) with onset of symptoms usually before the age of 40. The disease is reversible only if diagnosed at the early stage followed by lifelong abstinence from tobacco.

GROSS FINDINGS: Signs of lower and/or upper limb ischemia, beginning distally, frequently (40%) associated with Raynaud's phenomenon and migrating thrombophlebitis; characteristic angiographic pattern of arterial obstruction and collaterals and segmental thrombotic occlusions.

MICROSCOPIC FINDINGS: The disease is histologically diagnostic only at the early or acute stage with clinical evident thrombophlebitis: inflammatory thrombosis of the arteries and veins with endovascular (intraluminal) "microabscesses" or "granulomas," within the thrombus, and containing one or more multinucleated giant cells. The intermediate or subacute phase is less diagnostic, but the organizing thrombus tends to be more cellular with greater neoangiogenesis than the ordinary noninflammatory thrombosis. The chronic phase or end-stage is nondiagnostic with fibrotic-occluded blood vessels. The internal elastic lamina remains essentially intact or only minimally disrupted at all stages of the disease.

References

1. Lie JT. Thromboangiitis obliterans (Buerger's disease) revisited. *Pathology Annual* 1988;23(part 2): 257–291.

2. Shionoya S. *Buerger's disease: Pathology, diagnosis and treatment.* Nagoya, Japan, University of Nagoya Press, 1990.
3. Stahbens WE, Lie JT, eds. *Vascular pathology.* London, Chapman & Hall; 1995:657–678.

CAVERNOUS SINUS THROMBOSIS

Entry Author: Alan G. Rose

SYNONYM: Thrombotic occlusion of the cavernous sinus.

DEFINITION: Thrombosis occurring within the cavernous sinus of the skull.

GROSS FINDINGS: The cavernous sinus is completely or partially occluded by thrombus.

MICROSCOPIC FINDINGS: Fresh, organizing, or organized thrombus depending on its age.

SPECIAL PROCEDURES NEEDED FOR DIAGNOSIS: Open up the cavernous sinus at postmortem.

DIFFERENTIAL DIAGNOSIS: No specific differential diagnosis.

KEY DIAGNOSTIC CRITERIA: Mass of thrombus confined to the cavernous sinus.

POTENTIAL PITFALLS: Cavernous sinus thrombosis may be missed at autopsy unless the bony covering of the sinus is opened. The thrombosis may have significant etiological factors, e.g., infection of the mid-portion of the face, oral contraceptive therapy in women, etc.

CEREBRAL THROMBOSIS

Entry Author: Alan G. Rose

SYNONYM: Thrombosis of a cerebral artery.

DEFINITION: Thrombus formation within a cerebral artery in the subarachnoid space, usually on the basis of underlying atherosclerosis or hypercoagulable state.

GROSS FINDINGS: The artery is distended by a mass of thrombus which has a white fibrin-platelet head and a red (erythrocyte-rich) propagated portion. Atherosclerosis of the underlying vessel may be evident. Commonly affected are the middle cerebral artery and other components of the circle of Willis, or the basilar-vertebral system.

MICROSCOPIC FINDINGS: The usual finding is that of atherosclerosis with superimposed thrombosis. Signs of organization of the thrombus may be evident depending on the age of the thrombus.

SPECIAL PROCEDURES NEEDED FOR DIAGNOSIS: Injection of radiopaque contrast material into the cerebral arteries followed by radiography may demonstrate the occlusion in the brain at autopsy.

DIFFERENTIAL DIAGNOSIS: It may be impossible to differentiate *in situ* thrombosis from thromboembolism (see *Arterial embolus*). The underlying vessel wall may appear uninvolved by atherosclerosis in the latter condition, but this is not an absolute criterion, because causes of cerebral arterial thrombosis, e.g., polycythemia, may exist.

KEY DIAGNOSTIC CRITERIA: Platelet-fibrin thrombus in cerebral artery which is the seat of significant atherosclerosis. No obvious source of systemic thromboembolism.

POTENTIAL PITFALLS: As mentioned, thromboembolism may be difficult to distinguish from thrombosis.

CHILBLAINS

Entry Author: J. T. Lie

SYNONYM: Pernio; pernio syndrome.

DEFINITION: Painful erythema or a bluish-red discoloration of the skin associated with slight edema, following exposure to near-freezing temperature with high humidity.

GROSS FINDINGS: Acute pernio, if uninfected, will gradually clear up in 7–10 days, sometimes with a residual brownish pigmentation that may persist for several weeks. Chronic pernio results from repeated exposure to cold and is characterized by erythematous skin ulceration, particularly around the ankles and the lower part of the leg. The ulcers heal spontaneously, leaving a pigmented and sometimes a depressed scar in the skin.

MICROSCOPIC FINDINGS: Acute pernio is rarely biopsied and may show only focal edema and purpuric hemorrhage. The histopathology of chronic pernio is also nonspecific and may include (a) microvascular intimal proliferation, (b) perivascular chronic inflammatory infiltrate, and (c) evidence of microhemorrhage and necrotizing panniculitis. Evidence of secondary infection may be observed.

DIFFERENTIAL DIAGNOSIS: Acrocyanosis; frostbite; livido reticularis; advanced Raynaud's phenomenon.

Reference

1. Juergens JL, Spittell JA Jr, Fairbairn JF II (eds). *Allen-Barker-Hines peripheral vascular diseases, 5th ed.* Philadelphia, WB Saunders Co; 1980:587–595.

CHURG-STRAUSS SYNDROME

Entry Author: J. T. Lie

SYNONYMS: Allergic granulomatosis and angiitis.

DEFINITION: A subset or "overlap syndrome" of polyarteritis nodosa. The pathologic diagnostic criteria require systemic and pulmonary necrotizing vasculitis with an eosinophilic infiltrate and extravascular granulomas. The clinical diagnostic criteria consist of the triad of (a) history of asthma or allergy, (b) peripheral blood eosinophil counts of 10^9/L or greater, and (c) pulmonary and systemic vasculitis with eosinophil infiltrate.

GROSS FINDINGS: Variable, depending on the affected organ(s) and extent of involvement. Isolated forms of Churg-Strauss syndrome manifest as single organ or anatomically regional involvement only.

MICROSCOPIC FINDINGS: Pulmonary and systemic polyarteritis-type vasculitis with eosinophil infiltrate, with or without extravascular granulomas. When the vascular lesions are confined to or limited to an isolated organ system, the condition is known as a limited or isolated form of Churg-Strauss syndrome.

References

1. Churg J, Strauss L. Allergic granulomatosis, allergic angiitis, and periarteritis nodosa. *Am J Pathol* 1951;27:277–301.
2. Lie JT. The classification of vasculitis and a reappraisal of allergic granulomatosis and angiitis (Churg-Strauss syndrome). *Mount Sinai J Med* 1986;53:429–439.
3. Lie JT. Limited forms of Churg-Strauss syndrome (review). *Pathol Ann* 1993;28(part 2):199–220.

COARCTATION OF THE AORTA

Entry Author: Alan G. Rose

SYNONYMS: Congenital coarctation of the aorta; stenosis of the proximal descending thoracic aorta.

DEFINITION: A congenital localized stenosis of the proximal aorta just beyond the origin of left subclavian artery and usually close to the insertion of the ductus arteriosus.

GROSS FINDINGS: An infolding of media from the anterior, superior and posterior portions of the aorta narrows the aortic lumen. The exterior or the aorta also appears constricted.

MICROSCOPIC FINDINGS: A curtain-like fold of dysplastic fibromuscular proliferation of the intima from the anterior, superior, and posterior portions of the aorta.

DIFFERENTIAL DIAGNOSIS: Takayasu arteritis may lead to (multiple) stenoses of the aorta at any site as well as aneurysm formation. The latter is not a feature of coarctation.

KEY DIAGNOSTIC CRITERIA: Congenital narrowing at a specific site of the proximal thoracic aorta producing systemic hypertension in the upper limbs and normotension/hypotension in the lower limbs. Rib notching due to collaterals on chest radiography. Congenital bicuspid aortic valve may be associated.

COGAN SYNDROME

Entry Author: J. T. Lie

DEFINITION: Originally described in 1945 as a syndrome of nonsyphilitic interstitial keratitis and audiovestibular dysfunction, it is now considered to be a systemic disease in at least 50% of patients with a constellation of more serious forms of inflammatory eye disease; systemic vasculitis, aortitis and aortic valvular disease; gastrointestinal hemorrhage; lymphadenopathy; renal parenchymal disease; musculoskeletal disease. The syndrome predominantly affects young adults and older children with equal gender distribution.

GROSS FINDINGS: Nonspecific and variable according to the vascular bed and the blood vessel size involvement.

MICROSCOPIC FINDINGS: The medium-sized and small vessel involvement is usually polyarteritis-type vasculitis; whereas large vessel involvement is commonly an aneurysmal disease; the aortitis, when present, has a lymphoplasmacytic and occasionally may be granulomatous with a variable number of giant cells.

DIFFERENTIAL DIAGNOSIS: Other vasculitides; Behçet's disease.

References

1. Cheson BD et al. Cogan's syndrome: a systemic vasculitis. *Am J Med* 1976;60:549–555.
2. Haynes BF et al. Cogan syndrome: Studies in thirteen patients, long-term follow-up, and a review of the literature. *Medicine* 1980;59:426–441.
3. Vollertson RS. Vasculitis and Cogan's syndrome. *Rheum Dis Clin North Am* 1990;16:433–439.

CYSTIC MEDIONECROSIS

Entry Author: Alan G. Rose

SYNONYMS: Idiopathic medial degeneration (hypertension and aging-related medial degeneration is mild and is limited to the aorta).

DEFINITION: A degenerative process involving the aortic media and characterized by focal areas of loss of smooth muscle cells, elastin, and collagen. Because nature does not like a vacuum, the areas in question are occupied by acid mucopolysaccharide.

GROSS FINDINGS: The aorta may appear excessively dilated and structurally weakened in the absence of atherosclerosis. Evidence of previous incomplete tearing of the inner layers of focal areas of the aorta may be noted in some cases. Such areas may lead to saccular aneurysms. The condition predisposes to complete arterial dissection which may also be present.

MICROSCOPIC FINDINGS: There are focal areas of loss of smooth muscle cells, elastin, and collagen in the media, and such areas are occupied by pools of acid mucopolysaccharide. Normal aging may produce similar but usually less striking changes in the aorta. In Erdheim, Ehlers-Danlos, and Marfan syndromes the aorta and possibly other arteries show the most striking changes of the above. It has been claimed that in these conditions there is loss of elastic fibers diffusely in the media, i.e., including the areas intervening between the pools of acid mucopolysaccharide.

KEY DIAGNOSTIC CRITERIA: Focal zones within the aortic media of increased deposition of acid mucopolysaccharide associated with loss of smooth muscle cells, elastin and collagen.

SPECIAL PROCEDURES NEEDED FOR DIAGNOSIS: Elastic van Gieson stain or Movat's pentachrome for elastic tissue component. Alcian blue or the colloidal iron stain for mucopolysaccharide.

DIFFERENTIAL DIAGNOSIS: Cystic medionecrosis may produce saccular aneurysms of the aorta that may be confused with syphilitic aneurysms or aneurysms due to primary (Takayasu) arteritis.

POTENTIAL PITFALLS: Normal aging changes may be difficult to distinguish from cystic medionecrosis. Areas of intimal laceration following on incomplete dissection may develop secondary atherosclerosis.

DIEULAFOY'S VASCULAR MALFORMATION

Entry Author: J. T. Lie

SYNONYM: Dieulafoy's disease or Dieulafoy's ulcer of the gastrointestinal tract.

DEFINITION: Large, submucosal vascular malformation (angiodysplasia) of usually the upper gastrointestinal tract (80% of lesions within 6 cm of the gastroesophageal junction but lesions have been described in the jejunum and colon), often associated with erosion of the overlying mucosa causing massive and often fatal (60% mortality) hemorrhage.

GROSS FINDINGS: Those of a massive upper gastrointestinal hemorrhage associated with mucosal ulceration.

MICROSCOPIC FINDINGS: A peculiar regional type of angiodysplasia consisting of an entanglement of thick-walled and tortuous small arteries and veins as well as morphologically hybrid blood vessels. There is usually no evidence of direct arteriovenous communication ("fistulae"), vasculitis, aneurysmal disease, or atherosclerosis. The overlying (Dieulafoy's) ulcer lacks the intense inflammation typical of peptic ulcer disease. It is superficial without involvement of the muscularis propria or mural fibrosis.

DIFFERENTIAL DIAGNOSIS: Other organic causes of massive gastrointestinal hemorrhage including the more common type of angiodysplasia of the gut.

References

1. Juler GL et al. The pathogenesis of Dieulafoy's gastric erosion. *Am J Gastroenterol* 1984;79:195–200.
2. Veldhuyzen van Zanten SJO et al. Recurrent massive haematemesis from Dieulafoy vascular malformations—A review of 101 cases. *Gut* 1986;27:213–222.
3. Miko TL, Thomazy VA. The caliber persistent artery of the stomach: a unifying approach to gastric aneurysm, Dieulafoy's lesion, and submucosal arterial malformation. *Human Pathol* 1988;19: 914–921.
4. Eidus LB et al. Caliber-persistent artery of the stomach (Dieulafoy's vascular malformation). *Gastroenterology* 1990;99:1507–1510.
5. Kaufman Z et al. Masssive gastrointestinal bleeding caused by Dieulafoy's lesion. *Am Surgeon* 1995; 61:453–455.

DISSECTING ANEURYSM OF AORTA

Entry Authors: Alan G. Rose and J. T. Lie

SYNONYMS: Aortic dissection, dissecting aortic aneurysm, complete dissecting aneurysm, traveling intramural hematoma.

DEFINITION: An intramural hematoma of the aorta usually resulting from an internal tear through the intima and inner half to two thirds of the media. Anatomically, aortic dissections are classified as DeBakey types I, II (corresponding to Stanford type A), and III (Stanford type B): the intimal tears are in the ascending aorta for types I and II, with the dissection involving the entire aorta in the former and only the ascending aorta in the latter; the intimal tears are in the proximal descending thoracic aorta in type III and the dissection spares the ascending aorta.

GROSS FINDINGS: The commonest site for the internal entry of the hematoma is a transverse tear in the aorta about 2–4 cm above the aortic valve. The outline of the aorta is expanded due to the presence of the intramural hematoma. The extent of the distal dissection is variable. Side branches of the aorta may be occluded by the dissection, the false lumen may actually supply the branch or the latter may even be supplied by an internal re-entry tear far distal to the original entry tear that gave rise to the dissection. If cystic medionecrosis is present the aorta may appear dilated and more fragile than normal. Signs of previous incomplete dissection may also be noted.

MICROSCOPIC FINDINGS: The intima and inner half to two thirds of the media is displaced inward into the true aortic lumen by an intramural hematoma which, after dissolution, creates a false lumen and contains circulating blood if a re-entry tear occurs distally. Occasionally the hematoma may undergo organization with healing—this is the optimum outcome. The outer half to one third of the media plus the adventitia are displaced outward leading to widening of the aortic outline and the appearance of an aneurysm. Cystic medionecrosis may be present as the cause of dissection in heritable disorders of the connective tissue (e.g., Ehlers-Danlos and Marfan syndromes). Disruption of vasa vasorum by the dissection may lead to a band of acute necrosis (laminar necrosis) in the mid-portion of the media.

SPECIAL PROCEDURES NEEDED FOR DIAGNOSIS: Elastic and Alcian blue-PAS stains are absolutely essential.

DIFFERENTIAL DIAGNOSIS: Dissecting aneurysm has to be distinguished from other causes of thoracic aortic aneurysms, e.g., atherosclerosis, trauma, saccular aneurysm due to syphilis or local weakening due to a tear, and incomplete dissection.

KEY DIAGNOSTIC CRITERIA: Intramural hematoma in aorta, usually associated with intimal entry tear (hemorrhage from vasa may be the source of the bleeding sometimes).

POTENTIAL PITFALLS: Aging-related medial degeneration of the aorta may be mistaken for cystic medionecrosis.

DISSEMINATED VISCERAL GIANT CELL ANGIITIS (DVGCA)

Entry Author: J. T. Lie

DEFINITION: A very rare type of granulomatous vasculitis, possibly an unusual variant of giant cell arteritis (*vide infra*), involving arteries of all sizes (from the aorta down to arterioles), occasionally veins and venules and, rarely, pulmonary arteries. The entity was first described in 1978 and, to date, probably less than a dozen or so cases have been reported in the world literature. The patients were mostly men, between 30 and 70 years of age. The cause of DVGCA is unknown; none of the patients had sarcoidosis, connective tissue disease, or an infectious disease.

GROSS FINDINGS: As in other more common types of systemic vasculitis, such as polyarteritis nodosa or giant cell arteritis.

MICROSCOPIC FINDINGS: Granulomatous vasculitis with variable numbers of giant cells in a predominantly lymphoplasmacytic mixed-cell infiltrate. Rarely, there may be a co-existing myocarditis.

DIFFERENTIAL DIAGNOSIS: Other idiopathic or secondary systemic/pulmonary angiitis and granulomatosis.

References

1. Lie JT. Disseminated visceral giant cell arteritis: Histopathologic description and differentiation from other granulomatous vasculitides. *Am J Clin Pathol* 1978;69:299–305.
2. Elling H, Kristensen IB. Fatal renal failure in polymyalgia rheumatica caused by disseminated giant cell arteritis. *Scan J Rheumatol* 1980;9:206–208.
3. Morita T et al. Disseminated visceral giant cell arteritis. *Acta Pathol Jpn* 1987;37:863–870.
4. Grishman E. Disseminated giant cell arteritis. *Modern Pathol* 1993;6:633–636.

EHLERS-DANLOS SYNDROME (EDS)

Entry Author: J. T. Lie

DEFINITION: EDS is a heritable disorder of connective tissue of at least 11 subgroups with different clinical manifestations, biochemical defects, and inheritance patterns; vascular disease is a feature of type IV, the so-called "arterial-ecchymotic" variant, which is dominantly inherited with approximately half of the cases representing new mutations.

GROSS FINDINGS: Typically single or multiple arterial aneurysms, with or without rupture and with or without dissection as complications; aorta, peripheral, visceral, and pulmonary all may be involved, and the affected organs and viscera may also undergo hemorrhage and rupture.

MICROSCOPIC FINDINGS: Variable degrees of medial degeneration, morphologically indistinguishable from that of Marfan syndrome, Erdheim's cystic medionecrosis, and aging.

REMARKS: All arterial sections should be routinely stained for elastin and acid mucopolysaccharides, in addition to the hematoxylin-eosin sections. Confirmation of diagnosis depends on analysis of connective tissue for type III collagen (which is deficient in type IV EDS) and on demonstration of decreased production of type III procollagen by cultured fibroblasts.

DIFFERENTIAL DIAGNOSIS: Marfan syndrome, Erdheim's cystic medionecrosis, aging.

Reference

1. Royce PM, Steinmann B (eds). *Connective tissue and its heritable disorders: Molecular, genetic and medical aspects*. New York, Wiley-Liss; 1993:351–407.

ENDARTERITIS OBLITERANS

Entry Author: Alan G. Rose

SYNONYM: Arteriolosclerosis obliterans.

DEFINITION: Reactive intimal fibrosis in a small artery or arteriole stimulated by an adjacent inflammatory focus.

GROSS FINDINGS: The artery has a reduced lumen due to intimal thickening, but this external diameter is not increased.

MICROSCOPIC FINDINGS: Intimal fibrous thickening with a variable number of fibroblasts/smooth muscle cells.

DIFFERENTIAL DIAGNOSIS: Any cause of intimal fibroplasia, e.g., postcannulation injury, postirradiation change, graft arteriopathy.

KEY DIAGNOSTIC CRITERIA: Intimal fibroplasia occurring in an artery in the vicinity of an appropriate stimulus, e.g., at the base of a peptic ulcer.

POTENTIAL PITFALLS: Usually an isolated or localized lesion. Multiple arterial involvement would be unusual.

ERGOTISM

Entry Author: J. T. Lie

DEFINITION: A potentially reversible vasospastic occlusive disease from chronic use of ergot-containing drugs of the peripheral, visceral, and sometimes, coronary arteries that may lead to ischemia and infarction of affected organs and body parts.

GROSS FINDINGS: Irregular long and short segments of alternating stenoses and dilations in arteries free of atherosclerosis, angiographically mimicking angiitis.

MICROSCOPIC FINDINGS: The stenoses in irreversible, chronic arterial lesions consist of fibrous intimal proliferation, sometimes with elastica reduplication and rarely with foam cells accumulation, and medial hypertrophy, without an inflammatory infiltrate. The dilations are poststenotic.

REMARKS: The diagnosis of ergotism arterial disease is usually made angiographically in patients who take ergot-containing drugs and after the exclusion of other causes. Tissue (biopsy) is available for examination only from patients who underwent surgical intervention.

DIFFERENTIAL DIAGNOSIS: Vasculitis; postirradiation arteriopathy; methysergide toxicity; carcinoid syndrome arteriopathy.

References

1. Goldfischer JD. Acute myocardial infarction secondary to ergot therapy. Report of a case and review of the literature. *N Engl J Med* 1960;262:860–863.
2. Richter A, Banker V. Carotid ergotism. A complication of migraine therapy. *Radiology* 1973;106: 339–340.
3. Green FL et al. Mesenteric and peripheral vascular ischemia secondary to ergotism. *Surgery* 1977;81: 176–179.

ERYTHERMALGIA
(A VARIANT OF ERYTHROMELALGIA)

Entry Author: J. T. Lie

DEFINITION: Erythromelalgia is a self-limiting asymmetrical disorder associated with thrombocythemia, platelet-mediated inflammation, and circulatory changes, and is responsive to aspirin.

GROSS FINDINGS: Burning, painful, red, swollen, warm limbs of unknown cause.

MICROSCOPIC FINDINGS: There is a paucity of histologic features other than the nonspecific perivascular edema and cell infiltrate of postcapillary venules and arterioles. A more recent description of secondary erythermalgia in systemic lupus erythematosus suggests cutaneous vasculitis as a putative mechanism. The diagnosis is usually based on clinical criteria and the lesion is seldom biopsied.

DIFFERENTIAL DIAGNOSIS: Erythromelalgia.

REMARKS: Primary erythermalgia is rare. It begins in childhood or adolescence as bilateral symmetrical burning distress in the feet, ankles, and legs. Secondary erythermalgia occurs in association with gout, systemic lupus erythematosus, rheumatoid arthritis cryoglobulinemia, and selected vasculitides.

References

1. Brown GE. Erythromelalgia and other disturbances of the extremities accompanied by vasodilation and burning. *Am J Med Sci* 1932;183:468–485.
2. Michiels JJ, van Joost T. Primary and secondary erythermalgia, a critical review. *Neth J Med* 1988;33: 205–208.
3. Drenth JPH et al. Erythermalgia secondary to vasculitis. *Am J Med* 1993;94:93–94.

ERYTHROMELALGIA

Entry Author: J. T. Lie

DEFINITION: Erythromelalgia refers to a clinical syndrome of redness and congested limbs with raised skin temperature and painful burning sensations.

GROSS FINDINGS: Warm, red, and swollen limb.

MICROSCOPIC FINDINGS: The characteristic but nonspecific histopathologic findings are fibromuscular intimal proliferation and occlusive thrombosis of arterioles and digital arteries. The diagnosis is usually based on clinical criteria and the lesion is seldom biopsied.

DIFFERENTIAL DIAGNOSIS: Primary and secondary erythermalgia.

REMARKS: In contrast to Raynaud's disease, warmth intensifies the discomfort in erythromelalgia and cold provides relief. The relief of pain for several days after a single low dose of aspirin is specific for erythromelalgia and can be used as a diagnostic criterion. Erythromelalgia may occur without an underlying disease (primary form) or in association with a systemic disease (secondary form), most commonly thrombocythemia and myeloproliferative disorders.

References

1. Michiels JJ et al. Histopathology of erythromelalgia in thrombocythaemia. *Histopathology* 1984;8: 669–678.
2. Michiels JJ et al. Erythromelalgia caused by platelet-mediated arteriolar inflammation and thrombosis in thrombocythemia. *Ann Intern Med* 1985;102:466–471.
3. Drenth JPH, Michiels JJ. Three types of erythromelalgia. Important to differentiate because treatment differs. *Br Med J* 1990;301:454–455.

FATTY STREAK

Entry Author: Avrum I. Gotlieb

SYNONYM: Fatty dot.

DEFINITION: A collection of lipid-laden cells (foam cells) in the intima.

GROSS FINDINGS: Focal yellow color on lumenal surface characteristic of this nonelevated lesion.

MICROSCOPIC FINDINGS: Collection of foam cells with or without extracellular lipid. Foam cell usually has round dark nucleus with a pale foamy to finely granular cytoplasm. Very mild fibrous matrix.

SPECIAL PROCEDURES NEEDED FOR DIAGNOSIS: Fat stain for gross identification. Electron microscopy has been used to show that foam cells may be macrophages and/or smooth muscle cells.

DIFFERENTIAL DIAGNOSIS: Intimal hyperplasia.

KEY DIAGNOSTIC CRITERIA: Foam cells.

Reference

1. Stary HC et al. A definition of initial, fatty streak, and intermediate lesions of atherosclerosis. A report from the Committee on Vascular Lesions of the Council on Arteriosclerosis, American Heart Association (review). *Arterioscler Thromb* 1994;14:840–856.

FIBROMUSCULAR DYSPLASIA (FMD)

Entry Author: J. T. Lie

SYNONYM: Fibromuscular hyperplasia.

DEFINITION: Considered to be a developmental vascular anomaly of medium-sized and small arteries, and rarely veins, in which the vessel wall is altered by dysplasia, hypoplasia, and/or hyperplasia of the fibromuscular components usually in the media, rarely in the intima or adventitia (<5%), causing stenosis, aneurysm formation, or medial dissection. Three morphologic types are recognized: medial hyperplasia (about 95%), intimal fibroplasia (about 2%), and adventitial fibroplasia (about 2%). Fibromuscular dysplasia occurs most commonly in the renal arteries of young women, followed in frequencies by the internal carotid arteries, visceral arteries, and only rarely, the coronary arteries. More often than by chance, association of FMD with cerebral berry aneurysms has been described.

GROSS FINDINGS: Usually occurs in a segmental, irregular, string of beads or corkscrew configuration. May angiographically mimic vasculitis. Spontaneous medial dissection of the affected arteries, with rupture, is a serious and potentially catastrophic complication.

MICROSCOPIC FINDINGS: Irregular, alternating, hill-and-valley type corrugation deformity of the vessel wall that can be demonstrated best or only recognizable in longitudinal sections of the artery or vein in question. Less commonly, marked intimal or adventitial fibroplasia.

SPECIAL PROCEDURES NEEDED FOR DIAGNOSIS: Whenever possible, if FMD is suspected, the arterial specimen should be sectioned longitudinally to demonstrate the telltale hill-and-valley or corrugated configuration of the dysplastic artery which cannot be discerned or shown to advantage in the traditional cross-section sampling method. Elastic van Gieson or Movat's pentachrome stain is mandatory for the histologic evaluation of FMD, without exception.

DIFFERENTIAL DIAGNOSIS: Arteriosclerosis; vasculitis.

Reference

1. Lüscher TF, Lie JT, Stanson AW et al. Arterial fibromuscular dysplasia (review). *Mayo Clin Proc* 1987; 62:931–952.

FROSTBITE

Entry Author: J. T. Lie

DEFINITION: Frostbite is the actual freezing of tissues. Tissue changes associated with frostbite are not unlike those associated with burns and it has been customary to classify frostbite according to degrees of tissue damage: either in four degrees in ascending order of severity or in two categories, superficial and deep.

GROSS FINDINGS: Superficial frostbite affects only the skin and tissue immediately beneath it. The skin has a whitish and waxy appearance because of vasoconstriction. After rewarming, the injured area appears mottled blue or purple and loses sensation. Swelling and stinging or burning pain may follow. Blisters form in 24–36 hours in more severe cases. Deep frostbite is more serious and involves the skin, subcutaneous tissues, and even bone. Ischemia is severe and prolonged with thrombosis of the small arteries and arterioles resulting in gangrene. Tissue death may also be produced directly by freezing with crystallization and ice formation of the cellular fluids. Blisters continue to form for 3 days to 1 week and functional loss lasts for 1 month or longer. Discoloration of the injured part, from blue-violet and gray is common; the gray color indicates most severe injury.

MICROSCOPIC FINDINGS: The diagnosis is usually clinical; biopsies are rarely done.

Reference

1. Juergens JL, Spittell Jr JA, Fairbairns JF II, eds. *Allen-Barker-Hines peripheral vascular diseases, 5th ed.* Philadelphia, WB Sauders; 1980:595–601.

GIANT CELL ARTERITIS

Entry Author: J. T. Lie

SYNONYMS: Temporal arteritis; cranial arteritis; Horton's disease.

DEFINITION: Granulomatous arteritis of large, medium-sized, and small arteries, affecting most commonly the superficial temporal artery in persons 50 years of age or older. There is a 2 or 3 to 1 female to male predominance, a common association with the clinical syndrome of polymyalgia rheumatica, and Westergren erythrocyte sedimentation rate of greater than 50 mm/hr.

GROSS FINDINGS: The disease may be unilateral or bilateral and the affected temporal artery may be tender, red, swollen, and cord-like. It is often markedly stenotic with or without thrombosis.

MICROSCOPIC FINDINGS: The arteritis is usually focal and segmental with a transmural infiltrate that is maximal in the media. The infiltrate is predominantly lymphoplasmacytic, but a variable number of multinucleated giant cells is found at the intima-media junction in about 50% of positive temporal artery biopsies. There is usually intimal proliferation, irregular disruption of the internal elastic lamina, and adventitial fibrosis.

DIFFERENTIAL DIAGNOSIS: Takayasu arteritis; disseminated visceral giant cell angiitis.

REMARKS: Giant cell arteritis is a systemic disease. Extracranial giant cell arteritis occurs in 10–15% of patients with temporal arteritis most commonly involving the ascending aorta and aortic arch branches and only rarely the lower limb arteries. Complications include aortic aneurysm and dissection, myocardial infarction, and stroke.

References

1. Lie JT. The classification and diagnosis of vasculitis in large and medium-sized blood vessels. *Pathol Ann* 1987;22(part 1):125–162.
2. Lie JT. Diagnostic histopathology of major systemic and pulmonary vasculitic syndromes. *Rheum Dis Clin North Am* 1990;16:269–292.
3. Lie JT. Aortic and extracranial large vessel giant cell arteritis: A review of 72 cases with histopathologic documentation. *Semin Arthritis Rheum* 1995;24:422–431.

HEREDITARY HEMORRHAGIC TELANGIECTASIA

Entry Author: J. T. Lie

SYNONYM: Osler-Weber-Rendu disease; Rendu-Osler-Weber syndrome.

DEFINITION: An autosomal dominant mucocutaneous and visceral angiodysplasia, clinically suspected or recognized by the classic triad of telangiectasia, recurrent epistaxis, and a family history of the disorder; painless hematemesis has been reported to occur in 15–30% of patients.

GROSS FINDINGS: Evidence of mucocutaneous and visceral angiodysplasias: telangiectatic lesions have been described most commonly in the alimentary tract, skin, nose, lungs, liver, pancreas, spleen, genitourinary tract, brain and meninges, and bone, probably in that descending order.

MICROSCOPIC FINDINGS: The vascular lesions may be few and localized or generalized, involving different segments of blood vessels ranging in caliber from capillaries to large arteries and veins, as telangiectases, arteriovenous malformations, aneurysms, or a combination thereof. The individual lesions are specific but the aggregates are diagnostic.

REMARKS: It is essential to have complete clinical, angiographic, and other radiologic imaging findings, including the family history and genetic consultations, prior to the pathologic evaluations. All histologic sections must have, in addition to H&E, elastin and connective tissue-stained preparations.

DIFFERENTIAL DIAGNOSIS: Other types of angiodysplasia (see individual listings).

References

1. Lande A et al. The spectrum of arteriographic findings in Osler-Weber-Rendu disease. *Angiology* 1976;27:223–240.
2. Peery WH. Clinical spectrum of hereditary hemorrhagic telangiectasia (Osler-Weber-Rendu disease). *Am J Med* 1987;82:989–997.
3. Guttmacher AE et al. Hereditary hemorrhagic telangiectasia. *N Engl J Med* 1995;333:918–924.

HEYDE SYNDROME

Entry Author: J. T. Lie

DEFINITION: The peculiar unexplained association of gastrointestinal (GI) bleeding (with or without a known source) in patients with aortic stenosis. Aortic stenosis occurs in 15–25% of patients bleeding from intestinal angiodysplasia. Whereas 2.6% of patients with aortic stenosis have GI bleeding, the incidence in the general population is only about one tenth of this rate. The association was first described by Heyde in a 146-word short letter to the editor (*N Engl J Med* 1958;259:196). Resolution of the syndrome after aortic valve replacement has been reported.

GROSS FINDINGS: Findings related to gastrointestinal bleeding (with or without a known source) in a patient with aortic stenosis.

MICROSCOPIC FINDINGS: Localized and isolated GI angiodysplasia, usually in the colon, is the only known lesion found in these patients.

DIFFERENTIAL DIAGNOSIS: Gastrointestinal bleeding from other known organic causes.

References

1. Cody MC et al. Idiopathic gastrointestinal bleeding and aortic stenosis. *Am J Digest Dis* 1974;19: 393–398.
2. Shoenfeld Y et al. Aortic stenosis associated with gastrointestinal bleeding. A survey of 612 patients. *Am Heart J* 1980;100:179–182.
3. Cappell MS, Lebwohl O. Cessation of recurrent bleeding from gastrointestinal angiodysplasias after aortic valve replacement. *Ann Intern Med* 1986;105:54–57.
4. Scheffer SM, Leatherman LL. Resolution of Heyde's syndrome of aortic stenosis and gastrointestinal bleeding after aortic valve replacement. *Ann Thorac Surg* 1986;42:477–480.

HURLER SYNDROME

Entry Author: J. T. Lie

SYNONYM: Mucopolysaccharidosis I-H (MPS I-H).

DEFINITION: One of the three clinical subtypes of MPS-I. Mucopolysaccharidoses are characterized by deficiencies in lysosomal enzymes involved in degrading various acid mucopolysaccharides (AMP) or proteoglycans. The consequences of such deficiencies are: (a) intracellular accumulations of AMP within lysosomes and (b) complex abnormalities in the organization of connective tissue and, both, result in morphologic cardiovascular abnormalities.

GROSS FINDINGS: A variable expression of large and small vessel occlusive disease in childhood, including the aorta, coronary, and other arteries, superficially resembling premature atherosclerosis.

MICROSCOPIC FINDINGS: The aorta and large and small arteries, including the coronary arteries, are rigid and occasionally calcified, with raised, occlusive intimal plaques composed of vascular smooth muscle cells, some vacuolated (Hurler cells), granular cells, and abundant fibrous connective tissue, causing critical concentric stenosis. The thickened intimal stains intensely for acid mucopolysaccharides. Ultrastructurally, Hurler cells contain numerous electron-lucent cytoplasmic inclusions and lamellar bodies and only some peripherally located contractile elements.

REMARKS: Hurler syndrome (MPS I-H) is usually first diagnosed clinically. Patients with MPS I-H present with lumbar lordosis, stiffness of joints, hepatosplenomegaly, umbilical hernias, clawhand deformities, short stature, clouding of the corneas, prominent and disproportionately large forehead, coarse facies, macroglossia, and mental retardation (so-called "gargoylism").

DIFFERENTIAL DIAGNOSIS: Other vasculopathies of metabolic disorders; atherosclerosis.

References

1. Goldfischer JL et al. Lysosomes and the sclerotic arterial lesion in Hurler's disease. *Human Pathol* 1975;6:633–637.
2. Brosius FC, Roberts WC. Coronary artery disease in the Hurler syndrome. Qualitative and quantitative analysis of the extent of coronary narrowing at necropsy in six children. *Am J Cardiol* 1981;47:649–653.
3. Stehbens WE, Lie JT, eds. *Vascular pathology.* London, Chapman & Hall; 1995:129–173.

HYPERSENSITIVITY ANGIITIS

Entry Author: J. T. Lie

SYNONYMS: Allergic vasculitis; cutaneous vasculitis; leukocytoclastic vasculitis; small vessel vasculitis.

VARIANTS: Hypocomplementemic vasculitis; cryoglobulinemic vasculitis; eosinophilic vasculitis; Schönlein-Henoch syndrome or purpura.

DEFINITION: Originally defined as angiitis resulting from an allergic response attributable to a precipitating antigen such as foreign proteins (as in serum sickness), drugs, chemicals, vaccines, or microorganisms. The same term has also been used to refer to nonpolyarteritis small vessel vasculitis and cutaneous vasculitis. The vascular injury is believed to be triggered by the deposition of immune complexes in the vessel wall with activation of the complement cascade to explain the histologic changes observed.

GROSS FINDINGS: Cutaneous and/or visceral purpuric rash or petechiae; occasionally signs of visceral ischemia.

MICROSCOPIC FINDINGS: Basically, this is an immune-mediated small vessel vasculitis. The initial infiltrate of polymorphonuclear leukocytes attracted to the area release lysosomal enzymes that damage the vessel wall, leading to diapedesis of erythrocytes and fibrin deposition, in addition to the vessel wall necrosis. In the prenecrosis stage, the cell infiltrate of hypersensitivity angiitis is predominantly granulocytic or lymphocytic; the former is often associated with hypocomplementemic vasculitis while the latter is with cryoglobulinemic vasculitis. However, the variation in cell infiltrates may simply represent different evolutional stages of a common basic pathogenetic process.

DIFFERENTIAL DIAGNOSIS: Other forms of small vessel vasculitis, especially microscopic polyarteritis.

References

1. Winkelmann RK. The spectrum of cutaneous vasculitis. *Clin Rheum Dis* 1980;6:413–453.
2. Calabrese LH, Clough JD. Hypersensitivity vasculitis group (HVG). A case-oriented review of a continuing clinical spectrum. *Cleve Clin J Med* 1982;49:17–42.
3. Lie JT. Illustrated histopathologic classification criteria for selected vasculitis syndromes. American College of Rheumatology Subcommittee on Classification of Vasculitis. *Arthritis Rheum* 1990;33:1074–1087.
4. Calabrese LH et al. The American College of Rheumatology 1990 criteria for the classification of hypersensitivity vasculitis. *Arthritis Rheum* 1990;33:1108–1113.

HYPOTHENAR HAMMER SYNDROME

Entry Author: J. T. Lie

DEFINITION: A thrombotic vaso-occlusive disease of the superficial branch of the ulnar artery as it passes the hook of the hamate bone before penetrating the palmar aponeurosis of the hand in workers who repeatedly use the palm of the hand as a hammer to strike, push, or twist hard objects. It is considered an occupational disease.

GROSS FINDINGS: Coldness in the dominant hand so affected, with absence of triphasic color change and thumb involvement and sometimes, signs of digital ischemia. Angiography shows the typical findings of irregularity or occlusion of the ulnar artery, and downstream occluded digital arteries with possibly demonstrable intraluminal emboli at sites of distal obstruction.

MICROSCOPIC FINDINGS: Thrombosis at variable stages of organization and recanalization with a chronic inflammatory infiltrate and fibrosis of the vessel wall; not a true vasculitis.

DIFFERENTIAL DIAGNOSIS: Small vessel vasculitis; primary and secondary Raynaud's phenomena; Buerger's disease; connective tissue disease (e.g., scleroderma).

REMARKS: It is important to recognize the hypothenar hammer syndrome and distinguish it from vasculitis because the treatment is surgical resection of the affected segment of the artery, with or without revascularization, and avoidance of the repetitive aggravating conditions (occupational trauma), and not corticosteroids and other forms of immunosuppressive therapy.

References

1. Conn J et al. Hypothenar hammer syndrome: post-traumatic digital ischemia. *Surgery* 1970;68: 1122–1128.
2. Dubois P, Stephen D. Angiographic findings in the hypothenar hammer syndrome. *Aust Radiol* 1975; 19:370–380.
3. Pineda C et al. Hypothenar hammer syndrome. Form of reversible Raynaud's phenomenon. *Am J Med* 1985:79:561–570.

IDIOPATHIC LYMPHEDEMA

Entry Authors: Alan G. Rose and J. T. Lie

SYNONYMS: Primary lymphedema; hereditary lymphedema; Milroy disease; idiopathic elephantiasis.

DEFINITION: Familial and nonfamilial forms of painless massive edema, usually present at birth, involving part or all of one or more limbs, resulting from obstruction to lymphatic drainage of unknown cause.

GROSS FINDINGS: The affected part appears grossly enlarged due to severe, longstanding edema with induration of the tissues, resulting in a "pigskin-like" appearance. Puncture of the overlying skin leads to a prominent oozing of edema fluid. Ulcers and recurrent infection are uncommon.

MICROSCOPIC FINDINGS: Extreme dilation of lymphatic with massive interstitial edema of the tissues with separation of collagen and elastic fibers. The lymph may show positive staining of proteinaceous material.

SPECIAL PROCEDURES NEEDED FOR DIAGNOSIS: Lymphangiography during life.

DIFFERENTIAL DIAGNOSIS: Idiopathic lymphedema including those with a familial basis must be distinguished from obstructive lymphedema of known cause, e.g., surgery, filariasis, tumor infiltration, as well as from severe peripheral edema due to heart failure or local causes of edema.

KEY DIAGNOSTIC CRITERIA: Condition usually present at birth with or without a positive family history.

INFECTIVE ARTERITIS

Entry Author: Alan G. Rose

SYNONYMS: Mycotic aneurysm, bacterial arteritis, fungal arteritis.

DEFINITION: Arterial wall inflammation caused by an infective agent, most often bacterial or fungal in nature.

GROSS FINDINGS: Grossly there may not be much to see, especially if the artery is small. The wall may be thickened, and secondary mural or occlusive luminal thrombosis may be evident. Tuberculous arteritis may produce prominent fibrosis with great thickening and narrowing of the vessel lumen. Infective arteritis may lead to mycotic (usually false) aneurysm formation.

MICROSCOPIC FINDINGS: Features reflect the cause, e.g., bacterial infection may show numerous pus cells and bacteria in the wall of the artery. Fungal infection may show fungal elements within the vessel wall without any specific inflammatory response. If the hyphae are nonseptate, think of the Phycomycoses (Mucor, Rhizopus, etc.). Cytomegalovirus may produce inclusion bodies within vascular endothelial cells.

SPECIAL PROCEDURES NEEDED FOR DIAGNOSIS: Microbiological culture of samples of the infected artery. Appropriate histological stains for microorganisms (e.g., Gram and Ziehl-Neelsen stains). Polymerase chain reaction may be used to identify certain organisms including Mycobacterium tuberculosis and viruses. Results of serology for syphilis may be useful in suspected syphilitic aortitis.

DIFFERENTIAL DIAGNOSIS: Noninfective arteritis may mimic infective arteritis, e.g., Takayasu arteritis versus tuberculous or syphilitic aortitis.

KEY DIAGNOSTIC CRITERIA: The demonstration of infective microorganisms in the wall of the blood vessel and a source of infection is important.

POTENTIAL PITFALLS: Infective arteritis due to systemic spread of infection must be distinguished from local arteritis with incidental involvement of an artery by the focal lesion, e.g., an abscess.

IRRADIATION ARTERIOPATHY

Entry Author: J. T. Lie

DEFINITION: Occlusive arteriopathy attributed to therapeutic or accidental postirradiation injury.

GROSS FINDINGS: Bland, long or short segment, uniform narrowing or occlusion of the affected arteries.

MICROSCOPIC FINDINGS: Changes observed and attributed to post-irradiation include concentric or eccentric myointimal proliferation, with or without lipid-laden foam cells, elastica reduplication, medial hyalinization or, rarely, necrosis.

REMARKS: None of the morphologic changes is specific, especially the atheromata. However, the severity of the lesions, limited to the irradiated areas, lend support to the diagnosis, particularly in young people.

DIFFERENTIAL DIAGNOSIS: Atherosclerosis; arteriosclerosis obliterans; angiographically, vasculitis or chronic ergotism/methysergide-induced arteriopathy.

Reference

1. Fajardo LF. *Pathology of radiation injury.* New York, Masson Publishing Inc.; 1982:15–33.

JUVENILE TEMPORAL ARTERITIS

Entry Author: J. T. Lie

DEFINITION: An isolated, unilateral or bilateral nongiant cell arteritis of the superficial temporal artery which is not associated with a systemic disease or vasculitis, occurring in preteens, adolescents, and young adults. The entity was first described in 1975 and, to date, probably fewer than 10 cases have been reported in the literature, only one with bilateral disease.

GROSS FINDINGS: A cord-like artery adherent to the surrounding soft tissue as a nodular mass, the lumen may or may not be visibly patent.

MICROSCOPIC FINDINGS: A nongranulomatous and nonnecrotizing vasculitis of the temporal artery and its branches, with a lymphohistiocytic infiltrate and prominent eosinophils, focal disruption of the internal elastic lamina, and intimal angiomatoid proliferation.

REMARKS: Commonly presents as a localized tender nodule or swelling but the patient is otherwise totally asymptomatic and without a history of trauma to the temporal regions and there has been no known recurrence after a simple excisional biopsy.

DIFFERENTIAL DIAGNOSIS: Kimura's disease; angiolymphoid hyperplasia with eosinophilia [see separate listings].

References

1. Lie JT, Gordon LP, Titus JL. Juvenile temporal arteritis. Biopsy study of four cases. *JAMA* 1975;234: 496–499.
2. Bollinger A, Leu HJ, Brunner U. Juvenile arteritis of extracranial arteries with hypereosinophilia. *Klin Wochenschr* 1986;64:526–529.
3. Tomlinson FH, Lie JT, Nienhuis BJ et al. Juvenile temporal arteritis revisited. *Mayo Clin Proc* 1994; 69:445–447.
4. Lie JT. Bilateral juvenile temporal arteritis. *J Rheumatol* 1995;22:774–776.

KAWASAKI DISEASE

Entry Author: J. T. Lie

SYNONYM: Kawasaki syndrome; mucocutaneous lymph node syndrome.

DEFINITION: An infantile febrile illness of unknown origin, diagnosed clinically by the presence of 5 of the following criteria:
1. Fever persisting for 5 days or longer
2. Reddening of palms and soles with desquamation
3. Polymorphous exanthema
4. Bilateral conjunctivitis
5. Strawberry tongue, reddened lips and oropharyngeal mucosa
6. Acute nonsuppurative cervical lymphadenopathy

Patients with only 4 items can be diagnosed in the presence of coronary artery aneurysms or arteritis which occur in 20–25% of cases. Next to Schönlein-Henoch syndrome this is the commonest form of childhood vasculitis. Sudden death may occur in infancy at the acute phase of the disease or in adolescents/young adults as late sequelae of coronary arteritis/aneurysm and thrombosis.

GROSS FINDINGS: At autopsy, the 1–2% fatal cases show pathologic changes that are indistinguishable from the classic form of infantile polyarteritis. These fatal cases all show active or healed coronary arteritis and the resulting coronary artery aneurysms or aneurysmal dilation with or without thrombosis.

MICROSCOPIC FINDINGS: Cardiac and extra-cardiac polyarteritis type necrotizing vasculitis; coronary and extra-coronary arterial aneurysms, usually multiple; less commonly nonsuppurative myocarditis. Late changes include healed arteritis, thrombosed aneurysms, evidence of recent or healed myocardial infarction.

References

1. Fujiwara H. Hamashima Y. Pathology of the heart in Kawasaki disease. *Pediatrics* 1978;61:100–107.
2. Amano S et al. Pathology of Kawasaki disease: I. Pathology and morphogenesis of the vascular changes. *Jpn Circ J* 1979;43:633–643;741–748.
3. Tanaka N et al. Pathological study of sequelae of Kawasaki disease (MCLS). With special reference to the heart and coronary arterial lesions. *Acta Pathol Jpn* 1986;36:1513–1527.
4. Wortmann DW. Kawasaki syndrome. *Semin Dermatol* 1992;11:37–47.

KIMURA'S DISEASE

Entry Author: J. T. Lie

SYNONYM: Angiolymphoid hyperplasia with eosinophilia (see REMARKS).

DEFINITION: Kimura's disease is a peculiar angiolymphoid proliferative disorder of soft tissue associated with eosinophilia and elevated IgE. It is most commonly seen in young men and is apparently more prevalent among Orientals.

GROSS FINDINGS: It usually presents as a nodular subcutaneous swelling of variable size with a predilection for periauricular and submandibular regions.

MICROSCOPIC FINDINGS: The histopathology varies somewhat according to the location and duration of these lesions. Early lesions show a prominent vascular proliferation with plump atypical (histiocytoid) endothelial cells and a mixed-cell infiltrate of lymphocytes, histiocytes, plasma cells, and prominent eosinophils. In later stages, vascular proliferation is less conspicuous but lymphoid follicular aggregates and fibrosis become prominent.

REMARKS: The occasional occurrence of genuine Kimura's disease among the few Caucasians probably causes confusion with angiolymphoid hyperplasia with eosinophilia (ALHE) (see separate listing). Most investigators now consider Kimura's disease and ALHE as two distinct entities on the basis of demographic, clinical, and pathologic differences.

References

1. Olsen TG, Helwig EB. Angiolymphoid hyperplasia with eosinophilia. A clinicopathologic study of 116 patients. *J Am Acad Dermatol* 1985;12:781–796.
2. Kuo TT et al. Kimura's disease. Involvement of regional lymph nodes and distinction from angiolymphoid hyperplasia with eosinophilia. *Am J Surg Pathol* 1988;12:843–854.
3. Fetsch JF, Weiss SW. Observations concerning the pathogenesis of epithelioid hemangioma (angiolymphoid hyperplasia). *Mod Pathol* 1991;4:449–455.

KLIPPEL-TRENAUNAY SYNDROME

Entry Author: J. T. Lie

SYNONYM: Klippel-Trenaunay-Weber syndrome

DEFINITION: A clinical triad of:
1. Port wine stain hemangioma (nevus flammeus)
2. Unilateral varicose veins
3. Ipsilateral hypertrophy of soft tissue and bone resulting in an asymmetric overgrown limb

Arteriovenous communication or fistulas described by Weber were not included in the original Klippel-Trenaunay syndrome. Pulmonary hypertension occurs rarely.

GROSS FINDINGS: Cutaneous and visceral hemangiomas, varicosities and asymmetric osteohypertrophy of the affected limb(s).

MICROSCOPIC FINDINGS: The visceral or cutaneous hemangiomas are usually of the cavernous type that may be associated with skin and/or intestinal mucosal ulceration. The most prominent and consistent vascular lesions in an affected limb are venous fibromuscular dysplasia with absent or defective valves, and arterial/venous angiodysplasia (so-called "arteriovenous malformation"). True arteriovenous communication ("fistula") may rarely be demonstrable in the angiodysplastic lesions.

Reference

1. Lie JT. Pathology of angiodysplasia in Klippel-Trenaunay syndrome. *Path Res Pract* 1988;747–755.

KÖHLMEIER-DEGOS DISEASE

Entry Author: J. T. Lie

SYNONYMS: Degos disease; Degos syndrome; malignant atrophic papulosis.

DEFINITION: A progressive thrombosing vasculitis of small arteries and veins, arterioles and venules of unknown etiology, frequently presenting as cutaneous papular eruptions with central nervous system and gastrointestinal disorders. Necrotizing vasculitis is unusual in Köhlmeier-Degos disease but has been described.

GROSS FINDINGS: Papular skin eruptions, changes of ischemic bowel disease, and possibly multifocal cerebral necrosis and cavitation.

MICROSCOPIC FINDINGS: The cutaneous lesion is characterized by atrophic and hyperkeratotic epidermis that overlies a zone of pale avascular superficial dermal collagen. The margin of the lesion is elevated and contains numerous ectatic and congested superficial vessels with thrombotic occlusion of the deeper arterioles and venules, not infrequently with lymphocyte mediated necrotizing vasculitis or perivascular lymphocytic infiltrate. The visceral and cerebral vascular lesions consist of arterial and venous occlusive thrombosis with or without vasculitis.

DIFFERENTIAL DIAGNOSIS: Other vasculitides and thrombotic vaso-occlusive disease.

References

1. McFarland HR et al. Papulosis atrophicans maligna (Köhlmeier-Degos disease): A disseminated occlusive vasculopathy. *Ann Neurol* 1978;3:388–392.
2. Anonymous. Case records of the Massachusetts General Hospital. Weekly clinicopathological exercises. Case 44-1980, MGH. *New Engl J Med* 1980;303:1103–1111.
3. Su DWP et al. Clinical and histological findings in Degos' syndrome (malignant atrophic papulosis). *Cutis* 1985;35:131–138.

LIVIDO RETICULARIS

Entry Author: J. T. Lie

SYNONYMS: Livido racemosa; livido annularis; livido vasculitis.

DEFINITION: This cutaneous disorder is characterized by its gross features of and gross reddish-blue discoloration of the skin of the limbs with a net-like pattern of mottling, which may become purpuric macules with ulceration. Livido reticularis may be primary (idiopathic) or secondary to an underlying systemic disease (e.g., vasculitis, antiphospholipid syndrome) or a local vascular disorder (e.g., cholesterol atheroembolism). Ulceration may be observed in both primary and secondary livido reticularis.

MICROSCOPIC FINDINGS: In primary livido reticularis, the microvascular occlusive disease results from fibrous intimal proliferation or arteriolar hyalinosis. Perivascular nonspecific cell infiltrate may be observed but not true vasculitis. In secondary livido reticularis, the microvascular occlusive disease is due to thrombosis (as in the antiphospholipid syndrome) or embolism (cholesterol atheromatous debris, cardiac myxoma).

DIFFERENTIAL DIAGNOSIS: Cutaneous vasculitis; Schönlein-Henoch purpura; stasis dermatitis; acrocyanosis (clinically).

References

1. Bard JW, Winkelmann RK. Livedo vasculitis. Segmental hyalinizing vasculitis of the dermis. *Arch Dermatol* 1967;96:489–499.
2. Gibson LE. Cutaneous vasculitis: Approach to diagnosis and systemic associations. *Mayo Clin Proc* 1990;65:221–229.
3. Moreland LW, Ball GV. Cutaneous polyarteritis nodosa. *Am J Med* 1990;88:426–429.

MALIGNANT ANGIOENDOTHELIOMATOSIS (MAE)

Entry Author: J. T. Lie

SYNONYMS: Intravascular lymphomatosis; angiotropic lymphoma.

DEFINITION: MAE is an uncommon systemic lymphoproliferative disease of poor prognosis, characterized by the peculiar intravascular proliferation of malignant lymphoid cells in the skin, viscera, and central nervous system, usually without generalized lymphadenopathy.

GROSS FINDINGS: Those of a malignancy or a systemic disease of undetermined origin (before biopsies) that resembles a lymphoproliferative disorder or mimics vasculitis.

MICROSCOPIC FINDINGS: Microvascular and endovascular proliferation of large pleomorphic malignant lymphoid cells with irregular nuclei, prominent nucleoli, and frequent mitoses. The neoplastic cells are of B-lymphocyte lineage.

DIFFERENTIAL DIAGNOSIS: Other systemic malignancies; vasculitides, especially angiitis of the central nervous system.

References

1. Mori S et al. Cellular characteristics of neoplastic angioendotheliosis. An immunohistological marker study of 6 cases. *Virchows Arch Pathol Anat* 1985;407:167–175.
2. Wick MR et al. Reassessment of malignant "angioendotheliomatosis." Evidence in favor of its reclassification as "intravascular lymphomatosis." *Am J Surg Pathol* 1986;10:112–123.
3. Bhawan J. Angioendotheliomatosis proliferans systemisata: An angitropic neoplasm of lymphoid origin. *Semin Diagn Pathol* 1987;4:18–27.
4. Lie JT. Malignant angioendotheliomatosis (intravascular lymphomatosis) clinically simulating primary angiitis of the central nervous system. *Arthritis Rheum* 1992;35:831–834.
5. Glass J et al. Intravascular lymphomatosis. A systemic disease with neurologic manifestations. *Cancer* 1993;71:3156–3164.

MARFAN SYNDROME

Entry Author: J. T. Lie

DEFINITION: A heritable disorder of connective tissue, characterized by cardiovascular, ocular, and skeletal abnormalities with variable degrees of clinical expression; evidence of aortic root aneurysmal disease, with or without valvular insufficiency, is present in 60–80% patients; the same intrinsic defect of the aortic wall (medial degeneration) occurs less frequently in the coronary, pulmonary, and visceral arteries.

GROSS FINDINGS: The saccular or flask-shaped aneurysmal aortic wall is thinner and more fragile than normal, almost semi-translucent in appearance; the intimal surface is smooth, often shows multiple intimal tears or lacerations.

MICROSCOPIC FINDINGS: Medial degeneration ("cystic medionecrosis") consists of multifocal or diffuse disruption and loss of the musculoelastic lamellae with accumulation of acid mucopolysaccharides filling the acellular areas, which may appear vacuolated but are not true cysts nor is there evidence of true tissue necrosis.

REMARKS: In addition to the standard hematoxylin-eosin, all arterial sections should be routinely stained for elastin and acid mucopolysaccharides.

DIFFERENTIAL DIAGNOSIS: Medial degeneration of aging; idiopathic (Erdheim) medial degeneration and medial degeneration of other heritable connective tissue disorders, notably, Ehlers-Danlos syndrome type IV.

References

1. Roberts WC, Honig HS. The spectrum of cardiovascular disease in the Marfan syndrome: A clinico-morphologic study of 18 necropsy patients and comparison to 151 previously reported necropsy patients. *Am Heart J* 1982;104:115–135.
2. Schlatmann TJM, Becker AE. Pathogenesis of dissecting aneurysm of aorta. Comparative histopathologic study of significance of medial changes. *Am J Cardiol* 1977;39:21–26.
3. Hirst AE, Gore I. Editorial: Is cystic medionecrosis the cause of dissecting aortic aneurysm? *Circulation* 1976;53:915–916.
4. Takebayashi S et al. Ultrastructural and histochemical studies of vascular lesions in Marfan's syndrome, with report of 4 autopsy cases. *Acta Pathol Jpn* 1973;23:847–866.

MESENTERIC INFLAMMATORY VENO-OCCLUSIVE DISEASE (MIVOD)

Entry Author: J. T. Lie

SYNONYM: Idiopathic enterocoelic lymphocytic phlebitis.

DEFINITION: A peculiar, isolated, mesenteric and enterocoelic phlebitis, unassociated with a known underlying disorder that often presents clinically as ischemic bowel disease.

GROSS FINDINGS: Those of ischemic bowel associated with veno-occlusive disease.

MICROSCOPIC FINDINGS: Widespread inflammatory veno-occlusive disease in the mesentery and gut, the infiltrate may be predominantly lymphocytic, polymorphonuclear or granulomatous, and the phlebitis may be associated with occlusive myointimal hyperplasia of the affected veins and venules.

DIFFERENTIAL DIAGNOSIS: Other causes of ischemic bowel disease including thromboembolism and vasculitides.

References

1. Saraga EP, Costa J. Idiopathic entero-colic lymphocytic phlebitis. A cause of ischemic intestinal necrosis. *Am J Surg Pathol* 1989;13:303–308.
2. Haber MM, Burrell M, West AB. Enterocolic lymphocytic phlebitis. Clinical, radiologic, and pathologic features. *J Clin Gastroenterol* 1993;17:327–332.
3. Flaherty MJ, Lie JT, Haggitt RC. Mesenteric inflammatory veno-occlusive disease. A seldom recognized cause of intestinal ischemia. *Am J Surg Pathol* 1994;18:779–784.

MÖNCKEBERG'S (MEDIAL) SCLEROSIS

Entry Author: Alan G. Rose

SYNONYMS: Arteriosclerosis of Mönckeberg, age-related medial calcification of artery, Mönckeberg's sclerosis, Mönckeberg's medial calcification (calcinosis), arterial medial calcification.

DEFINITION: Dystrophic calcification of the hyalinized media of aged medium-sized artery.

GROSS FINDINGS: Pipestem-like thickened, calcified, rigid arteries.

MICROSCOPIC FINDINGS: The aged medium-sized artery shows dystrophic calcification within its hypocellular, hyalinized media. Because the condition is a medial change the intima is not affected by the process, and the lumen is not reduced by Mönckeberg's sclerosis.

SPECIAL PROCEDURES NEEDED FOR DIAGNOSIS: Radiography will confirm the calcification in excised arterial segments. Stains for phosphate, e.g., von Kossa or Alizarin-red stains will confirm the calcification histologically.

DIFFERENTIAL DIAGNOSIS: Calcification of intimal plaques in atherosclerosis.

KEY DIAGNOSTIC CRITERIA: Calcification, rarely ossification, within an aged arterial media. No intimal lesion forms a component of this entity.

POTENTIAL PITFALLS: Atherosclerosis and Mönckeberg's sclerosis often coexist in elderly persons; ischemia must not be attributed to Mönckeberg's sclerosis.

MONDOR'S DISEASE

Entry Author: J. T. Lie

DEFINITION: Superficial thrombophlebitis of the thoracoepigastric vein and its branches, usually unilateral, of unknown cause. It is a benign and self-limiting condition. The phlebitis resolves spontaneously within weeks or months.

GROSS FINDINGS: Linear cord-like lesions on the anterolateral chest wall in patients who are otherwise in good health, though some may have a history of minor trauma of undetermined significance that antedated the onset of phlebitis. Pain may be the only symptom.

MICROSCOPIC FINDINGS: Early biopsies reveal a nonspecific sclerosing endophlebitis and periphlebitis. Most biopsies done later in the course of the disease show a fibrous cord of the occluded veins.

DIFFERENTIAL DIAGNOSIS: Malignancy-induced skin puckering; malignancy-associated thrombophlebitis; subcutaneous lymphangitic metastases.

REMARKS: Mondor's disease is uncommon, with perhaps fewer than 250 cases reported in the world literature since its first description by Henri Mondor in 1939. The gender ratio, M/F = 3/1, and the age range is 30–60 years. There has been virtually no reports of this condition since 1965.

References

1. Bircher J et al. Mondor's disease, a vascular rarity. *Mayo Clin Proc* 1962;37:651–656.
2. Hogan GF. Mondor's disease. *Arch Intern Med* 1964;113:881–885.
3. Hatteland K, Kluge T. Mondor's disease. A subcutaneous form of periarteritis nodosa? *Acta Chir Scand* 1965;129:67–71.

MOYAMOYA DISEASE

Entry Author: J. T. Lie

DEFINITION: A peculiar cerebral vaso-occlusive disease of unknown etiology, initially described and defined in Japan, and it remains much more common there than in Western countries. The condition is quite often familial, and it may occur in infants and children as well as in adults, commonly under 50 years of age.

The term "moyamoya" was derived from the unusual angiographic appearance of profuse basal collateral vessels resembling "a puff of smoke floating in the air."

The disease typically presents as repetitive episodes of transient or irreversible cerebral ischemia or as a subarachnoid hemorrhage.

GROSS FINDINGS: The main features are angiographic evidence of bilateral stenosis of the internal carotid artery bifurcation and basal telangiectasias comprising dilated collateral lenticulostriate and thalamoperforating arteries.

MICROSCOPIC FINDINGS: The basic light microscopic features are occlusive intimal hyperplasia, tortuosity, and disorganization of the internal elastic lamina and medial fibrosis. Stainable lipids and inflammatory infiltrate are not present. Ultrastructural and immunohistochemical studies IgG, IgM-C3-positive granules on the endoplasmic reticulum of intimal vascular smooth muscle cells.

DIFFERENTIAL DIAGNOSIS: Atherosclerosis, vasculitis, fibromuscular dysplasia.

References

1. Suzuki J. *Moyamoya disease*. Berlin/Heidelberg. Springer-Verlag; 1986.
2. Takebayashi S et al. Ultrastructural studies of cerebral arteries and collateral vessels in moyamoya disease. *Stroke* 1984;15:728–732.
3. Bruno A et al. Cerebral infarction due to moyamoya disease in young adults. *Stroke* 1988;19:826–833.
4. Li B et al. A histological, ultrastructural and immunohistochemical study of superficial temporal arteries and middle meningeal arteries in moyamoya disease. *Acta Pathol Jpn* 1991;41:521–530.

MYCOTIC ANEURYSM

Entry Author: Alan G. Rose

SYNONYM: Infective aneurysm.

DEFINITION: An aneurysm of an artery, cardiac chamber, or vein graft that arises due to local weakening of the vascular structure by infection. A septic embolus is a common cause.

GROSS FINDINGS: The unruptured aneurysm is likely to be small, and the wall is apt to be discolored and yellowish in appearance due to the presence of infection and neutrophilic infiltration. Rupture is likely to occur before the aneurysm reaches a diameter of several centimeters.

MICROSCOPIC FINDINGS: The arterial wall will show local destruction, polymorphonuclear leukocytic infiltration, and bacterial or fungal proliferation. Luminal thrombosis is commonly seen within the aneurysm. Specific forms of infection, e.g., tuberculosis, may produce a granulomatous inflammatory response.

SPECIAL PROCEDURES NEEDED FOR DIAGNOSIS: Gram stain for bacteria, Ziehl-Neelsen stain for acid fast bacilli, and Grocott methenamine silver stain for fungi.

DIFFERENTIAL DIAGNOSIS: At times, particularly if antibiotics have been given, it may be difficult to distinguish treated septic from noninfective thromboemboli.

KEY DIAGNOSTIC CRITERIA: The development of one or more arterial aneurysms in a patient with a known source of sepsis (e.g., infective endocarditis). The aneurysm usually has inflammatory cells and the causative microorganism in its wall.

POTENTIAL PITFALLS: The infective nature of the aneurysm may be missed, particularly if antibiotics have been given. The condition may lead to fatalities (due to aneurysmal rupture) long after the causative infective endocarditis and infection in the aneurysmal wall have been eliminated.

NECROTIZING SARCOID GRANULOMATOSIS (NSG)

Entry Author: J. T. Lie

DEFINITION: An uncommon pulmonary granulomatous disease with vasculitis of unknown etiology that resembles sarcoidosis but its relationship with sarcoidosis is uncertain. First described in 1973 by Liebow, to date only about 100 additional cases have been reported in the literature. The prognosis is extremely favorable.

GROSS FINDINGS: The majority of patients with NSG have pulmonary symptoms but they tend not to have other clinical features of sarcoidosis. The lung lesions are usually multiple and bilateral with nodular chest radiographic appearance with or without signs of pleural effusion. Extrapulmonary lesions are extremely rare. Women outnumber men by about 2:1, with a mean age of 48 (range: 12 to 72 years).

MICROSCOPIC FINDINGS: There are three major elements: (a) granulomatous pneumonitis with many and often confluent sarcoid-like nodules; (b) variable extent of necrosis but usually less widespread and severe than in Wegener's granulomatosis; (c) vasculitis of the lung parenchymal arteries and veins, which may be granulomatous or necrotizing or both.

DIFFERENTIAL DIAGNOSIS: Classic pulmonary sarcoidosis; Wegener's granulomatosis; fungal or mycobacterial infection.

References

1. Liebow AA. The J. Burns Amberson lecture: Pulmonary angiitis and granulomatosis. *Am Rev Respir Dis* 1973;108:1–18.
2. Churg A et al. Necrotizing sarcoid granulomatosis. *Chest* 1979;406–413.
3. Lie JT. Classification of pulmonary angiitis and granulomatosis: Histopathologic perspectives. *Semin Respir Med* 1989;10:111–121.

NEOINTIMA

Entry Authors: Avrum I. Gotlieb and J. T. Lie

SYNONYMS: Intimal hyperplasia; diffuse intimal thickening; intimal thickening; intimal cushion.

DEFINITION: Fibrocellular proliferation as a healing-repair response of injured artery or vein, e.g., postendarterectomy; healing arterial dissection; postangioplasty; bypass vein grafts.

GROSS FINDINGS: Not distinguishable from the original, native intima.

MICROSCOPIC FINDINGS: Proliferation of vascular smooth muscle cells, commonly in a loose mucoid-appearing matrix rich in acid mucopolysaccharides, with or without surface endothelialization, scanty macrophages, and other inflammatory cells may be present; hypocellular sclerosis is the late change, with or without atherosclerosis.

SPECIAL PROCEDURES NEEDED FOR DIAGNOSIS: Immunofluorescence microscopy may be used to identify smooth muscle cells, macrophages, lymphocytes; trichrome stain to identify fibrous tissue, Alcian blue-PAS stain to identify mucopolysaccharides, and Movat's pentachrome or Verhoeff-Van Gieson stain will identify elastic tissue.

DIFFERENTIAL DIAGNOSIS: Native intimal hyperplasia and atherosclerosis.

KEY DIAGNOSTIC CRITERIA: Fibrocellular proliferation in a loose, mucoid matrix; known vascular injury, traumatic, surgical, or iatrogenic.

NEUROFIBROMATOSIS, VASCULOPATHY OF

Entry Author: J. T. Lie

SYNONYMS: von Recklinghausen disease; neurofibromatosis, type 1.

DEFINITION: Vascular lesions associated with neurofibromatosis, type 1.

GROSS FINDINGS: Occlusive arterial disease affecting most commonly the abdominal aorta and renal arteries in children and young adults, as a cause of renovascular hypertension and, occasionally, renal infarction; rarely, other visceral and peripheral arteries are affected with ischemic complications.

MICROSCOPIC FINDINGS: Three histologic types were described by Reubi in 1944: (a) Intimal proliferation of vascular smooth muscle cells. (b) Intimal proliferation associated with aneurysm formation. (c) Adventitial nodules.

DIFFERENTIAL DIAGNOSIS: Congenital abdominal coarctation; vasculitis.

References

1. Salyer WR, Salyer DC. The vascular lesions of neurofibromatosis. *Angiology* 1974;25:510–519.
2. Schürch W et al. Arterial hypertension and neurofibromatosis: Renal artery stenosis and coarctation of abdominal aorta. *Can Med Assoc J* 1975;113:879–885.
3. Elias DK et al. Renovascular hypertension complicating neurofibromatosis. *Am Surgeon* 1985;51: 97–106.

PHLEGMASIA ALBA DOLENS

Entry Author: J. T. Lie

SYNONYMS: Deep thrombophlebitis of the limbs; deep venous thrombosis.

DEFINITION: Thrombosis involving one or more deep calf veins of the limbs, with pallor of the affected limbs.

GROSS FINDINGS: Thrombosis usually originates in the venous valve pockets and often involves one or more perforating veins. It has the potential of causing pulmonary embolism, especially in the early stages before the thrombosis is firmly attached. Postphlebitic disease is a common late sequela.

MICROSCOPIC FINDINGS: Typical venous thrombosis with histologic features corresponding to the stages of thrombosis at the time of examination. True inflammatory reaction is absent.

Reference

1. Browse NL, Burnand KG, Thomas ML. *Diseases of the veins: Pathology, diagnosis and treatment.* London, Edward Arnold, 1988:278,475,477.

PHLEGMASIA CERULEA DOLENS

Entry Author: J. T. Lie

SYNONYM: Cyanotic ischemic thrombophlebitis.

DEFINITION: Extensive deep vein thrombosis, usually involving the common, external, and internal iliac veins.

GROSS FINDINGS: Edematous and cyanotic limb, covered by taut, shiny skin with small petechiae, blebs, or even gangrene. Gross dissection will show the extensive large pelvic vein thrombosis.

MICROSCOPIC FINDINGS: Extreme venous congestion and thrombosis is the hallmark. Arterial insufficiency, when present, is due to multiple factors including mechanical compression and vasospasm. Arterial thrombus is seldom found at post mortem study.

References

1. Browse NL, Burnand KG, Thomas ML. *Diseases of the veins: pathology, diagnosis and treatment.* London, Edward Arnold, 1988:278,475,477.
2. Juergens JL, Spittel JA Jr, Fairbairn JF II, eds. *Allen-Barker-Hines Peripheral Vascular Diseases, 5th ed.* Philadelphia, WB Saunders; 1980:741.

POLYARTERITIS NODOSA

Entry Author: J. T. Lie

SYNONYMS: Periarteritis nodosa; polyarteritis (classic and microscopic).

DEFINITION: Necrotizing vasculitis of medium-sized and small arteries, less commonly arterioles and only rarely venules. Involvement of the aorta and other elastic arteries is unknown; involvement of pulmonary arteries is infrequent. Focal, segmental necrotizing glomerulonephritis with or without concomitant arteriolar vasculitis is considered a renal-limited variant, or as the microscopic form of polyarteritis.

GROSS FINDINGS: In the classic form of polyarteritis, virtually any and usually multiple organs and tissues may be involved. In descending order in adults are the kidneys, muscles, and nerves, viscera, heart, and others. The heart is the most commonly involved organ in infantile and childhood polyarteritis. Classic nodular lesions are seldom seen but microaneurysms may be discernible.

MICROSCOPIC FINDINGS: Focal segmental necrotizing vasculitis with fibrinoid necrosis is the histologic hallmark of acute or active phase lesions, together with a mixed-cell infiltrate with prominent macrophages and a propensity for microaneurysm formation. The healing or healed lesions are characterized by vascular wall sclerosis with less intense infiltrate which is almost entirely mononuclear. The characteristic and diagnostic feature of polyarteritis is coexisting acute necrotizing lesions and healing/healed lesion, or with a segment of normal artery in different tissues or different parts of the same tissue.

Reference

1. Lie JT. Systemic and isolated vasculitis. A rational approach to classification and pathologic diagnosis (review). *Pathol Ann* 1989;24(Part 1):25–114.

POPLITEAL ARTERY
ENTRAPMENT SYNDROME

Entry Author: J. T. Lie

SYNONYM: Entrapment of the popliteal artery.

DEFINITION: Compression of the popliteal artery resulting from an anomaly where the artery assumes a position medial to the medial head of the gastrocnemius muscle. With motion of the leg, the artery becomes entrapped by the tendon of the abnormally inserted muscle with the ensuing ischemia to the affected limb.

GROSS FINDINGS: Signs of limb ischemia with angiographic evidence of partial or complete occlusion of the proximal popliteal artery, and identification of abnormally inserted muscle at exploratory surgery.

MICROSCOPIC FINDINGS: Nonspecific histologic changes of varying degrees of intimal and adventitial fibrosis with or without superimposed thrombosis.

REMARKS: This is an uncommon syndrome, first described in 1965, with probably fewer than 100 reported cases in the literature up until 1994.

DIFFERENTIAL DIAGNOSIS: Arteriosclerosis obliterans; thrombosis; thromboangiitis obliterans (Buerger's disease); adventitial cystic disease.

References

1. Collins PS et al. Popliteal artery entrapment: An evolving syndrome. *J Vasc Surg* 1989;10:484–490.
2. Zünd G, Brunner U. Surgical aspects of popliteal artery entrapment syndrome: 26 years of experience with 26 legs. *VASA* 1995;24:29–33.

PRIMARY ANGIITIS OF THE CENTRAL NERVOUS SYSTEM (CNS)

Entry Author: J. T. Lie

SYNONYMS: Granulomatous angiitis of the CNS; isolated angiitis of the CNS.

DEFINITION: Unless otherwise specified, angiitis of the CNS refers to primary angiitis of the CNS (PACNS). PACNS is unassociated with a known underlying systemic disease or infection, seldom (<5%) has extracranial involvement and usually has a poor prognosis. The diagnosis may be suspected clinically by a process of elimination and angiographically by the characteristic (but not specific) string of beads or tubular stenosis. Brain biopsy is required for confirmation of diagnosis.

GROSS FINDINGS: Those of focal or diffuse cerebral infarcts.

MICROSCOPIC FINDINGS: The histopathology of PACNS is typically focal and segmental (therefore, a single, small, negative biopsy does not rule out the disease), and typically a granulomatous (giant cell) angiitis of the leptomeningeal and cortical small blood vessels, which may coexist, side-by-side with normal blood vessels or blood vessels with necrotizing (PAN type) or lymphocytic angiitis. Thrombosis in the cerebral microvasculature is common in PACNS.

References

1. Lie JT. Primary (granulomatous) angiitis of the central nervous system: A clinicopathologic analysis of 15 new cases and a review of the literature (review). *Hum Pathol* 1992;23:164–171.
2. Calabrese LH et al. Primary angiitis of the central nervous system: diagnostic criteria and clinical approach (review). *Cleve Clin J Med* 1992;59:293–306.

PSEUDOXANTHOMA ELASTICUM

Entry Author: J. T. Lie

SYNONYM: Grönblad-Strandberg syndrome

DEFINITION: An autosomal recessive heritable systemic disease characterized by a widespread degeneration of elastic tissue fibers affecting primarily the ocular, cutaneous, and cardiovascular systems.

GROSS FINDINGS: Angioid streaks in the fundi and skin lesions aid clinical diagnosis of the disease, usually presenting in adolescence or early childhood, with a slight female predominance. The patient may present with gastrointestinal hemorrhage.

MICROSCOPIC FINDINGS: Nonspecific, and may include premature occlusive fibroelastosis of the affected and blood vessels, resembling hypertensive arteriosclerosis, with or without microcalcification. The diagnosis is usually reinforced or confirmed by extra-cardiac and extravascular findings.

References

1. Goodman RM et al. Pseudoxanthoma elasticum: a clinical and histopathological study. *Medicine* 1963; 42:297–334.
2. Bardsley JL, Koehler PR. Pseudoxanthoma elasticum: Angiographic manifestations in abdominal vessels. *Radiology* 1969;93:559–562.
3. Mendelsohn G et al. Cardiovascular manifestations of Pseudoxanthoma elasticum. *Arch Pathol Lab Med* 1978;102:298–302.
4. Stehbens WE, Lie JT, eds. *Vascular Pathology*. London, Chapman & Hall; 1995:153–154.

PULMONARY PLEXOGENIC ARTERIOPATHY (PPA)

Entry Author: J. T. Lie

SYNONYM: Primary pulmonary hypertension.

DEFINITION: Pulmonary plexogenic arteriopathy (PPA) refers to a unique and characteristic type of hypertensive pulmonary vascular disease that was initially recognized in patients with congenital heart disease but also occurs as an idiopathic or primary form or in association with other recognized causes (see below). The six morphologic types of PPA: medial hypertrophy, cellular intimal proliferation, concentric laminar intimal fibrosis, plexiform lesions, dilation lesions, and arteritis with fibrinoid necrosis are indicative of progressively more severe PPA and correspond with the Heath-Edwards Grade 1–6 lesions, respectively.

GROSS FINDINGS: In longstanding and severe pulmonary hypertension, typical atherosclerotic plaques may be present in the elastic and larger muscular pulmonary arteries. The normally inconspicuous small peripheral muscular arteries become more prominent, but the most striking gross finding is the pulmonary artery, right atrial and ventricular dilation, and hypertrophy with the right ventricular wall thickness approaching or equal that of the left, and leftward flattening of the ventricular septum in transverse sections of the heart.

MICROSCOPIC FINDINGS: The histologic evaluation of all hypertensive pulmonary vascular disease must include (in addition to H&E) elastic stain sections. Medial hypertrophy is the most common form and earliest manifestation of PPA; the medial thickening appears roughly proportional to pressure and resistance in the pulmonary circulation, normally in the range of 4–5% of the external diameter may increase to ≥20%. Cellular intimal proliferation of myofibroblasts (altered vascular smooth muscle cells) may be associated with concentric laminar intimal fibrosis and obstruct the vessel lumen almost completely. Plexiform lesions, the hallmark of PPA, is usually located in a pulmonary arterial branch shortly after its origin from a larger artery, ranging in size from 200 μm to 400 μm but may be smaller. The classic form consists of a plexus of capillary-like small blood vessels within a focal dilation of the arterial branch and separated by proliferating myofibroblasts/smooth muscle cells. The media is scanty or absent in part/in whole and the elastic laminae are rarely intact. Distal to the plexiform lesion, the arterial branch together with its ramifications is thin-walled and becomes dilation lesions of PPA. Arteritis with fibrinoid necrosis occurs in sustained severe pulmonary hypertension, characteristically observed in a branch close to its origin from a larger artery and over a short distance. In all pulmonary hypertension of varying severity, more than one Heath-Edwards grade of lesions may be observed and it is the highest grade observed that determines the histologic grade of hypertension.

REMARKS: Plexogenic arteriopathy in pulmonary hypertension includes but is not synonymous with plexiform lesions that occur only in the final stages of pulmonary hypertension and are usually considered irreversible. PPA is essentially a disease of peripheral (muscular) pulmonary arteries and pulmonary veins are usually not involved. PPA is not exclusive to primary pulmonary hypertension and occurs in a variety of conditions of different causes (see Table 1). Thrombotic or thromboembolic lesions are common in adult patients with PPA due to congenital cardiac shunts or in its primary form and found increasingly with age in various forms of pulmonary hypertension. They complicate patterns of PPA rather than being an integral part of PPA in pulmonary hypertension.

TABLE 1. *Causes of Pulmonary Plexogenic Arteriopathy**

1. Congenital heart disease with a left-to-right shunt:
    atrial septal defect
    ventricular septal defect (VSD)
    atrioventricular septal defect
    transposition of great arteries with VSD
    truncus arteriosus
    patent ductus arteriosus
    aorto-pulmonary window
2. Congenital heart disease without shunt: transposition of great arteries without VSD
3. Acquired cardiac left-to-right shunt
    surgical shunt for tetralogy of Fallot
4. Hepatic disease with portal hypertension
5. Schistosomiasis
6. Anorexigens (dietary pulmonary hypertension)
7. Spanish toxic-oil-syndrome
8. Rheumatic connective tissue diseases, including eosinophilia-myalgia (l-tryptophan toxicity)
    syndrome
9. Intravenous cocaine drug abuse
10. Primary (idiopathic) pulmonary hypertension

*Modified and expanded from Wagenenvoort CA, Mooi WJ. *Biopsy pathology of the pulmonary vasculature.* London, Chapman & Hall, 1989: 1997.

Vasoconstriction is considered a key factor in the pathogenesis of PPA, but how constriction of pulmonary arteries is brought about remains unresolved.

References

1. Hatano S, Strasser T eds. *Primary pulmonary hypertension: Report of Committee, World Health Organization.* Geneva, 1975.
2. Wagenvoort CA, Wagenvoort N. *Pathology of pulmonary hypertension.* New York: John Wiley; 1977.
3. Wagenvoort CA. Plexogenic arteriopathy. *Thorax* 1994;49:S39–S45.

RAYNAUD'S PHENOMENON, PRIMARY AND SECONDARY

Entry Author: J. T. Lie

SYNONYMS: Raynaud's disease; Raynaud's syndrome.

DEFINITION: A reversible vasospastic disorder of unknown cause, seen principally in young healthy women (F/M = 4/1), usually between 15 and 45 years of age, who show episodic digital ischemia from an exaggerated reaction to cold in otherwise normal digital vessels. The cause may be unknown (primary) or related to an underlying systemic disease (secondary).

GROSS FINDINGS: The reversible vasospasm is characterized by blanching or cyanosis of the digits (usually the fingers and toes in about 40%) on exposure to cold, and a red, reactive hyperemia phase may occur when the attack ends. The arteriograms are usually normal but may show stenosis or occlusion in chronic and severe cases. Trophic changes of the digits occur in less than 10%. Ulceration and gangrene, when present, strongly suggest an underlying connective tissue disease.

MICROSCOPIC FINDINGS: Digital arteries, and only rarely arterioles, are involved. In mild cases, there are no pathologic changes. In severe cases, there may be intimal hyperplasia adventitial fibrosis and thrombosis, resulting in stenosis or occlusion of the digital arteries. Inflammatory infiltrate is absent.

REMARKS: Endothelin-1 (ET-1) is a novel endothelium-derived vasoactive peptide with the most potent vasoconstrictive effect known to date. Plasma ET-1 immunoreactivity levels increase markedly in patients with Raynaud's phenomenon just after immersion of their hands in cold water. The reported prevalence of Raynaud's phenomenon in the general population ranges from 4.6–30%. A recent comparative study (Maricq) calculated a prevalence of 5.0% in a moderate climate and 16.8% in a cold climate. Secondary Raynaud's phenomenon is associated with a variety of underlying systemic disorders.

Common Causes:
1. Connective tissue diseases (e.g., scleroderma and CREST)
2. Arterial occlusion (e.g., Buerger's disease, thromboemboli)
3. Drug therapy (e.g., ergot, methysergide, chemotherapy)
4. Carpal tunnel or thoracic outlet syndromes
5. Traumatic vasospastic disease (e.g., vibrational tool)

Uncommon Causes:
1. Cryoglobulinemias
2. Cold agglutinins
3. Polycythemia
4. Vasculitis
5. Paraneoplastic syndrome

References

1. Birnstingl M. The Raynaud syndrome (review). *Postgrad Med J* 1971;47:297–310.
2. Coffman JD. *Raynaud's phenomenon.* New York, Oxford University Press; 1989.
3. Coffman JD. Raynaud's phenomenon: An update. *Hypertension* 1991;17:593–602.
4. Maricq HR et al. Geographic variation in the prevalence of Raynaud's phenomenon: Charleston, SC, USA, vs. Tarentaise, Savoie, France. *J Rheumatol* 1993;20:70–76.

RENOVASCULAR HYPERTENSION

Entry Author: J. T. Lie

DEFINITION: Systemic hypertension due to renal arterial or parenchymal diseases.

GROSS FINDINGS: Changes of hypertension in general and with angiographically definable extra- or intra-renal vascular/glomerular lesions.

MICROSCOPIC FINDINGS: The histopathology depends on the vascular/glomerular lesions in question, which may be one or more of the following:
1. Arteriosclerosis and atherosclerosis
     stenosis or occlusion (including ostial lesions)
     aneurysm and/or arterial dissection
     thromboembolism including atheroembolism
2. Fibromuscular dysplasia
     stenosis or occlusion
     aneurysm and/or arterial dissection
     thromboembolism
3 Takayasu arteritis
     stenosis, less commonly aneurysm
     arterial dissection or perforation
4. Hereditary and rare disorders
     Ehlers-Danlos syndrome
     Marfan syndrome
     neurofibromatosis, type 1
     angiodysplasia
5. Renal parenchymal disease

Reference

1. Lüscher TF, Lie JT, Sheps SG. In: Lüscher TF, Kaplan NM, eds. *Renovascular and renal parenchymatous hypertension.* Berlin, Springer-Verlag; 1992:73–106.

SCHÖNLEIN-HENOCH SYNDROME
(OR PURPURA)

Entry Author: J. T. Lie

SYNONYMS: Anaphylactoid purpura; Henoch-Schönlein purpura

DEFINITION: This is the most common form of vasculitis in children and adolescents but it also occurs in adults, characterized by a purpuric skin eruption, fever, arthralgia, and visceral symptoms, and it has a seasonal incidence that peaks in winter. Renal involvement occurs in one third to one half of patients.

The eponym *Schönlein-Henoch* is preferred to *Henoch-Schönlein* because Schönlein's description of the disease (1837) predated that of Henoch (1874).

GROSS FINDINGS: Skin purpura; hemorrhagic bowel and/or kidney; lung hemorrhage.

MICROSCOPIC FINDINGS: The extrarenal lesions are essentially a small vessel necrotizing vasculitis, histologically indistinguishable from small vessel forms of polyarteritis. The renal lesions are focal proliferative or necrotizing glomerulonephritis. IgA is the most common type of immune deposit detectable in the affected tissue. Capillaritis and lung hemorrhage also occur.

DIFFERENTIAL DIAGNOSIS: Other forms of small vessel vasculitis.

References

1. Cream JJ et al. Schönlein-Henoch purpura in the adult. A study of 77 adults with anaphylactoid or Schönlein-Henoch purpura. *Q J Med* 1970;39:461–484.
2. Meadow SR et al. Schönlein-Henoch nephritis. *Q J Med* 1972;41:241–258.
3. Lie JT. Illustrated histopathologic classification criteria for selected vasculitis syndromes. American College of Rheumatology Subcommittee on Classification of Vasculitis. *Arthritis Rheum* 1990;33: 1074–1087.
4. Mills JA. The American College of Rheumatology 1990 criteria for the classification of Henoch-Schönlein purpura. *Arthritis Rheum* 1990;33:1114–1121.

SEGMENTAL MEDIOLYTIC ARTERIOPATHY

Entry Author: J. T. Lie

SYNONYMS: Segmental mediolytic arteritis; arterial mediolysis.

DEFINITION: A peculiar noninflammatory lesion of the visceral arteries and, rarely, coronary arteries, that is characterized by focal lytic changes (vacuolation, mucoid degeneration) of the arterial wall that may result in arterial wall hemorrhage or dissection and thrombosis.

GROSS FINDINGS: Changes of ischemic bowel disease, visceral or myocardial necrosis/infarction associated with (or related to) arterial dissection, aneurysm formation, and rupture.

MICROSCOPIC FINDINGS: Focal, segmental, medial lytic changes (vacuolation, mucoid degeneration) of the arteries that may result in arterial wall hemorrhage or dissection and thrombosis, and ischemic necrosis of organs subserved by the affected arteries.

REMARKS: The pathogenesis of this arterial lesion is unknown and the two opposing views are (a) inappropriate vasospastic response to shock or severe hypoxemia, and (b) a variant of arterial fibromuscular dysplasia.

References

1. Slavin RE. Segmental mediolytic arteritis. A clinicopathologic and ultrastructural study of two cases. *Am J Surg Pathol* 1989;13:558–568.
2. Lie JT. Segmental mediolytic arteritis. Not an arteritis but a variant of arterial fibromuscular dysplasia (editorial). *Arch Pathol Lab Med* 1992;116:238–241.
3. Leu HJ. Spontaneous dissecting aneurysms of arteries of muscular composition due to mucoid media degeneration (mediolytic arteriopathy) (German). *Pathology* 1993;14:325–329..
4. Slavin RE et al. Segmental arterial mediolysis: A precursor to fibromuscular dysplasia? *Modern Pathol* 1995;8:287–294.

SNEDDON SYNDROME

Entry Author: J. T. Lie

DEFINITION: An unusual neurocutaneous disorder first described by Sneddon in 1965. The combination of ischemic cerebrovascular disease and livido reticularis (racemora) is known as *Sneddon syndrome*. It is characterized by a violaceous network patterning of the skin and a wide variety of neurologic symptoms ranging from transient ischemic attacks, sensory dysfunctions, seizures, psychiatric disturbances, or intellectual impairment to full-blown ischemic stroke. Sneddon syndrome is now considered as a manifestation of the antiphospholipid syndrome.

GROSS FINDINGS: Cutaneous lesions described above and changes reflecting cerebrovascular disease.

MICROSCOPIC FINDINGS: Thrombotic, small and medium-sized, arterial and venous vaso-occlusive disease of the brain (leptomeningeal and parenchymal) and skin (most often at the dermis-subcutis boundary). The vaso-occlusion may be associated with a variable intensity of mixed-cell infiltrate but no true vasculitis has been observed.

REMARKS: About 50% of patients with Sneddon syndrome are hypertensive. The expanded Sneddon syndrome may include (in addition to the classic neurocutaneous disorder) cardiac pathology (vaso-occlusive and valvular heart disease), visceral and peripheral arterial and venous thromboses, thrombocytopenia, recurrent fetal loss, and pulmonary thromboembolism and hypertension.

References

1. Kalashnikova LA et al. Sneddon's syndrome: Cardiac pathology and antiphospholopid antibodies. *Clin Exp Rheumatol* 1991;9:357–361.
2. Zelger B et al. Life history of cutaneous vascular lesions in Sneddon's syndrome (see comments). *Hum Pathol* 1992;23:668–675.
3. Hughson MD et al. Thrombotic cerebral arteriopathy in patients with the antiphospholipid syndrome. *Modern Pathol* 1993;6:644–653.

SUPERIOR MEDIASTINAL SYNDROME

Entry Author: Alan G. Rose

SYNONYMS: Thoracic outlet disease; thrombosis or extreme compression of the superior vena cava; superior vena cava syndrome.

DEFINITION: A syndrome resulting from obstruction to venous drainage into the thorax via the superior mediastinum.

GROSS FINDINGS: The patient has congestive features in the face, neck and upper limbs and chest (i.e., the upper half of the body) due to interference with proper venous drainage into the chest from these sites. Venous distention is noted in the areas concerned. Important collaterals include the azygous vein, the internal mammary veins, the lateral thoracic route, and the vertebral route.

MICROSCOPIC FINDINGS: Histological examination of a biopsy from the upper half of the body reveals congestion and possible edema of the affected tissues, and rarely, tissue necrosis.

SPECIAL PROCEDURES NEEDED FOR DIAGNOSIS: Lymph node biopsy from the neck or mediastinum may reveal the cause, e.g., lymphoma or metastatic carcinoma. Mediastinal fibrosis may also be detected on biopsy.

DIFFERENTIAL DIAGNOSIS: Generalized edema due to congestive heart failure should not be confused with the superior mediastinal syndrome. Constrictive pericarditis may also cause obstruction of the superior vena cava as, too, may an intrathoracic aneurysm.

KEY DIAGNOSTIC CRITERIA: Edema, congestion, and venous distention in the drainage distribution of the superior vena cava.

POTENTIAL PITFALLS: Mediastinal fibrosis produces compression rather than thrombosis of the superior vena cava.

SYPHILITIC AORTITIS

Entry Author: J. T. Lie

DEFINITION: A tertiary form of cardiovascular syphilis affecting typically the ascending and descending thoracic aorta.

GROSS FINDINGS: The aorta is usually aneurysmal, may be associated with aortic insufficiency and/or involvement of the coronary ostia, and the proximal ends of coronary arteries. The age-related atherosclerosis often will obscure the classic "tree bark" wrinkled appearance of the thickened intima; calcification of the aorta, often visible radiologically, occurs in about two thirds of the cases.

MICROSCOPIC FINDINGS: It is typically a chronic mesaortitis with multifocal patchy destruction of the medial musculoelastic lamellae and replacement by vascularized scar tissue. Endarteritis obliterans commonly involved the vasa vasorum with lymphoplasmacytic infiltrate and adventitial fibrosis. Microgummas may be found in the media in about 20% of cases, but giant cells and the spirochetes are seen only very rarely, if at all.

REMARKS: The morphologic changes of syphilitic aortitis are characteristic but not specific and positive serology is required for confirmation of diagnosis. As is in all other instances of the histopathologic evaluation of the vascular lesions, elastin stain sections are mandatory.

DIFFERENTIAL DIAGNOSIS: Atherosclerosis; primary (idiopathic) lymphoplasmacytic aortitis; Takayasu aortitis.

References

1. Heggtveit HA. Syphilitic aortitis. A clinicopathologic autopsy study of 100 cases. *Circulation* 1964; 29:346–355.
2. Heggtveit HA. In: Silver MD, ed. *Cardiovascular pathology, 2nd ed.* New York, Churchill Livingstone; 1991:307–340.

TAKAYASU ARTERITIS

Entry Author: J. T. Lie

SYNONYMS: Aortic arch syndrome; aortitis syndrome; idiopathic aortitis; nonspecific aortoarteritis; primary aortitis/arteritis; occlusive thromboarteriopathy; pulseless disease; Takayasu's disease.

DEFINITION: Takayasu arteritis is a chronic inflammatory disease of the aorta and its aortic arch and other major branches and of the elastic pulmonary arteries. It occurs most commonly in women of reproductive age (15–45 years), with an overall gender ratio of F/M = 8/1. It has a worldwide distribution but with greatest prevalence in the Orient, Latin America, and Eastern Europe.

GROSS FINDINGS: The four anatomic types of involvement are: (I) aortic arch and arch vessels; (II) thoracoabdominal aorta; (III) the entire aorta; (IV) pulmonary arteries. Although it is classically known as a stenotic lesion, aortic aneurysmal disease and aortic insufficiency occur in 15–30% of cases.

MICROSCOPIC FINDINGS: Acute or active phase is characterized by a granulomatous panarteritis with or without identifiable giant cells in the lymphoplasmacytic infiltrate, morphologically indistinguishable from extracranial giant cell arteritis. Healed lesions show progressive intimal and adventitial fibrosis difficult to distinguish from end-stage arteriosclerosis.

REMARKS: Type III Takayasu arteritis is an important and common cause of renovascular hypertension affecting adolescents in the Orient and Southeast Asia.

References

1. Lie JT. Takayasu arteritis. In: Churg A, Churg J, eds. *Systemic vasculitides.* New York: Igaku Shoin; 1991:159–179.
2. Numano F, Lee KT, Hong CY (eds). Takayasu arteritis. *Heart Vessels* 1992;Suppl 7:1–179.

VARICOSE VEIN

Entry Author: Alan G. Rose

SYNONYMS: Varix; varices; varicocele; varicosities; venous ectasia.

DEFINITION: Dilation and tortuosity of a segment of a vein due to an increase in the pressure of blood within the vein, e.g., due to venous valvular incompetence.

GROSS FINDINGS: The vein appears excessively dilated and tortuous due to elongation. The dilation may be irregular with nodular zones of greater ectasia. The venous diameter is so increased that the venous valves are not able to maintain competence. Esophageal varices are located in the submucosa of the lower end of the esophagus.

MICROSCOPIC FINDINGS: The affected vein has a greatly dilated lumen and the intima may show fibrous thickening with increased elastin (phlebosclerosis).

SPECIAL PROCEDURES NEEDED FOR DIAGNOSIS: In order to demonstrate esophageal varices at autopsy the esophagus should be everted, the lower end tied with a circumferential ligature and the blood milked down the esophagus to fill the varices.

DIFFERENTIAL DIAGNOSIS: Varicose veins are not easily confused with other conditions. Esophageal varices are maximal at the lower end of the esophagus in patients with portal hypertension due to cirrhosis. The varices may become ulcerated. This ulceration may occur in a similar situation to that of a reflux ulcer.

KEY DIAGNOSTIC CRITERIA: Dilation and tortuosity of a vein, particularly involving the veins of the lower limb, gastroesophageal junction, or pampiniform plexus.

POTENTIAL PITFALLS: Varices of the esophagus may be missed at autopsy unless special dissection procedures are used (see above).

VENO-OCCLUSIVE DISEASE

Entry Author: J. T. Lie

DEFINITION: A predominantly or exclusively venous and venular fibrous occlusive disease occurring most commonly in the lungs and liver, of unknown cause in some cases (primary) and, in others, associated with toxins and drugs, irradiation, and as a graft-versus-host reaction, especially after allograft bone marrow transplantation (secondary).

GROSS FINDINGS: In the lungs, the gross changes are those of hypertensive pulmonary vascular disease, including right ventricular hypertrophy and dilation; in the liver, the gross changes are congestion with or without fibrosis and evidence of both old and recent venous thrombosis and sclerosis.

MICROSCOPIC FINDINGS: In both lung and liver, venous and venular obstruction is caused by progressive intimal fibrosis, with "arterialization" changes and later, complete luminal occlusion. At the early stage, there may be initially phlebitis and venulitis and, in the late stage, there is usually some secondary occlusive arterial changes and dilated lymphatics, as well as plentiful hemosiderin-laden macrophages.

REMARKS: As in studying all vascular diseases, it is mandatory that elastic stain be routinely used in addition to the hematoxylin-eosin stain.

DIFFERENTIAL DIAGNOSIS: In the lungs, other causes of primary or secondary pulmonary hypertension and, in the liver, other causes of hepatic and/or portal vein thrombosis (e.g., Budd-Chiari syndrome, and antiphospholipid syndrome).

References

1. Wagenvoort CA, Wagenvoort N. The pathology of pulmonary veno-occlusive disease. *Virchows Arch Pathol Anat* 1974;364:69–79.
2. Ludwig J et al. Classification of hepatic venous outflow obstruction: Ambiguous terminology of the Budd-Chiari syndrome. *Mayo Clin Proc* 1990;65:51–55.

VENOUS GANGRENE

Entry Author: Alan G. Rose

SYNONYMS: Infarction due to (total) venous obstruction.

DEFINITION: Venous gangrene is a form of gangrene resulting from severe venous obstruction which grossly impedes the blood flow through the tissue in question but allows arterial blood to enter the organ for a period during the evolving infarct.

GROSS FINDINGS: The infarcted organ is intensely congested and hemorrhagic. Venous occlusion may be due to torsion (e.g., of the gut mesentery, the ovary or testis).

MICROSCOPIC FINDINGS: The infarcted tissue is stuffed with extravasated erythrocytes following the subtotal venous obstruction which brought the local circulation to an end (whereas the arteries continued to pump blood into the organ) and finally led to infarction.

DIFFERENTIAL DIAGNOSIS: Infarction due to arterial occlusion usually is not as hemorrhagic as infarction due to total venous obstruction. The central vein of the adrenal gland has noncircumferential smooth muscle to prevent the possibility of venous gangrene in this vital organ. Hemorrhagic infarction of the adrenal gland in meningococcal septicemia due to a Schwartzman-type reaction may mimic venous gangrene.

KEY DIAGNOSTIC CRITERIA: Hemorrhagic infarction of a tissue or organ resulting from total or near total venous obstruction that brings the blood supply to a halt. Microscopic features of infarction are associated with massive extravasation of erythrocytes.

POTENTIAL PITFALLS: Autolysis of the bowel may yield a discolored appearance that may be confused with venous infarction. Venous infarction of the brain is usually secondary to local sepsis, dehydration or trauma.

VENOUS THROMBOSIS

Entry Author: Alan G. Rose

SYNONYMS: Phlebothrombosis, thrombophlebitis.

DEFINITION: Thrombosis occurring within a vein.

GROSS FINDINGS: Fibrin-platelet head of thrombus starts initially within a venous valve pocket and the thrombus extends to occlude the venous segment. More proximal extension of the original thrombus consists of propagated red thrombus. The white thrombus distends the vein and has a dry appearance.

MICROSCOPIC FINDINGS: A mass of fibrin with entrapped platelets constitutes the head of the thrombus. Propagated thrombus consists of numerous erythrocytes entrapped in fibrin. Signs or organization of the thrombus may be present and the presence of a noninfected thrombus per se invokes an inflammatory reaction in the wall of the vein. This response may not be detected in deep venous thrombosis (phlebothrombosis) but may be clinically evident in thrombosis of a superficial vein (thrombophlebitis). In addition, an inflammatory process involving the wall of a vein may lead to venous thrombosis, and this is also termed *thrombophlebitis.*

SPECIAL PROCEDURES NEEDED FOR DIAGNOSIS: Martius scarlet-blue stain for fibrin. Gram stain to demonstrate microorganisms.

DIFFERENTIAL DIAGNOSIS: Phlebothrombosis and thrombophlebitis have been artificially separated (see above). True primary thrombophlebitis is a rare event. Thrombophlebitis migrans refers to multiple, repetitive episodes of thrombosis of peripheral arm or leg veins.

KEY DIAGNOSTIC CRITERIA: Mass of fibrin, platelets, and erythrocytes within a vein.

POTENTIAL PITFALLS: Thromboembolism may lead to a vein which is found to be devoid of thrombus. The degree of adhesion of a recent thrombus to the vein wall is an unreliable criterion for distinguishing it from a postmortem clot, because both may be quite adherent.

WEGENER'S GRANULOMATOSIS

Entry Author: J. T. Lie

DEFINITION: A necrotizing granulomatous disease of unknown etiology that, in its classic form, affects the upper and lower respiratory tract and the kidneys but various other organs may also be involved infrequently. A limited form of the disease, without renal involvement, has also been described. About 75% of the classic form are c-ANCA (anti-neutrophil cytoplasmic antibody) positive.

GROSS FINDINGS: As determined by the location of the disease and extent of involvement.

MICROSCOPIC FINDINGS: The extrarenal lesions of Wegener's granulomatosis have three basic histopathologic components: a geographic pattern tissue necrosis often with microabscesses; granulomatous inflammation with giant cells; and vasculitis. All three components are present in about 40–60% of the pulmonary lesions and only 20–30% of extrapulmonary lesions (e.g., nasal, sinus, and orbital biopsies). Capillaritis occurs in up to 30% of pulmonary lesions and may be the only biopsy abnormality. The renal lesion is typically a focal segmental necrotizing glomerulonephritis with or without extraglomerular vasculitis.

DIFFERENTIAL DIAGNOSIS: Churg-Strauss syndrome and other pulmonary angiitides and granulomatose; granulomatous infectious diseases.

References

1. Lie JT. Systemic and isolated vasculitis. A rational approach to classification and pathologic diagnosis (review). *Pathol Annual* 1989;24(Part 1):25–114.
2. Lie JT. Classification of pulmonary angiitis and granulomatosis: Histopathologic perspectives. *Semin Resp Med* 1989;10:111–121.

WILLIAMS SYNDROME

Entry Author: J. T. Lie

SYNONYM: Williams-Beuren syndrome

DEFINITION: Supravalvular aortic stenosis and mental retardation associated with a typical facie in children 1 month to 15 years of age at time of diagnosis.

GROSS FINDINGS: Peripheral arteriopathy and pulmonary artery stenosis associated with supravalvular aortic stenosis.

MICROSCOPIC FINDINGS: Arterial medial hypertrophy and intimal fibrosis without an inflammatory component or calcification; mosaic pattern of dysplastic musculoelastic lamellae of the aortic wall.

DIFFERENTIAL DIAGNOSIS: Idiopathic arterial calcification of infancy; fibromuscular dysplasia in children and infants.

References

1. O'Connor WN et al. Supravalvular aortic stenosis\Clinical and pathologic observations in six patients. *Arch Pathol Lab Med* 1985;109:179–185.
2. Zalstein E et al. Spectrum of cardiovascular anomalies in Williams-Beuren syndrome. *Pediatr Cardiol* 1991;12:219–223.
3. Rein AJJT et al. Generalized arteriopathy in Williams syndrome: An intravascular ultrasound study. *J Am Coll Cardiol* 1993;21:1727–1730.

Section 4

Diseases of the Pericardium and Epicardium

Section Editor: Jagdish W. Butany
Editorial Assistance: Malcolm D. Silver and Francesca V. Lobo

CHYLOUSPERICARDIUM

Entry Author: Jagdish W. Butany

DEFINITION: The accumulation of chylous fluid in the pericardial sac. Usually idiopathic but may be secondary to surgery or trauma to the thoracic duct.

GROSS FINDINGS: Accumulation of milky, viscous fluid in the pericardial sac.

MICROSCOPIC FINDINGS: Nonspecific. The parietal and visceral pericardium may be mildly thickened and the lining mesothelial cells flattened and stretched. The lining layer may show the accumulation of macrophages, many of which have a foamy appearance. The surrounding tissue may show focal areas of chronic inflammation. Marginal areas may show fibrous adhesions.

SPECIAL PROCEDURES NEEDED FOR DIAGNOSIS: Echocardiography and demonstration of localized/general accumulation of fluid. Aspiration of pericardial fluid.

DIFFERENTIAL DIAGNOSIS: Pericardial cysts; acquired or congenital.

KEY DIAGNOSTIC CRITERIA: Accumulation of milky fluid in the pericardial space, with/without history of surgery or trauma.

CONGENITAL ABSENCE OF PERICARDIUM

Entry Author: Jagdish W. Butany

DEFINITION: Partial or complete absence of the parietal pericardium. Partial absence may result in pleuropericardial defects. Approximately 1/3 of these congenital anomalies are associated with congenital anomalies of the left side of the heart and/or lungs, including patent ductus arteriosus, atrial septal defects, mitral stenosis, and bronchogenic cysts.

GROSS FINDINGS: No significant clinical abnormality. At one time, the diagnosis was made only at autopsy. Today diagnosis is often made at surgery or by echocardiography and MRI. In partial absence of the parietal pericardium there may be fibrous adhesions between the pleura and the epicardium.

MICROSCOPIC FINDINGS: The findings are nonspecific. Residual pericardium, if any, is likely structurally normal. The epicardial surface shows mesothelial cells that may be hyperplastic because of friction and adhesions with the parietal pleura.

REMARKS: Congenital pericardial absence, partial or complete, is exquisitely rare. Its absence does not appear to make a significant difference to cardiac function.

The etiology of pericardial defects is not definitely established. Embryologically they (and pleural defects) may result from the premature atrophy of the duct of Cuvier, with resulting loss of blood supply to the pleuropericardial membrane, which also gives rise to the myocardium. Hence, approximately one third of cases are associated with congenital anomalies of the left side of the heart and/or lungs.

DIFFERENTIAL DIAGNOSIS: Partial pericardial absence following open heart procedures. Obviously, clinical information regarding previous operative procedures would help exclude this.

KEY DIAGNOSTIC CRITERIA: 1. Partial or complete absence of pericardium on gross inspection.
2. Echocardiographic or MRI finding of pericardial absence.

References

1. Baille M. On the want of a pericardium in the human body. *Trans Soc Improve Med Chir Knowl* 1793; 1:91.
2. Saint-Pierre A, Fremont R. Absences totales et partialles du pericardes. *Arch Mal Coeur* 1970;63:638.
3. Butany J. The pericardium and its diseases. In: Silver MD, ed. *Cardiovascular pathol, 2nd ed.* Churchill-Livingstone, New York, 1996.

CONGENITAL CYSTS

Entry Author: Jagdish W. Butany

DEFINITION: Cysts found inside the pericardial sac, either at open heart surgery or at autopsy. They are thin walled, filled with clear serous fluid, and may have a lining of cells having an enteric or bronchial somatotype. They usually produce no symptoms.

GROSS FINDINGS: Thin-walled cysts of varying size, weighing up to 300 g and measuring up to 25.0 × 37.0 cm in diameter.

MICROSCOPIC FINDINGS: Cysts of variable size, filled with clear or serous fluid. The wall is lined by a single layer of flattened cells, similar to bronchial mucosal/intestinal mucosal cells. The wall itself is comprised of fibrous connective tissue.

SPECIAL PROCEDURES NEEDED FOR DIAGNOSIS: A loculated effusion, as may occur after surgery, does not have a cyst wall. The wall of a pericardial diverticulum should have all layers of the pericardial wall. Furthermore, it should communicate freely with the pericardial cavity (a true cyst should not communicate directly with the pericardial cavity). The two terms should not be used interchangeably.

REMARKS: Small cysts are easily missed, especially if there are fibrous pericardial adhesions in adjacent tissues. Larger cysts are easier to appreciate and are today fairly easily diagnosed on 3-D echocardiography.

DIFFERENTIAL DIAGNOSIS: A loculated effusion, as may occur after surgery, does not have a cyst wall. The wall of a pericardial diverticulum should have all layers of the pericardial wall. Furthermore, it should communicate freely with the pericardial cavity (a true cyst should not communicate directly with the pericardial cavity). The two terms should not be used interchangeably.

KEY DIAGNOSTIC CRITERIA: The gross finding of a cyst of varying size within the pericardial sac.

POTENTIAL PITFALLS: Postoperative loculated collections of fluid in the pericardium may be mistaken for congenital pericardial cysts. However, history of surgery and evidence of adjacent fibrous adhesions should allow easy differentiation.

PERICARDIAL EFFUSION

Entry Author: Jagdish W. Butany

DEFINITION: The accumulation of fluid (serous, purulent, serosanguinous, or sanguinous) in the pericardial sac. This may be slow and progressive or rapid and catastrophic, in which case it presents as cardiac tamponade and electromechanical dissociation on ECG. A cardiac tamponade may be the first indication of cardiac-pericardial metastases.

GROSS FINDINGS: The features depend on the cause of the effusion. Following acute injury, the pericardium reacts with congestion and a clear serous effusion. In inflammatory conditions, e.g., viral pericarditis, there is an initial serous effusion and the pericardium shows minimal to mild thickening. This may be patchy or more extensive. The mesothelial cells may show reactive changes.

Malignant tumors (primary or metastatic) involving the pericardium, the tumor itself would usually be evident in the pericardium and the pericardial fluid likely be serosanguinous.

If the effusion is due to an inflammatory condition, especially a bacterial inflammation, the fluid is likely to be purulent. Traumatic injury can lead to a bloody effusion/hemopericardium.

MICROSCOPIC FINDINGS: The pericardium in this case gets significantly thickened and shows increasing deposition of a variable thickness, layer of fibrin, with necrotic debris, inflammatory cells, and microorganisms. Sanguinous effusions are usually associated with trauma (especially automobile accidents with chest injury), following open heart surgery, and myocardial rupture following acute myocardial infarction. The pericardial findings will be discussed further in the appropriate sections. The common denominator would be variable degrees of pericardial thickening, the presence of inflammatory cells, and the fluid in the pericardial sac.

REMARKS: Complications of pericardial effusion: A slow and gradual accumulation of pericardial fluid may remain asymptomatic for significant periods of time. Up to 1 and occasionally 2 liters of fluid may accumulate gradually without significant elevation of intrapericardial pressure or alteration of cardiac function. Such volumes may be tolerated for months, even years. However, the acute accumulation of even 250–300 ml of fluid leads to significant cardiac decompensation and the clinical syndrome of cardiac tamponade. This is associated with electromechanical disassociation on electrocardiography and if not treated on an emergent basis results in sudden cardiac death. This is usually associated with a ruptured acute myocardial infarction or trauma.

DIFFERENTIAL DIAGNOSIS: Any of the causes of the effusion listed above must be considered and excluded.

KEY DIAGNOSTIC CRITERIA: 1. History. This should suggest the underlying cause.
2. Microscopic features will help differentiate between the different etiologies.

References

1. Fadouach S et al. Cardiac tamponade disclosing neoplasm: Apropos of 23 cases. *Arch des Maladies du Coeur et des Vaisseaux* 1994;87:1333–1338.

PERICARDITIS

Entry Author: Jagdish W. Butany

Pericarditis or inflammation of the pericardium may be due to numerous causes including infectious, idiopathic, or iatrogenic. It may also be associated with systemic diseases or associated with malignant neoplasms.

Infectious pericarditis may be bacterial, fungal, viral, protozoal, or associated with the immunodeficiency syndrome or Lyme disease.

The establishment of a specific etiology for pericarditis is often difficult. Primary acute pericarditis is not a common condition. The use of a pericardial tissue sample, i.e., histopathology-alone, is often insufficient for making a specific etiologic diagnosis. Utilization of a diagnostic protocol including clinical data, data from therapeutic pericardiocentesis, and diagnostic pericardiocentesis are much more likely to yield positive results!

References

1. Zayas R et al. Incidence of specific etiology and role of methods for specific etiologic diagnosis of primary acute pericarditis. *Am J Cardiol* 1995;75(5):378–382.
   The incidence of pericarditis and its management has remained fairly unchanged. A surgical management review of 86 cases showed that pericarditis was associated with effusion in 41 patients, calcific in 33, and fibrous in 12. The etiologic factors were nonspecific in 36 and specific in the rest.
2. Anyanwu GH et al. Pericarditis a persisting surgical problem. *Cardiovascular Surg* 1994;2:711–715.

PERICARDITIS, AIDS-ASSOCIATED

Entry Author: Jagdish W. Butany

DEFINITION: A mild often patchy pericarditis in patients with Acquired Immune Deficiency Syndrome (AIDS), usually with no microorganisms demonstrable. Rarely, organisms have been demonstrated and these include CMV, *Rhodococcus equi, Toxoplasma M. kansasii.*

GROSS FINDINGS: The pericardium shows focal mild thickening, fibrosis, and a minimal to mild effusion. The heart is usually mildly enlarged with four chamber dilation (AIDS-associated cardiomyopathy). No microorganisms are demonstrable. It is almost invariably associated with a mild myocarditis.

MICROSCOPIC FINDINGS: Mild nonspecific pericardial thickening. No evidence of microorganisms. Focal pericarditis with a mild infiltrate of mononuclear cells, mostly lymphocytes.

SPECIAL PROCEDURES NEEDED FOR DIAGNOSIS: Clinically, echocardiography would demonstrate the pericardial effusion. However, the effusion is usually small, not very significant clinically. In addition, the patient is usually so ill from other HIV-related problems that this takes fairly low priority. In some series, up to 30% of patients develop cardiac tamponade. Simultaneous pericardial involvement by mycobacterium avium intracellulare and/or Kaposi's sarcoma may occur.

DIFFERENTIAL DIAGNOSIS: Other causes of chronic nonspecific pericarditis. The pericardium usually shows a mild infiltrate of lymphocytes with abundant plasma cells.

KEY DIAGNOSTIC CRITERIA: 1. HIV positive status—Diagnosis of AIDS.
2. Features of AIDS-associated dilated cardiomyopathy.
3. Morphological features alone are nonspecific.

References

1. Lee-Chiong T et al. Case reports, pericarditis and lymphadenitis due to *Rhodococcus equi. Am J Med Sc* 1995;310:31–33.

2. Guerot E et al. *Toxoplasma* pericarditis in acquired immunodeficiency syndrome. *Intensive Care Medicine* 1995;21:229–230.
3. Moreno F et al. *Mycobacterium kansasii* pericarditis in patients with AIDS. *Clin Inf Dis* 1994;19:967–969.
4. Decker CP et al. *Staph. aureus* pericarditis in HIV-infected patients. *Chest* 1994;105:615–616.

PERICARDITIS, BACTERIAL

Entry Author: Jagdish W. Butany

SYNONYM: Purulent pericarditis.

DEFINITION: Infection of the pericardial sac by gram-positive or gram-negative microorganisms resulting in inflammation and a purulent effusion. This may be associated with infection of adjacent structures.

GROSS FINDINGS: Variable accumulation of clear or turbid fluid in the pericardial sac. Pericardial thickening (visceral and parietal). Presence of acute inflammatory cells in the pericardial sac and covering of the pericardium by a fibrinopurulent exudate. The exudate contains polymorphonuclear leukocytes. In untreated cases, the microorganisms may be demonstrable in the exudate and in the wall.

MICROSCOPIC FINDINGS: Congestion and inflammatory changes in the pericardium, microorganisms (bacteria) may be demonstrated on special stains (e.g., Gram stain). A thick layer of fibrin with acute inflammatory cells and microorganisms is seen. Deeper layers of fibrin will show evidence of organization with large, pleomorphic fibroblasts and endothelial cells evident.

DIFFERENTIAL DIAGNOSIS: Other causes of pericarditis such as viral infections or parasitic infections.

KEY DIAGNOSTIC CRITERIA: 1. Presence of acute inflammatory infiltrate.
2. Demonstration of microorganisms.
3. Thickening of pericardium.
4. Constitutional symptoms.

POTENTIAL PITFALLS: The possibility of an associated infective endocarditis must be kept in mind. Especially in the presence of prosthetic heart valves, an annular abscess may have led to the pericarditis.

The diagnosis is confirmed by demonstration of microorganisms on special stains (Gram, PAS, GMS). Whereas gram-positive organisms are the common cause, gram-negative microorganisms and fungi may also be the underlying cause.

Reference

1. Friedland IR, du Plessis J, Ciliers A. Cardiac complications in children with staphylococcus aureus bacteremia. *J Pediatrics* 1995;127:746–748.

PERICARDITIS, CHOLESTEROL-ASSOCIATED

Entry Author: Jagdish W. Butany

DEFINITION: Pericarditis due to accumulation of cholesterol or cholesterol "crystals" in the pericardial space and in the thickened pericardium. It may be idiopathic or associated with chronic inflammatory (usually granulomatous) diseases such as tuberculosis, rheumatoid arthritis, hypothyroidism. Hypercholesterolemia of any cause may lead to it. It may occasionally be associated with pericardial hemorrhage and breakdown of red blood cells with release of cholesterol and lipids.

GROSS FINDINGS: A mild pericardial effusion rich in cholesterol is present. The cause of this cholesterol-rich effusion is usually not established. The pericardium is thickened with fibrosis and fibrous adhesions may be present. However, in the presence of a significant exudate, pericardial adhesions may be seen only in the basal regions of the heart. The two layers of pericardium may show thickening due to significant inflammatory reactions.

MICROSCOPIC FINDINGS: Pericardial fibrosis and thickening, significant accumulation of cholesterol crystals, and a marked cellular reaction with mononuclear cells and macrophages. A late, though rare, result may be constrictive pericarditis. The cause is not established. It may be due to necrosis of cell membranes in an inflammatory exudate.

KEY DIAGNOSTIC CRITERIA: 1. History of one of the associated/underlying conditions, listed above.
2. The finding of significant amounts of cholesterol in the pericardial exudate.
3. The presence of pericardial fibrosis and the inflammatory infiltrate.

PERICARDITIS, CONSTRICTIVE

Entry Author: Jagdish W. Butany

DEFINITION: Constrictive pericarditis is a clinical phenomenon associated with parietal pericardial thickening its adhesion to the epicardium and constriction of the ventricular chambers due to this pericardial fibrosis. Clinically, it is characterized by minimal to occasionally significant change in ventricular contraction/emptying. The symptoms are usually rapidly reversed by surgical pericardiectomy.

GROSS FINDINGS: Marked thickening of the parietal pericardium with extensive, fibrous pericardial adhesions. The pericardial sac may show significant amount of fluid which has accumulated rapidly and led to mechanical compression of the cardiac chambers, especially the ventricles. If fluid is present, the accumulation is generally greater than 250–300 ml, over a short period of time. The myocardial chambers, especially the ventricles, are significantly smaller than usual.

MICROSCOPIC FINDINGS: The parietal pericardium shows marked fibrosis, variable calcification, and mild chronic inflammatory infiltrate. The epicardium usually shows similar changes and the underlying myocardium may not show any significant abnormality, or if the constriction is secondary to a hemopericardium (trauma or postoperative), tissues may also show hemosiderin laden macrophages. Microorganisms must be stained for, especially *Mycobacterium tuberculosis.*

SPECIAL PROCEDURES NEEDED FOR DIAGNOSIS: Clinical echocardiography will usually help demonstrate the thickened pericardium and the small cardiac chambers, especially the ventricles.

REMARKS: The pericardium shows a thickening due to fibrosis. Many cases used to be due to tuberculous involvement of the pericardium. Today, a majority of cases show no microorganisms and often only a mild, nonspecific, chronic inflammation. Variable areas of calcification are often present. An occasional case may be related to Mitomycin C given for malignant pericardial effusion.

DIFFERENTIAL DIAGNOSIS: 1. Causes of chronic pericarditis.

KEY DIAGNOSTIC CRITERIA: 1. Marked thickening of the pericardium with fibrosis.
2. Fibrous pericardial adhesions.
3. Compression of the ventricles and atria by the fibrous pericardial adhesions.
4. History of trauma to chest, pervious surgery.
5. Clinical features of biventricular equalization of pressures, elevated JVP, etc.
6. Enlarged congested liver.
7. Hypoperfused lungs.

Reference

1. Lin MT et al. Constrictive pericarditis after sclerosing therapy with Mitomycin C for malignant pericardial effusion. *J Formosan Med Assn* 1994;93:250–252.

PERICARDITIS, FUNGAL

Entry Author: Jagdish W. Butany

DEFINITION: Infection of the pericardium with fungi, most commonly *Candida* (*C. albicans*) species, associated with inflammation and at times an effusion.

GROSS FINDINGS: The pericardium is thickened and shows an abundant and thick layer of soft, pale pink, fibrinoid material.

MICROSCOPIC FINDINGS: In addition to *Candida*, histologic examination shows thickening of the pericardium, and special stains show fungi (Gomori methenamine silver). Fungi commonly associated with pericarditis are *Histoplasma*, *Aspergillus*, *Cryptococcus*, and *Coccidioides*. Occasionally *Nocardia* and other fungi may also lead to pericarditis.

Histoplasma pericarditis: Rare except in endemic areas. Patient generally young. Associated with pulmonary/disseminated infection and serosanguinous effusion.

Effusion: Contains mixed inflammatory cells.

Histology: Granulomata with or without necrosis. Fibrosis and calcification occur late. Constrictive pericarditis may develop.

Candida pericarditis: *Candida* causes disease in susceptible, i.e., immunodeficient/immunosuppressed, individuals with depressed T-cell function and in those with *Candida* endocarditis (usually with prosthetic valves). Purulent pericarditis due to *Candida* species generally has a poor prognosis.

DIFFERENTIAL DIAGNOSIS: Other causes of pericarditis are ruled out, and the fungal etiology established, when microorganisms are demonstrated in routine sections or by special stains.

KEY DIAGNOSTIC CRITERIA:
1. Demonstration of the microorganisms on light microscopy.
2. An infection with the fungus in an adjacent organ.
3. History of immunosuppression and/or depressed T-cell functions.

Reference

1. Hormick P, Harris P, Smith P. *Nocardia asteroides* purulent pericarditis. *Eur J Cardiothoracic Surg* 1995;9:468–470.

PERICARDITIS, IDIOPATHIC

Entry Author: Jagdish W. Butany

SYNONYMS: Benign, relapsing, or primary pericarditis.

DEFINITION: Mild pericardial inflammation, usually patchy, with no demonstrable microorganisms. Probably associated with previous viral infection and rarely with familial Mediterranean fever.

GROSS FINDINGS: Patchy whitish areas of pericardial thickening, usually epicardial. In somewhat more severe pericarditis, patchy fibrous adhesions may be seen (disease primarily of men).

MICROSCOPIC FINDINGS: The findings are nonspecific. The pericardium is thickened due to fibrosis. The underlying tissue shows focal aggregates of lymphocytes. Special stains do not show microorganisms. Reactive mesothelial cells may be present, especially adjacent to areas of fibrous adhesions.

Early: Pericardium usually congested with a mixed inflammatory infiltrate. Serous effusion may be present.

REMARKS: A new tool that may help make definitive diagnoses easier is pericardioscopy-assisted pericardial biopsy.

DIFFERENTIAL DIAGNOSIS: Other causes of pericarditis. In the early stages these can be differentiated by the use of special stains.

KEY DIAGNOSTIC CRITERIA: Focal and mild nature of lesions. Incidence rises during epidemics of viral disease. Etiologic factor difficult to diagnose. Viral antigens may be demonstrated in the pericardium. In tropical countries this is second only to purulent pericarditis as far as frequency is concerned. A history of preceding U.R.I. followed by symptoms and signs of CHF, is generally available. Often associated with myocarditis.

References

1. Tauber T et al. Recurrent pericarditis in familial Mediterranean fever. *Harefuah* 1995;128:611–612, 672 (Hebrew).
2. Maisch B et al. Pericardioscopy and epicardial biopsy—New diagnostic tools in pericardial and perimyocardial disease. *Eur Heart J* 1994;15 Suppl C:68–73.

PERICARDITIS, LYME DISEASE-ASSOCIATED

Entry Author: Jagdish W. Butany

DEFINITION: Pericardial inflammation and associated changes in a patient with Lyme disease, i.e., infection with *Borrelia burgdorferi*. (Transmitted by Ixodes dammini ticks in the USA and Ixodes ricinus in Europe).

GROSS FINDINGS: The pericardium may show mild thickening due to fibrosis, and there may be mild pericardial effusion. It may be associated with *cardiomegaly* (dilation or hypertrophy or both).

MICROSCOPIC FINDINGS: The heart shows a pancarditis. There may at times be a mild chronic pericarditis alone. Pericardial involvement is the major cardiac involvement in most cases. Mild pericardial fibrosis and patchy mild infiltrate of lymphocytes may at times be the only evidence of Lyme disease. The microorganism is *Borrelia burgdorferi,* a spirochete associated with ticks (Ixodes dammini in North America, and Ixodes ricinus in Europe). Occasionally Lyme disease may be associated with an acute myopericarditis.

DIFFERENTIAL DIAGNOSIS: Other causes of pericarditis, such as bacteria, fungi, and parasites.

KEY DIAGNOSTIC CRITERIA: History of exposure to ticks (Ixodes dammini). The microorganism may be demonstrable. History of travel in wooded areas (Massachusetts—commonly).

The associated skin lesion—erythema migrans may be helpful in making a diagnosis. The morphologic features themselves are nonspecific and mild. The presence of cardiac dysrhythmias and demonstration of *Borrelia burgdorferi,* history of tick bites are helpful in confirming the etiology.

Demonstration of antibodies to *B. burgdorferi.* Majority of patients seropositive within first month of illness.

References

1. Horowitz HW, Belkin RN. Acute myopericarditis resulting from Lyme disease. *Am Heart J* 1995;130: 176–178.
2. Bruyn GA et al. Lyme pericarditis leading to tamponade. *Br J Rheumatology* 1994;33:862–866.

PERICARDITIS, MALIGNANT NEOPLASM-ASSOCIATED

Entry Author: Jagdish W. Butany

DEFINITION: Inflammation of the pericardium associated with malignant neoplasms involving the pericardial sac including pericardial tumors.

GROSS FINDINGS: The pericardium often shows a serous or, more commonly, a serosanguinous effusion. The pericardial surfaces are thickened, rough, and shaggy. Single or usually multiple sites are covered by grayish-white to hemorrhagic areas of tumor. Usually associated with a serosanguinous effusion.

MICROSCOPIC FINDINGS: Demonstration of metastatic tumors consistent with the known primary (occasionally primary sarcoma of the heart or mesothelioma) with pericardial effusion (cytologic examination positive for malignant cells). Adjacent uninvolved surfaces show fibrinous and/or fibrous adhesions and a mild to moderate infiltrate of chronic inflammatory cells in the subepicardial tissues.

Occasionally patients with neoplasms have pericarditis but without actual demonstrable involvement of the pericardium.

DIFFERENTIAL DIAGNOSIS: Other causes of pericarditis, pericardial thickening.

KEY DIAGNOSTIC CRITERIA: History of a primary tumor at another site. Whereas virtually any tumor may metastasize to the heart (and pericardium) involvement by lymphomas, melanomas and neoplasms arising from adjacent structures is most common (seen in up to 13.9% of cases in one series).

PERICARDITIS, MYCOBACTERIAL

Entry Author: Jagdish W. Butany

DEFINITION: Pericardial infection with *Mycobacterium tuberculosis* (occasionally infection with other mycobacteria, especially *Mycobacterium avium-intracellulare*—in HIV positive individuals). Invariably secondary to tubercular involvement elsewhere in the body.

GROSS FINDINGS: In the early active stages, the pericardium is thickened and covered by a shaggy layer of fibrin and shows extensive adhesions. The thickened pericardium may show nodularity.

MICROSCOPIC FINDINGS: The pericardium may show acute, subacute, or chronic involvement with fibrosis and scattered necrotizing granulomas. Special stains for mycobacterium should demonstrate the microorganism. (Occasionally, the pericardial infection with *Mycobacterium chelonei* have been reported).
Acute Stage: Fibrinous and effusive (serosanguinous) stages. Inflammatory cells present. Effusion may occasionally be massive (to 200 ml of serous, serosanguinous, or bloody fluid).
Subacute Stage: Characterized by granulomas with or without caseation and mycobacteria demonstrable on special stains.
Chronic Stage: Fibrosis and thickening of the pericardium (both layers), virtual obliteration of the cavity and constriction may result. Mononuclear cells may be seen. Calcification is usually seen.

DIFFERENTIAL DIAGNOSIS: Other causes of chronic pericarditis.

KEY DIAGNOSTIC CRITERIA: The presence of necrotizing granulomas and the demonstration of mycobacterium on special stains, (demonstration of *Mycobacterium tuberculosis* in the pericardium or in the primary focus, i.e., in other organs—usually the lungs).

PERICARDITIS, MYOCARDIAL INFARCTION-ASSOCIATED

Entry Author: Jagdish W. Butany

DEFINITION: A mild, nonspecific usually localized pericarditis seen following a transmural myocardial infarction. The fibrinous exudate and inflammation are believed to be secondary to increased permeability of blood vessels. (This condition has become much less common in recent years. Thrombolytic therapy appears to be associated with an even lower incidence).

GROSS FINDINGS: Patchy pericardial fibrinous, later fibrous, adhesions. A mild pericardial effusion may be present.

MICROSCOPIC FINDINGS: Mild, nonspecific acute inflammation (later chronic) of the pericardium associated with edema and thickening of the parietal and of the visceral pericardium. The adjacent myocardium shows features of a transmural myocardial infarction.

At later stages, there may be patchy fibrous adhesions and mild nonspecific mononuclear cell infiltrate, associated with aneurysm formation.

DIFFERENTIAL DIAGNOSIS: Other causes of pericarditis. The associated myocardial ischemic damage would generally exclude all other causes. Also, the inability to demonstrate any microorganisms would confirm the nonspecific nature of the pericarditis.

KEY DIAGNOSTIC CRITERIA: The presence of transmural myocardial infarction in the adjacent tissue.

References

1. Widimsky P, Gregor P. Pericardial involvement during the course of myocardial infarction. *Chest* 1995; 108:89–93.
2. Cheng TO. Disappearance of the Dressler syndrome. *Cardiology* 1994;85:255–258.
3. Shahar A, Hod H, Barabash GM, Kaplinsky E, Motro M. Disappearance of a syndrome. Dressler's syndrome in the era of thrombolysis. *Cardiology* 1995;86:444.

PERICARDITIS, NONINFLAMMATORY

Entry Author: Jagdish W. Butany

SYNONYM: Pericarditis associated with systemic disease.

DEFINITION: A usually nonspecific pericarditis associated with other conditions such as rheumatic fever, collagen vascular diseases, and radiation exposure. (Operative procedures and self-induced trauma or injury may result in a similar very mild pericarditis). More rarely it may be associated with *Legionella* infection or myxedema.

GROSS FINDINGS: In virtually any one of these conditions, the cardiac size is usually normal. The pericardium shows patchy mild fibrous adhesions. In the early or acute stages, however, some (e.g., rheumatic fever) are associated with prominent fibrinous "bread and butter" pericarditis.

MICROSCOPIC FINDINGS: These are nonspecific and are comprised largely of fibrous adhesions with a mild mononuclear cell infiltrate. The pericardium may in the early stages have a thick layer of fibrin on its surface (rheumatic fever). The pericarditis may be patchy, that is involving only part of the pericardial sac. In rheumatoid pericarditis the typical nodules are seldom found.

DIFFERENTIAL DIAGNOSIS: Other conditions associated with pericardial adhesions and fibrosis. Attempts must be made to demonstrate microorganisms and rule out infectious causes. At times a history of preexistent collagen vascular disease or rheumatic fever (valvulitis) or exposure to radiation may be obtainable and helpful in making the diagnosis.

Bacterial pericarditis can normally be ruled out because of the lack of a purulent exudate and demonstrable organisms. However, the distinction can be difficult if antibiotic treatment is begun before the diagnosis is established as cultures and special stains fail to demonstrate microorganisms.

Rheumatoid pericarditis may be excluded by the absence of the diagnostic rheumatoid nodules. It is more helpful to assess the sedimentation rate, serum levels of immunoglobulins (G, M&A), analysis of rheumatoid factor, C3 or C4 components, and positive ANA.

References

1. Alusik S, Skalicka H, Vencovsky J, Kohoutova M. Rheumatoid pericarditis: Correlation with immunologic parameters. *Vnitrni Lekarstvi* 1995;41:764–766.
2. Allessandri JL et al. Myxedematous pericarditis in a child (letter) (French). *Archives de Pediatrie* 1995;2:382–383.
3. Benof LJ, Schweitzer P. Radiation therapy induced cardiac injury. *Am Heart J* 1995;129:1193–1196.
4. Moroni G et al. Cardiologic abnormalities in patients with long term lupus nephritis. *Clin Nephrology* 1995;43:20–28.
5. Travaglio-Encinoze A et al. Rheumatoid pericarditis: New immunopathological aspects. *Clin Expt Rheumatol* 1994;12:313–316.

PERICARDITIS, PARASITIC, NOS

Entry Author: Jagdish W. Butany

DEFINITION: A pericarditis associated with protozoa or other parasites. Uncommon as a group, the parasites seen include *Entamoeba histolytica, Toxo-*

plasma gondii, Trypanosoma cruzi, and *Echinococcus granulosus.* Of these the commonest are amoebae (*Entamoeba histolytica*) with thickening of the pericardium associated with variable degrees of pericardial exudate. The exudate varies with the microorganism. In *Entamoeba histolytica* infection, pericardial involvement is invariably secondary to rupture of an amoebic liver abscess into the pericardial space through the diaphragm.

MICROSCOPIC FINDINGS: The pericardium shows fibrosis and thickening. In Entamoeba infections a thick "anchovy sauce" type of fluid may be present. The parasites can be demonstrated in smears of this fluid.

DIFFERENTIAL DIAGNOSIS: Other pericarditides associated with pericardial thickening.

KEY DIAGNOSTIC CRITERIA: Demonstration of *Entamoeba histolytica* (or other parasites) in the pericardial exudate and the pericardium. A history of amoebic liver abscess with clinical features of rupture into the pleural and pericardial spaces. Clinical features of other parasitic infestation may be available or a history of travel to or origin from an endemic area should raise the appropriate suspicion.

PERICARDITIS, SYSTEMIC DISEASE-ASSOCIATED

Entry Author: Jagdish W. Butany

DEFINITION: This is a nonspecific pericarditis associated with many collagen vascular diseases.

GROSS FINDINGS: Pericardium shows patchy thickening. Fibrous adhesions are usually absent though focal areas may show some adhesions. A mild pericardial effusion is usually present.

MICROSCOPIC FINDINGS: Nonspecific and generally with patchy areas of pericardial fibrosis. A mild infiltrate of mononuclear inflammatory cells may be seen in the subepicardium or focally in the parietal pericardium. Stains for microorganisms are negative.

DIFFERENTIAL DIAGNOSIS: Other causes of nonspecific pericarditis. A history of an underlying systemic disease is also helpful. Infiltrative processes such as amyloidosis may be established by special stains.

KEY DIAGNOSTIC CRITERIA: 1. A history of systemic disease and demonstration of the lesions of systemic disease in other organs.
2. Demonstration of the definitive lesions, as in amyloidosis.

PERICARDITIS, UREMIA-ASSOCIATED

Entry Author: Jagdish W. Butany

SYNONYM: Uremic pericarditis.

DEFINITION: A fibrinous pericarditis associated with uremia. Pathogenesis unknown but presumably related to altered permeability of capillaries permitting leakage of fibrinogen into the pericardial sac, together with its conversion into fibrin.

GROSS FINDINGS: The pericardium is thickened but more striking is the amount of fibrinous material between the pericardial layers, which is very significant. This is first noted as easily broken "fibrinous adhesions" between the visceral and parietal layers. The fibrin-covered pericardium is nonreflective and rough, with shaggy and easily removed fibrin strands. It has the classical shaggy "bread and butter" appearance. The fibrin itself is usually relatively colorless, as compared to such an exudate in other conditions, in which case it may be sanguinous or purulent. There is usually little effusion.

MICROSCOPIC FINDINGS: Thick layer of fibrinous material on the pericardial surface. Mild nonspecific inflammatory infiltrates may also be evident. Deep layers may show evidence of organization. No microorganisms seen or demonstrable.

KEY DIAGNOSTIC CRITERIA: 1. Fibrinous pericarditis with evidence/ history of uremia.
2. No microorganisms seen/demonstrated.
Pericardial Effusions: These may be acute or chronic accumulations of fluid in the pericardial space. The mesothelial lining shows reactive changes. Occasionally the fluid may get infected. Pericardial effusions may be seen with myocardial infarction or following open heart surgery.

PERICARDITIS, VIRAL

Entry Author: Jagdish W. Butany

DEFINITION: The inflammatory changes involving the pericardium and their sequelae, secondary to a viral infection. It is assumed that the virus has directly damaged the pericardial mesothelium, but this is unproven. The virus is generally not morphologically demonstrable in the pericardium nor recoverable from it by culture. The morphological changes are generally nonspecific. Viruses commonly associated with pericarditis include Coxsackie A and B, ECHO virus, and poliomyelitis viruses. However, a wide variety of viruses may be implicated as etiologic agents. (A subset of sudden infant deaths is associated with myoperi-carditis. Molecular diagnostic techniques may help identify the causative virus).

GROSS FINDINGS: Mild pericardial fibrosis, mild pericardial effusion, and in the late stages, mild pericardial fibrous adhesions. The virus is invariably not demonstrable or culturable. A specific viral etiology is difficult to establish.

MICROSCOPIC FINDINGS: Mild pericardial fibrosis. The organism is neither demonstrable (light or electron microscopy) nor grown on culture. Virtually any virus associated with common viral infections may be associated with viral pericarditis. A focal, generally mild, lymphocytic infiltrate, is usually present in the thickened epicardium. A myocarditis is also generally seen.

DIFFERENTIAL DIAGNOSIS: Other causes of nonspecific pericarditis, including those associated with collagen vascular diseases.

KEY DIAGNOSTIC CRITERIA:
1. The absence of any demonstrable organisms.
2. The absence of any symptoms or signs of collagen vascular diseases.
3. A history of preceding viral illness.
4. Very rarely, demonstration of the virus in the tissues or demonstration of seropositivity or rising viral time.
5. History of an acute exanthematous illness.

Reference

1. Shimuzu C et al. Molecular identification of viruses in sudden death associated with myocarditis and pericarditis. *Ped Inf Dis J* 1995;1497:584–588.

ACQUIRED TUFTED ANGIOMA (ANGIOBLASTOMA, PROGRESSIVE CAPILLARY HEMANGIOMA)

Entry Authors: Allen P. Burke and Elizabeth A. Montgomery

DEFINITION: Enlarging cutaneous vascular tumor composed of scattered nodules of capillary-sized vessels that protrude into vascular spaces imparting the appearance of vascular "tufts."

GROSS FINDINGS: Multiple small firm, dark nodules, often painful, that grow slowly before stabilizing. Common locations are neck, upper chest, and shoulder.

MICROSCOPIC FINDINGS: Tightly packed clusters of capillaries with a rounded or ovoid appearance, concentrated in the mid- and deep dermis and arranged in a "cannonball" distribution. Vascular tufts contain plump or spindled endothelium, pericytes, and occasional smooth muscle cells. Capillary spaces are usually collapsed and slit-like. Intervening stroma lacks inflammation and consists of dense fibrous tissue.

DIFFERENTIAL DIAGNOSIS: Capillary hemangioma lacks mature intervening stroma and "cannonball" appearance of angioblastoma, and generally has larger tumor lobules. Pyogenic granuloma is more polypoid and contains inflammation and the stroma is more fibromyxoid. Angiosarcoma contains anastomosing channels with atypical cells and mitotic figures. Kaposi sarcoma contains a prominent spindled element, PAS-positive globules, and hemosiderin.

KEY DIAGNOSTIC CRITERIA: Absolute requirements for diagnosis: "Cannonball" distribution of aggregates of proliferating capillaries. Well-formed capillaries with supporting elements, e.g., pericytes. Aggregates of capillary-sized vessels compress larger, ectatic, crescent-shaped vessels.

Items incompatible with diagnosis: Extensive inflammation. Frequent mitotic figures. Deep extension into subcutaneous tissue.

ANGIOSARCOMA

Entry Authors: Allen P. Burke and Elizabeth A. Montgomery

DEFINITION: Malignant mesenchymal tumor, the cells of which show endothelial differentiation by histologic, immunohistochemical, and/or ultrastructural techniques. Often separated clinically into cutaneous angiosarcoma, deep angiosarcoma of soft tissue, angiosarcoma of specific organs (e.g., heart, breast), and secondary angiosarcoma (lymphedema-associated angiosarcoma, postirradiation angiosarcoma, foreign body-associated angiosarcoma, angiosarcoma associated with exposure to thorium, vinylchloride, arsenical compounds).

GROSS FINDINGS: Cutaneous angiosarcoma: Wide variety of appearances, usually in white patients over 60 years of age, resembling hemangioma, scarring, alopecia, pigmented lesion, or carcinoma. They may be well marginated, ill defined, solitary, multifocal, elevated, nodular, or cystic. Most are red or bluish-purple. Ulceration usually occurs late in the course.

Lymphedema-associated angiosarcoma: Pitting, indurated, pachydermatous skin with red or bluish-purple fungating lesions that are solitary or multicentric, occurring 1–24 years after mastectomy. A dominant mass with multiple satellite lesions may occur.

Angiosarcoma of breast parenchyma: Painless, soft mass with bluish-red discoloration of overlying skin.

MICROSCOPIC FINDINGS: Wide variety of appearances. A well-differentiated angiosarcoma may appear similar to hemangioma, but areas show anastomosing and infiltrating cords, with areas of nuclear hyperchromasia, piling up of endothelium, or papillations. Poorly differentiated angiosarcoma shows large areas of spindle cell sarcoma reminiscent of fibrosarcoma. Areas with endothelial structures (anastomosing cords or intracytoplasmic vacuoles containing red blood cells) may be present. In epithelioid angiosarcoma there are sheets of epithelioid cells with abundant cytoplasm, prominent nucleoli.

Areas of lumen formation will identify the lesion as angiosarcoma. Epithelioid tumors are more likely to occur in the deep soft tissue and endocrine organs (thyroid, adrenal).

SPECIAL PROCEDURES NEEDED FOR DIAGNOSIS: Reticulin stain may highlight tube-like vascular growth that may not be apparent in hematoxylin and eosin stains. Immunohistochemistry is useful in detecting endothelial markers. (Factor VIII-related antigen is quite specific for endothelial differentiation, CD34, and Ulex europaeus agglutinin I are more sensitive but less specific. Often a panel of markers is helpful). Cytokeratin is often positive in epithelioid angiosarcoma, but unlike carcinoma, epithelial membrane antigen is negative, and endothelial markers are positive.

DIFFERENTIAL DIAGNOSIS: Hemangioma (well-differentiated angiosarcoma); fibrosarcoma or poorly differentiated spindle-cell sarcoma (poorly differentiated angiosarcoma); metastatic carcinoma (epithelioid angiosarcoma).

KEY DIAGNOSTIC CRITERIA: Absolute requirements for diagnosis: Well-differentiated and poorly differentiated angiosarcoma—anastomosing vascular spaces, endothelial atypia, or intracytoplasmic lumina.

Epithelioid angiosarcoma: Positivity for factor VIII-related antigen, QBend, or Ulex europaeus. Lack of primary carcinoma.

Items incompatible with diagnosis: Positivity for epithelial membrane antigen.

ANGIOSARCOMA (HEART/PERICARDIUM)

Entry Author: Allen P. Burke

DEFINITION: Sarcoma demonstrating areas of endothelial differentiation.

GROSS FINDINGS: Usually right-sided tumors, especially right atrium. Pericardial extension common. Pericardium may be sole site of tumor. Tumor is typically dark, hemorrhagic, and infiltrative.

MICROSCOPIC FINDINGS: Diagnostic patterns include anastomosing channels lined by atypical endothelial cells, papillary structures lined by atypical endothelial cells, intracellular endothelial-lined vacuoles that may contain red blood cells. Extensive areas of spindled cells with a hemorrhagic background may be present. Epithelioid variant of angiosarcoma has not yet been described in the heart.

SPECIAL PROCEDURES NEEDED FOR DIAGNOSIS: Immunohistochemical stains for endothelial markers will often be positive in tumor cells. Factor VIII related antigen will be positive in a diffuse punctate distribution in about

50% of cases. Other endothelial markers, such as CD34, may be more sensitive but lack specificity. Ultrastructural analysis will show the presence of Weibel-Pallade bodies in a minority of cases.

DIFFERENTIAL DIAGNOSIS: Spindle cell sarcoma: A hemorrhagic spindle cell tumor may lack diagnostic areas of angiosarcoma. Hemangioma with papillary endothelial hyperplasia: There are few mitotic figures, little cellular atypia, and areas of typical benign hemangioma.

KEY DIAGNOSTIC CRITERIA: Absolute requirements for diagnosis: Papillary endothelial-lined structures, anastomosing vascular channels, intracytoplasmic vacuoles containing red cells, or positivity for factor VIII related antigen in tumor cells. Mitotic figures and/or necrosis.

Items incompatible with diagnosis: Presence of other types of sarcoma (e.g., osteosarcoma, chondrosarcoma, rhabdomyosarcoma, liposarcoma, leiomyosarcoma) indicate the diagnosis of malignant mesenchymoma.

ARTERIOVENOUS MALFORMATION (HEMANGIOMA)

Entry Authors: Allen P. Burke and Elizabeth A. Montgomery

SYNONYMS: Arteriovenous malformation, cirsoid aneurysm, racemose aneurysm, arteriovenous aneurysm.

DEFINITION: Acquired (traumatic) or congenital lesion consisting primarily of an arteriovenous anastomosis with secondary vascular proliferation. May be a component of Parkes-Weber syndrome or Klippel-Trenaunay-Weber syndromes.

GROSS FINDINGS: Irregular mass that is often spongy with grossly apparent vessels, that may be pulsatile if superficial, and occasionally associated with soft tissue and skeletal hypertrophy or port wine stains of the skin.

MICROSCOPIC FINDINGS: Mixture of arteries and veins. The latter will often appear "arterialized," that is, there will be fibrointimal proliferation, medial hypertrophy, and thickening of the internal elastic lamina. Only occasionally will a direct anastomosis between an artery and vein be apparent.

SPECIAL PROCEDURES NEEDED FOR DIAGNOSIS: Radiologic evaluation is often helpful in diagnosis. Arteriography demonstrates presence of arteriovenous anastomosis.

DIFFERENTIAL DIAGNOSIS: Angiomatosis lacks arterialized veins, but diagnosis is best confirmed by arteriographic studies.

KEY DIAGNOSTIC CRITERIA: Absolute requirements for diagnosis: Veins and arteries, mass lesion. Evidence of arteriovenous connection, either histologic, radiologic, or clinical (pulsatile mass, high output congestive heart failure).

BACILLARY ANGIOMATOSIS

Entry Authors: Allen P. Burke and Elizabeth A. Montgomery

DEFINITION: Reactive vascular proliferation secondary to infection by intracytoplasmic rickettsial-like organisms (*Bartonella* [formerly *Rochalimaea*] *henselaea* and possibly others), seen most commonly in immunocompromised patients.

GROSS FINDINGS: Multiple cutaneous erythematous nodules. Systemic infection with hemorrhagic nodules of lymph nodes, bone marrow, spleen, liver, and mucosal surfaces may occur.

MICROSCOPIC FINDINGS: Lobulated proliferation of capillaries, with aggregates of neutrophils and extracellular debris.

SPECIAL PROCEDURES NEEDED FOR DIAGNOSIS: Warthin Starry silver stain (pH 4.0) will demonstrate numerous small curved rods measuring 0.5–1.0 microns in length, in areas of neutrophils and extracellular debris.

DIFFERENTIAL DIAGNOSIS: Pyogenic granuloma will lack neutrophilic abscesses and organisms. Lesions are usually solitary. Kaposi sarcoma is often in the clinical differential diagnosis of multiple cutaneous lesions in an immunocompromised individual. Abscesses and organisms are lacking, and a spindle cell proliferation is usually present. Carrion's disease is seen almost exclusively in South America (see entry), and only skin lesions are present in tissue phase, sparing deep organs.

KEY DIAGNOSTIC CRITERIA: Absolute requirements for diagnosis: Presence of Warthin-Starry-positive bacteria.
Items incompatible with diagnosis: Extensive spindle cell proliferation.

BENIGN FIBROUS HISTIOCYTOMA

Entry Author: Allen P. Burke

DEFINITION: Benign neoplasm of myofibroblastic origin. If there is a prominent inflammatory infiltrate, the term *inflammatory fibrous histiocytoma* (or inflammatory myofibroblastic tumor, plasma cell granuloma, inflammatory pseudotumor) has been used.

GROSS FINDINGS: There is no site predilection in the heart. Because of their extreme rarity, few generalizations about their gross appearance can be made. In general, they are infiltrating, whitish-tan fibrous masses that show little hemorrhage or cavitation.

MICROSCOPIC FINDINGS: There is a proliferation of compact spindled cells with intermingled xanthoma cells or histiocytic-appearing cells that have abundant cytoplasm, foamy lipid-rich cytoplasm, and occasionally multiple nuclei. Some tumors are indistinguishable from nodular fasciitis. If there is a prominent infiltrate of lymphocytes, plasma cells, and eosinophils, the term inflammatory fibrous histiocytoma is used. The immunohistochemical profile is nonspecific, with positivity for muscle specific actin and vimentin.

DIFFERENTIAL DIAGNOSIS: Fibromas lack xanthoma cells and inflammation is restricted to a few cells in a perivascular location or at the periphery of the tumor. Clinically, hypergammaglobulinemia and fever favor inflammatory fibrous histiocytoma. Histologically, there is a diffuse background of lymphocytes and histiocytes, often with numerous plasma cells.

CAPILLARY HEMANGIOMA

Entry Authors: Allen P. Burke and Elizabeth A. Montgomery

SYNONYMS: Juvenile (capillary) hemangioma (hemangioendothelioma).

DEFINITION: Proliferation of capillaries, usually in the skin, generally present in infants in the first weeks of life as a lesion that expands for several months and later regresses in several years.

GROSS FINDINGS: Soft, red, lobulated tumor or tumors that may reach a large size, most often present in the head or neck region (strawberry nevus).

MICROSCOPIC FINDINGS: Lobular proliferation of capillary vessels, similar in appearance to pyogenic granuloma. However, surface ulceration and inflammation is usually absent. In early lesions, the capillary channels are collapsed, mitoses are frequent, and fibroblasts and other supporting cells, such as pericytes, may be present. In later lesions, lumina open, first at the periphery, and vascular lobules are accentuated by ingrowth of fibrous septa.

DIFFERENTIAL DIAGNOSIS: Nevus flammeus (port wine stain); clinically these are red patches present at birth that only occasionally become raised lesions. Histologically, there is not a proliferation of capillaries but rather a dilation of dermal capillaries and venules (telangiectasia) and clinically these stains do not typically regress.

CARDIAC CALCIFIED AMORPHOUS TUMOR

Entry Author: Allen P Burke

DEFINITION: Non-neoplastic calcified masses that occur on the endocardial surfaces, possibly are organizing thrombi.

GROSS FINDINGS: Occur on the endocardial surface of any cardiac chamber, are whitish yellow, calcified masses with an irregular bosselated surface, occasionally with surface thrombi, that on section are homogeneous and diffusely calcified (generally needing decalcification before sectioning).

MICROSCOPIC FINDINGS: Degenerating fibrin, microcalcification, occasionally surface fibrin thrombi.

SPECIAL PROCEDURES NEEDED FOR DIAGNOSIS: Electron microscopy has demonstrated material similar to degenerated fibrin.

DIFFERENTIAL DIAGNOSIS: Myxoma, organizing thrombus.

KEY DIAGNOSTIC CRITERIA: Absolute requirements for diagnosis: Calcium, intracavitary location. Items incompatible with diagnosis: Myxoma cells.

CARDIAC FIBROMA

Entry Author: Allen P. Burke

DEFINITION: Benign tumor composed of fibrocytes, collagen, and sometimes elastic fibers occurring within the myocardium; status as true neoplasm or fibromatosis-like process uncertain.

GROSS FINDINGS: Bulging whorled well-circumscribed tumor, often reminiscent of uterine "fibroid," located within the ventricular myocardium and often extending partly into the lumen. On sections, fibromas are firm or rubbery, without cysts, hemorrhage, or necrosis. Calcifications are common and are occasionally grossly evident. Tumors are always single, range from 2–>10 cm.

MICROSCOPIC FINDINGS: Findings depend partly on the age of the patient. In infants, fibromas are quite cellular with little collage and may have rare mitoses. In adults, the tumors are composed predominantly of collagen. Numerous elastic fibers, identifiable with special stains, are found in over 50%

of cases. Foci of calcification, and less commonly ossification, are seen in about 50% of cases. Small groups of lymphocytes and mononuclear inflammatory cells may be present, especially around vessels and at the junction of normal myocardium in tumors from younger individuals. Inflammation is never diffuse or prominent. Margins of fibromas are usually microscopically infiltrating. Hemosiderin is absent.

DIFFERENTIAL DIAGNOSIS: Inflammatory pseudotumor: these rare cardiac masses show diffuse inflammation, numerous plasma cells, reactive myofibroblastic cells with abundant amphophilic cytoplasm. Healed infarct: present in hearts with severe coronary artery disease, do not bulge on section, hemosiderin present. Organized thrombus: these are mural lesions with prominent hemosiderin, do not infiltrate muscle. Scarred myxomas: contain prominent hemosiderin, are mural, not intramyocardial. Fibrosarcoma: these tumors may be confused with cellular fibromas. However, the latter occur exclusively in newborns or infants (<6 months), and fibrosarcomas are tumors of adults, occasionally children and adolescents.

KEY DIAGNOSTIC CRITERIA: Absolute requirements for diagnosis: Grossly bulging tumor; presence of collagen, fibrocytes.

Items incompatible with diagnosis: Necrosis, cellular pleomorphism, numerous plasma cells, inflammatory cells.

CARDIAC MYXOMA

Entry Author: Allen P. Burke

DEFINITION: Benign neoplasm of cardiac endocardium with unknown histogenesis.

GROSS FINDINGS: Smooth-surfaced or friable intracavitary masses that are attached to the endocardium without any infiltration of the underlying tissues. Most common location is the left atrium (75%) and right atrium (majority of remainder).

MICROSCOPIC FINDINGS: Myxomas are composed of myxoma cells, which often form syncytia, cords, and rings that are typically infiltrated by lymphocytes and histiocytes. Hemosiderin is present within histiocytes and some myxoma cells. Myxoma cells have an ovoid nucleus with inconspicuous or large nucleoli, abundant eosinophilic cytoplasm, and indistinct cell borders. Myxoma cells appear to emanate from capillaries when ring structures are present. Fibrosis, Gamna-Gandy bodies, thrombosis, and calcification are common. Extramedullary hematopoiesis is present in about 10% of cases. A myxoid background is present in areas without fibrosis.

DIFFERENTIAL DIAGNOSIS: Myxoid sarcoma: Lack of hemosiderin deposits, thrombosis, and myxoma cells. Myxoid hemangioma: Lack of myxoma cells, inflammation.

KEY DIAGNOSTIC CRITERIA: Absolute requirements for diagnosis: Myxoma cell, hemosiderin, prominent vascularity.

Items incompatible with diagnosis: Infiltration of underlying myocardium, cellular areas of spindle cells.

CARRION'S DISEASE (VERRUGA PERUANA)

Entry Authors: Allen P. Burke and Elizabeth A. Montgomery

DEFINITION: Oroya fever, or Carrion's disease, is a febrile illness characterized by cutaneous lesions in the tissue phase, which occurs about 2 months after the systemic or hematic phase of disease. The etiologic agent is *Bartonella bacilliformis,* a hemotropic, motile, pleomorphic gram-negative bacterium that elaborates an angiogenesis factor *in vitro*, and presumably *in vivo*.

GROSS FINDINGS: Nodules in the dermis and subcutaneous regions that measure from <1 mm to several cm in size.

MICROSCOPIC FINDINGS: Multinodular, lobulated nodules of capillaries lined by atypical endothelial cells (verruga cells). Areas of acute and chronic inflammation may be present, with necrosis. Organisms may be identified as Rocha-Lima inclusions, granular structures that stain positive for the Giemsa reagent, and weakly with Warthin Starry silver stain.

SPECIAL PROCEDURES NEEDED FOR DIAGNOSIS: Giemsa, Warthin Starry stain.

DIFFERENTIAL DIAGNOSIS: Kaposi sarcoma, pyogenic granuloma, bacillary angiomatosis.

KEY DIAGNOSTIC CRITERIA: Absolute requirements for diagnosis: Rocha-Lima inclusions or appropriate clinical setting (endemic area of South America, often recent febrile illness).

CAVERNOUS HEMANGIOMA

Entry Authors: Allen P. Burke and Elizabeth A. Montgomery

DEFINITION: Benign vascular tumors of children and adults, often occurring in the skin or liver, although many organs may be involved.

GROSS FINDINGS: Soft, blue or purple masses that blanch with pressure (cutaneous lesions).

MICROSCOPIC FINDINGS: Localized, moderately circumscribed mass of thin-walled vessels with dilated lumina. A component of capillary hemangioma may be present.

DIFFERENTIAL DIAGNOSIS: Spindle cell hemangioendothelioma contains a spindle-cell component. Arteriovenous hemangioma features thick-walled vessels and may have arterialized veins.

KEY DIAGNOSTIC CRITERIA: Absolute requirements for diagnosis: Thin-walled vascular channels filled with blood.

Items incompatible with diagnosis: Presence of muscularized vessels within the lesion. Spindled cells.

CYSTIC TUMOR OF THE ATRIOVENTRICULAR NODE

Entry Author: Allen P. Burke

DEFINITION: Multicystic inclusions in the area of the atrioventricular node that are most likely endodermal rests present from birth.

GROSS FINDINGS: In about 50% of cases, the heart is grossly normal. The inclusions are not visible with the naked eye. In the remainder of cases, the cysts are grossly evident, either as one dominant cyst that may be filled with inspissated fluid or multiple smaller cysts. The cysts are always in the location of the membranous septum and near the inferior interatrial septum.

MICROSCOPIC FINDINGS: The cysts are lined by cuboidal ciliated cells, stratified squamous cells, or a combination of both. Often the lining cells appear transitional and the nuclei may have a "coffee bean" appearance. A dual population of cells is often apparent. The lumina of the cysts are either apparently empty or filled with proteinaceous material that is PAS-positive, diastase resistant. Occasionally, there are nests of cells without cystic lumina; these nests are usually transitional in appearance. The location of the cysts is invariably in the area of the atrioventricular node and they never extend inferior to the central fibrous body in the ventricular septum. They may extend into the inferior atrial septum and are most numerous on the right atrial side of the interatrial septum.

SPECIAL PROCEDURES NEEDED FOR DIAGNOSIS: Ultrastructurally, the cells are epithelial, possess intercellular tight junctions and true desmosomes, and cilia or micro villi. Immunohistochemically, the cells strongly express cytokeratins, and variably express carcinoembryonic antigen, B72.3 antigen, BER-EP4 antigen. In some cysts there is a small population of endocrine cells which possess dense core granules ultrastructurally and express chromogranin immunohistochemically.

DIFFERENTIAL DIAGNOSIS: Some cases of atrioventricular nodal tumors have been mistaken for metastatic adenocarcinoma. Unlike metastatic adenocarcinoma, there is no extracardiac malignancy, there are no mitoses, and no cellular atypia. Rarely, atrioventricular nodal tumors have been mistaken for cardiac myxoma with glandular structures. There is no myxoid matrix and no luminal component in atrioventricular nodal tumors. Cardiac teratoma may occasionally occur in the atrioventricular nodal area. These tumors contain, in addition to endodermal cysts, mesodermal and ectodermal structures. Bronchogenic cysts may occasionally be located within the myocardium. In contrast to tumors of the atrioventricular node, the location is not near the membranous septum, and microscopically, there is a well-developed muscular layer surrounding the cyst.

KEY DIAGNOSTIC CRITERIA: Absolute requirements for diagnosis: Location in the atrioventricular nodal area; nests or cysts lined by epithelial cells.

Items incompatible with diagnosis: Cellular pleomorphism and atypia; presence of immature cell types, mesodermal structures, or ectodermal structures.

"DABSKA" TUMOR (MALIGNANT ENDOVASCULAR PAPILLARY ANGIOENDOTHELIOMA)

Entry Authors: Allen P. Burke and Elizabeth A. Montgomery

DEFINITION: Extremely rare, cutaneous vascular tumor of possible low-grade malignancy that usually occurs in infants and children. The histologic features are typical and define the process.

GROSS FINDINGS: Superficial cutaneous or dermal tumors that may eventually grow into underlying bone or muscle and capable of lymph node spread.

MICROSCOPIC FINDINGS: Capillary and cavernous vascular tumor with areas of atypical endothelial cells forming papillary tufts with a central avascular hyaline core. The endothelial cells lining the papillae have eccentricity located nuclei that line the luminal aspect of the tuft. Intravascular lymphocytes may be prominent. Lymphoid aggregates, foci of hemorrhage, cholesterol clefts, and siderophages may be noted. Epithelioid endothelial cells with vacuoles may be present.

SPECIAL PROCEDURES NEEDED FOR DIAGNOSIS: Electron microscopy demonstrates that the hyaline core consists of basal lamina-like material.

DIFFERENTIAL DIAGNOSIS: Spindle cell hemangioma may also show vacuolated endothelial cells but will not form papillary structures.

KEY DIAGNOSTIC CRITERIA: Absolute requirements for diagnosis: Papillary tufts within dilated vascular channels.

Items incompatible with diagnosis: Necrosis, large numbers of mitotic figures.

EPITHELIOID HEMANGIOMA

Entry Authors: Allen P. Burke and Elizabeth A. Montgomery

DEFINITION: A proliferation of benign-appearing, capillary-sized vessels lined by plump epithelioid (histiocytoid) endothelial cells, typically associated with eosinophils and lymphocytes.

GROSS FINDINGS: Small, single mass (usually <3 cm) that is well demarcated and frequently attached to a damaged artery.

MICROSCOPIC FINDINGS: Muscular artery with focal medial disruption. Intraluminal proliferation of immature uncanalized capillaries. Endothelial cells have an epithelioid appearance. Process may extend into the adventitia and surrounding soft tissue, inciting an inflammatory response that may contain lymphoid follicles and an eosinophilic infiltrate. A less circumscribed, dermal form of epithelioid hemangioma without attachment to a muscular artery has been described.

DIFFERENTIAL DIAGNOSIS: Pyogenic granuloma has a lobulated growth pattern. Kimura's disease (see entry) is a predominantly fibroinflammatory process without significant vascular proliferation. Epithelioid hemangioendothelioma is infiltrative and consist of more atypical cells with intracytoplasmic lumina.

KEY DIAGNOSTIC CRITERIA: Items incompatible with diagnosis: Microabscesses. Irregular extension and infiltration of surrounding soft tissue. Significant cytologic atypia.

EPITHELIOID HEMANGIOENDOTHELIOMA

Entry Authors: Allen P. Burke and Elizabeth A. Montgomery

DEFINITION: Low- or intermediate grade malignant vascular tumor of adults with a characteristic histologic appearance. Older names include intravascular bronchoalveolar tumor (for those occurring in the lung), and sclerosing cholangiocarcinoma (for liver lesions). It is unclear what proportion of pulmonary and hepatic epithelioid hemangiomas, which are typically multiple, represent metastases from occult soft tissue primaries.

GROSS FINDINGS: Multilobular tumor, often associated with a medium-sized vein, with a propensity for the subcutis or deep soft tissue of the extremities. Tumors are typically whitish-tan, well marginated, firm and rubbery, or cartilaginous.

MICROSCOPIC FINDINGS: Epithelioid endothelial cells are organized in cord-like arrangements or clusters within a myxohyaline or chondromyxoid matrix. Neoplastic cells contain prominent cytoplasmic vacuoles. Atypia is usually mild, although more cytologically pleomorphic and bizarre areas suggestive of epithelioid angiosarcoma may be found. The neoplastic cells do not organize into well-formed vessels.

SPECIAL PROCEDURES NEEDED FOR DIAGNOSIS: Immunohistochemical stains demonstrate factor VIII-related antigen, as well as other endothelial markers, such as CD34.

DIFFERENTIAL DIAGNOSIS: Carcinoma: Many examples of epithelioid hemangioendothelioma are initially considered to be carcinoma because of the epithelioid appearance of the cells. Presence of intracytoplasmic vacuoles, association with a vein, and immunohistochemical expression of endothelial markers are consistent with a vascular tumor. It is prudent to perform a battery of immunohistochemical stains when considering this diagnosis. Epithelioid angiosarcoma (see entry for *Angiosarcoma*) is in the differential diagnosis if there is significant pleomorphism and prominent irregular, eosinophilic nucleoli. There may be a biologic continuum between these two entities.

KEY DIAGNOSTIC CRITERIA: Absolute requirements for diagnosis: Intracytoplasmic vacuoles. Expression of endothelial marker(s). Epithelioid appearance of neoplastic cells.

Items incompatible with diagnosis: Expression of multiple epithelial markers (cytokeratin may be expressed). Diffuse pleomorphism with anastomosing vascular channels. Prominent, irregular nucleoli.

FIBROSARCOMA

Entry Author: Allen P. Burke

DEFINITION: Sarcoma composed of spindled fibroblast-like cells often arrayed in a herringbone pattern.

GROSS FINDINGS: Cardiac fibrosarcomas are usually relatively well demarcated. Endocardial-based tumors of the left atrium, that are generally myxoid, homogeneous, and often infiltrate surrounding myocardium.

MICROSCOPIC FINDINGS: Relatively bland proliferation of spindled cells usually with myxoid background. Densely cellular areas with a "herringbone" pattern are classically described. Fibrosis is common with areas of mild cellular pleomorphism and crowding.

SPECIAL PROCEDURES NEEDED FOR DIAGNOSIS: Immunohistochemical studies demonstrate that the tumor cells do not express desmin, S-100 protein, or cytokeratin. There is usually smooth muscle and muscle-specific actin expression.

DIFFERENTIAL DIAGNOSIS: Lesion may be misdiagnosed as myxoma (see entry, *Cardiac myxoma*) if there is a prominent myxoid background. the inflammatory background and hemosiderosis typical of myxoma are absent. Myxoma cells and their characteristic structures are absent. Malignant fibrous histiocytoma may be considered in the spectrum of fibrosarcoma and is the preferred diagnosis if there are tumor giant cells and a storiform growth pattern.

KEY DIAGNOSTIC CRITERIA: Absolute requirements for diagnosis: Spindled cells, monomorphic growth, foci of atypia, or mitotic activity.

Items incompatible with diagnosis: Marked pleomorphism or tumor giant cells. Areas of osteoid or chondrosarcoma. Expression of desmin. Structure characteristic of myxoma or abundant hemosiderin.

GLOMERULOID HEMANGIOMA

Entry Authors: Allen P. Burke and Elizabeth A. Montgomery

DEFINITION: Small, usually multifocal hemangiomas of the skin that are part of the POEMS syndrome (polyneuropathy, organomegaly, endocrinopathy, monoclonal protein, and skin lesions).

GROSS FINDINGS: Pin- to pea-sized papules.

MICROSCOPIC FINDINGS: Dilated, ectatic vessels with intraluminal capillary proliferation architecturally resembling renal glomeruli. There may be intervening stromal cells with clear cytoplasm and PAS-positive diastase resistant globules that are believed to represent phagocytosed immunoglobulin.

DIFFERENTIAL DIAGNOSIS: Kaposi sarcoma has a spindled component and is not intravascular.

KEY DIAGNOSTIC CRITERIA: Absolute requirements for diagnosis: Intravascular proliferation. Presence of one or more stigmata of POEMS syndrome.

GRANULAR CELL TUMOR

Entry Author: Allen P. Burke

DEFINITION: Benign neoplasm of nerve sheath origin composed of homogeneous granular cells.

GROSS FINDINGS: Epicardial nodule, usually single, at the base of the heart and often overlying an epicardial coronary artery. On section, granular cell tumors are firm, homogeneous, whitish-tan.

MICROSCOPIC FINDINGS: There is monotonous proliferation of polygonal cells with abundant cytoplasm and small ovoid nuclei. The cytoplasm contains numerous granules that are weakly PAS-positive with little staining change after diastase pretreatment. S-100 protein is immunohistochemically demonstrable. Ultrastructurally, the granules consist of membrane-bound autophagic vacuoles containing cellular debris of mitochondria, rough endoplasmic reticulum, and myelinated and nonmyelinated structures resembling axons.

DIFFERENTIAL DIAGNOSIS: Histiocytoid (oncocytic) cardiomyopathy (Purkinje cell hamartoma): these are multiple, intramural and subendocardial, and found in infants. They are PAS-negative and S-100 negative and ultrastructurally show numerous mitochondria. Rhabdomyoma: These are intramural and usually multiple. Histologically, they are PAS-positive, contain large clear vacuoles, and ultrastructurally contain abundant glycogen. Whipple's disease: Microscopic infiltrates of histiocytes that contain strongly PAS-positive intracellular bacteria.

KEY DIAGNOSTIC CRITERIA: Absolute requirements for diagnosis: Epicardial location, S-100-positivity, presence of weakly PAS-positive granules.

HAMARTOMA

Entry Author: Allen P. Burke

DEFINITION: A benign, presumably congenital, non-neoplastic proliferation of mature tissue of a type that is normally found in the heart, forming a mass fairly distinct from surrounding normal tissue.

Specific definitions: Two cardiac masses defined elsewhere in this book are hamartomas—see *Rhabdomyoma, Purkinje cell hamartoma* (histiocytoid [oncocytic] cardiomyopathy). Other lesions of uncertain nature are variably considered hamartomas—see *Fibrosarcoma, Lipomatous hypertrophy, Papillary fibroelastoma, Hemangioma.*

Nonspecific hamartomas: Occasionally a cardiac mass is identified that does not fit a specific definition but has characteristics of a hamartoma. For example, discrete masses of disorganized myocardium have been described in the right ventricle that histologically resemble the myofiber disarray seen in cases of hypertrophic cardiomyopathy.

HEMANGIOMA

Entry Authors: Allen P. Burke and Elizabeth A. Montgomery

DEFINITION: A benign proliferation of blood vessels. May be composed of various proportions of capillaries, arteries, and veins. May be subclassified by vascular component into capillary, cavernous, arteriovenous, or mixed types.

GROSS FINDINGS: There are two varieties: those that are endocardial-based lesions and those that are intramural hemangiomas. Endocardial hemangiomas are well circumscribed, variably myxoid, soft masses. Intramural hemangiomas are often poorly circumscribed, spongy masses that appear variably hemorrhagic or congested.

MICROSCOPIC FINDINGS: Endocardial hemangiomas are usually capillary or mixed cavernous-capillary hemangiomas. There is often a myxoid stroma with a sparse inflammatory background. The capillaries are lined by a single layer of endothelial cells without significant atypia. Intramural hemangiomas are histologically diverse and may be capillary or cavernous hemangiomas that are fairly circumscribed. Intramural hemangiomas may also be composed of thick walled dysplastic arteries, vein-like vessels, and capillaries. Unlike endocardial hemangiomas, intramural cardiac hemangiomas may contain other tissue elements, especially fat, and occasionally fibrous tissue. In this regard, intramural cardiac hemangiomas resemble intramuscular hemangiomas of soft tissue.

DIFFERENTIAL DIAGNOSIS: Myxoma: Endocardial hemangiomas are typically misdiagnosed as myxoma (see entry, cardiac myxoma). Unlike myxoma, there are no myxoma cells. Endothelial structures are lined by a single layer of cells. There are no cords or ring structures that are infiltrated by lymphocytes and they are more likely ventricular in location than atrial. Angiosarcoma: Necrosis, cellular atypia, anastomosing vascular structures, mitotic figures, and pericardial infiltration are typical of angiosarcoma and lacking in hemangioma. If there is papillary endothelial hyperplasia in an otherwise typical hemangioma, angiosarcoma may be more difficult to exclude. Lipoma: If there is a prominent fatty background, the differential diagnosis includes lipoma. However, thick-walled vessels and areas of capillary or cavernous hemangioma are generally present. Angiolipoma: A rare entity that may exist in the heart. The vascular component is composed of capillary-sized vessels that infiltrate the fat but areas of solid hemangioma, fibrosis, and thick-walled arterial vessels are absent.

INFANTILE KAPOSIFORM HEMANGIOENDOTHELIOMA

Entry Authors: Allen P. Burke and Elizabeth A. Montgomery

DEFINITION: Rare, locally aggressive, distinctive vascular tumor of infants and children, which is typically deep-seated and has histologic features that overlap with Kaposi sarcoma. Believed by some to be an aggressive variant of juvenile capillary hemangioma. These may be locally aggressive but metastases have not been reported.

GROSS FINDINGS: Large, infiltrative reddish-brown mass that occurs most often in the retroperitoneum. May infiltrate adjacent organs resulting in jaundice or intestinal obstruction. Tumors that occur in the extremities, scalp, and neck may be less infiltrative at the time of diagnosis.

MICROSCOPIC FINDINGS: Infiltrative lesion composed of lobules of well-formed capillaries, often with fibrin thrombi, separated by intervening fibrous septa. the capillaries are intermixed with spindled cells with slit-like lumina that may be reminiscent of Kaposi sarcoma.

DIFFERENTIAL DIAGNOSIS: Kaposi sarcoma is generally a tumor of immunosuppressed adults and is multifocal and nonlobulated. In contrast to Kaposiform tumor of infancy, Kaposi sarcoma possesses a greater inflammatory reaction, lacks pericytic cells, and contains more hyaline globules. Angiosarcoma lacks a lobulated growth pattern, possesses interanastomosing vascular patterns, and cytologic atypia. Cellular capillary hemangioma lacks spindled endothelial cells.

KEY DIAGNOSTIC CRITERIA: Absolute requirements for diagnosis: Presence of mixture of capillaries and spindled cells. Occurrence in the pediatric age group.

Items incompatible with diagnosis: Necrosis, cellular atypia.

INTRAVASCULAR FASCIITIS

Entry Authors: Allen P. Burke and Elizabeth A. Montgomery

DEFINITION: Nodular fasciitis occurring within a blood vessel.

GROSS FINDINGS: Nodular, attached to a vein, or less commonly, an artery, usually in the arms, head, or neck.

MICROSCOPIC FINDINGS: Intravascular multinodular or plexiform proliferation of spindled cells. Spindled cells have a feathery or tissue culture appearance and have the histologic and immunohistochemical features of myofibroblasts. Mitoses may be plentiful.

DIFFERENTIAL DIAGNOSIS: Epithelioid hemangioendothelioma will possess more infiltrating margins and intracytoplasmic vacuoles (rudimentary vascular lumina). Tumor cells are positive for factor VIII-related antigen and CD34. Vascular smooth muscle tumors will have more compact fascicular growth, may have paranuclear vacuoles and longitudinal cytoplasmic striations as seen on Masson trichrome stain, and may express immunoreactive desmin.

KEY DIAGNOSTIC CRITERIA: Absolute requirements for diagnosis: Location in or near vessel. Spindle cell growth.

Items incompatible with diagnosis: Intracytoplasmic vacuoles, positivity for factor VIII-related antigen, nuclear pleomorphism.

INTRAMUSCULAR HEMANGIOMA

Entry Authors: Allen P. Burke and Elizabeth A. Montgomery

DEFINITION: Benign vascular proliferation occurring within skeletal muscle.

GROSS FINDINGS: Infiltrating whitish-tan to reddish-brown mass occurring within skeletal muscle. Dilated vascular channels may or may not be grossly identified. Fat may be grossly visible. Ossified lesions may be gritty on section.

MICROSCOPIC FINDINGS: There are a variety of histologic appearances, compatible with capillary hemangioma, cavernous hemangioma, arteriovenous hemangioma. Often there is a combination of angiomatous patterns. Overgrowth of adipose tissue is common, and ossification is sometimes present.

DIFFERENTIAL DIAGNOSIS: Angiosarcoma demonstrates an interanastomosing sinusoidal pattern with pleomorphism and atypical mitotic activity, and is rare within skeletal muscle. Intramuscular lipoma does not contain areas of capillary proliferation or the gaping vasculature present in most intramuscular hemangiomas. Liposarcoma will contain lipoblasts absent in intramuscular hemangioma.

KEY DIAGNOSTIC CRITERIA: Absolute requirements for diagnosis: Location in skeletal muscle. Presence of either capillary, cavernous, or arteriovenous hemangioma.

KAPOSI SARCOMA

Entry Authors: Allen P. Burke and Elizabeth A. Montgomery

DEFINITION: Multifocal vascular tumor associated with immunosuppression that characteristically evolves through several stages.

GROSS FINDINGS: Early lesions are cutaneous purple patches, followed by plaques and nodules that may coalesce and ulcerate. Individual lesions may regress. The skin is the most common site, but mucosal and visceral lesions, especially in the late stages of disease, may occur.

MICROSCOPIC FINDINGS: Early lesions (patch stage) show a proliferation of capillaries, often ectatic or angulated, around preexisting dermal vessels and adnexa. Atypia is mild. A "promontory" sign, i.e., protrusion of proliferating cells into a larger dermal vessel, is a helpful diagnostic sign. There may be a lymphocytic or lymphoplasmacytic inflammatory infiltrate, and hemosiderin deposition with PAS-positive diastase-resistant hyaline globules.

In plaque lesions, the spindled component becomes prominent within dermal collagen and around a network of new vessels. Slit-like spaces appear that contain red blood cells. Plasma cells and hemosiderin deposits become more obvious. One to seven micron eosinophilic hyaline globules appear that may form grape-like agglomerations.

In nodular lesions, the spindle-cell proliferation predominates, and may suggest leiomyosarcoma of fibrosarcoma. Extravasated red blood cells, a peripheral lymphoplasmacytic infiltrate, hyaline globules, and single cell necrosis may still be present.

DIFFERENTIAL DIAGNOSIS: Early lesion: Hemangioma—angiodermatitis secondary to chronic venous insufficiency. Targetoid hemosiderotic hemangioma (usually solitary). Bacillary angiomatosis.

Late lesion: Fibrosarcoma, leiomyosarcoma.

KEY DIAGNOSTIC CRITERIA: Absolute requirements for diagnosis: Early lesion—High clinical index of suspicion, unless promontory sign, hemosiderin deposits with PAS-positive globules, or areas of spindle cell proliferation are present.

Absolute requirements for diagnosis: Late lesion—Proliferation of spindle cells. PAS-positive, diastase-resistant globules, hemosiderin deposits, slit-like spaces with red blood cells.

KAPOSI SARCOMA
(PERICARDIUM/EPICARDIUM)

Entry Author: Allen P. Burke

DEFINITION: Atypical multinodular proliferation of spindled mesenchymal cells arranged in fascicles and separated by slit-like spaces containing erythrocytes and hyaline globules. Presumably a neoplasm. Virtually all accepted cases of cardiac Kaposi sarcoma have occurred in patients with underlying immunosuppression.

GROSS FINDINGS: Multiple hemorrhagic nodules in the pericardium. May superficially invade myocardium or result in tamponade. Kaposi sarcoma of skin and viscera almost always present.

MICROSCOPIC FINDINGS: Proliferation of atypical spindled cells with slit-like vascular spaces. Hemosiderin deposition. PAS-positive, diastase-resistant hyaline globules typically present.

DIFFERENTIAL DIAGNOSIS: Angiosarcoma. Invades myocardium. Hyaline globules and hemosiderin unusual. Not present in immunocompromised patients.

KEY DIAGNOSTIC CRITERIA: Requirements for diagnosis: History of immunosuppression a virtual requirement.

KIMURA'S DISEASE

Entry Authors: Allen P. Burke and Elizabeth A. Montgomery

DEFINITION: Fibroinflammatory subcutaneous mass, usually in the head and neck that may be multifocal or bilateral associated with lymphadenopathy and peripheral eosinophilia that possesses typical histologic features.

GROSS FINDINGS: Poorly circumscribed subcutaneous process, single or multinodular, ranging in size from a few millimeters to several centimeters.

MICROSCOPIC FINDINGS: Fibroinflammatory lesion with minimal vascular proliferation, eosinophils (including eosinophilic microabscesses), lymphocytes, and fibrosis.

DIFFERENTIAL DIAGNOSIS: Epithelioid hemangioma is often associated with an artery and consists of a proliferation of epithelioid endothelial cells.

KEY DIAGNOSTIC CRITERIA: Absolute requirements for diagnosis: Occurrence in endemic location (China, Japan, and neighboring countries), subcutaneous location, lymphoid aggregates, or follicles, eosinophilic infiltrate (in early stages of lesion).

Items incompatible with diagnosis: Occurrence near muscular artery, epithelioid appearance of vascular proliferation.

LEIOMYOSARCOMA

Entry Author: Allen P. Burke

DEFINITION: Sarcoma of smooth muscle cells.

GROSS FINDINGS: Endocardial-based tumor, usually of the left atrium, may have smooth endocardial surface but typically infiltrates the myocardium. Cut surface may be homogeneous or show areas of hemorrhage and necrosis.

MICROSCOPIC FINDINGS: Densely cellular tumor of perpendicularly oriented fascicles of spindled cells. Perinuclear vacuoles are occasionally present. Longitudinal fuchsinophilic striations may be seen. Intracytoplasmic glycogen may be noted as a diffuse punctate positivity by PAS stain. Myxoid areas may occur and foci of epithelioid and rounded cells may be present. Areas of pleomorphism reminiscent of malignant fibrous histiocytoma may occur.

SPECIAL PROCEDURES NEEDED FOR DIAGNOSIS: Immunohistochemical stains for desmin show tumor cell expression in 50% or more cases.

DIFFERENTIAL DIAGNOSIS: Rhabdomyosarcoma: Rhabdomyoblasts are absent. Fibrosarcoma: Fascicles are arranged in a herringbone pattern rather than perpendicularly and collagen deposition is more prominent. Nuclei of leiomyosarcoma are usually more blunt-ended. Malignant fibrous histiocytoma possesses more haphazard fascicles which may have a storiform pattern. Fascicular growth, desmin positivity, and perinuclear vacuoles are absent.

KEY DIAGNOSTIC CRITERIA: Absolute requirements for diagnosis: Typical histologic features (see above) or positivity for desmin. Occasionally, the distinction between leiomyosarcoma and undifferentiated sarcoma or malignant fibrous histiocytoma may be difficult.

Items incompatible with diagnosis: Presence of rhabdomyoblasts. Diffuse positivity for epithelial markers.

LIPOMA

Entry Author: Allen P. Burke

DEFINITION: Like lipomas of extracardiac soft tissue, lipomas of the heart are benign neoplasms of adipose tissue.

GROSS FINDINGS: Circumscribed, spherical or elliptic mass of homogeneous yellow fat. Nearly all cardiac lipomas are epicardial lesions that may occur at any site on the atrial or ventricular surface. Most reported cases have been single, although multiple lipomas have been reported in patients with congenital heart defects, tuberous sclerosis, and rarely in an otherwise normal heart.

MICROSCOPIC FINDINGS: Histological findings: Cardiac lipomas are composed of mature adipocytes, although there may be entrapped myocytes at the base of the tumor. A capsule is usually present, although it may be focally absent or attenuated.

DIFFERENTIAL DIAGNOSIS: Lipomatous hypertrophy has an interatrial location and shows the presence of fetal fat and/or hypertrophic myocytes within the tumor. In hemangioma with fatty stromal overgrowth there are blood vessels of various sizes, often dysplastic vessels, and a lack of circumscription.

LIPOMATOUS HYPERTROPHY

Entry Author: Allen P. Burke

DEFINITION: Lipomatous hypertrophy of the atrial septum is a nonencapsulated proliferation of mature fat, adipose cells resembling fetal fat cells, and enlarged cardiac myocytes. Any deposit of fat in the atrial septum at the level of the fossa ovalis that exceeds 2 cm in transverse dimension is diagnostic of lipomatous hypertrophy. The upper limit of normal has alternately been defined as 1.5 cm in young adults, with increasing limits as age progresses. The increase in mass in the atrial septum is likely secondary to an increased number of fat cells, as opposed to hypertrophied myocytes. Therefore, the word "hypertrophy" in lipomatous hypertrophy of interatrial septum is a misnomer.

GROSS FINDINGS: The atrial septum is thickened up to several centimeters, and the fatty mass generally extends into the right atrium. The thickness of the atrial septum cephalad to the fossa ovalis is always greater than that of the atrial septum caudal to the fossa ovalis. These tumors can achieve great dimensions, occasionally attaining a size of 15 cm. There can be involvement of the entire septum, and occasionally the bulk of the tumor is attached to the atrial surface. Although histologically the lesions are infiltrating, they can occasionally appear circumscribed grossly because of the bulging of the endocardial surfaces. Usually, the fossa ovalis is spared, although there can be mild fatty infiltration at this site.

MICROSCOPIC FINDINGS: There is a mixture of fat and cardiac myocytes. At least some of the fat will show vacuolization with centrally placed nuclei. These cells resemble fetal fat and fat cells that are present in malnourished or starving patients. In most cases, the interspersed cardiac myocytes will be bizarre and greatly enlarged. However, mitoses are absent, distinguishing this lesion from a malignancy.

DIFFERENTIAL DIAGNOSIS: The differential diagnosis of lipomatous hypertrophy includes liposarcoma and other sarcomas, especially if there is a large mass resected surgically. The "fetal" fat cells in lipomatous hypertrophy are sometimes mistaken for lipoblasts. Unlike lipoblasts, fat cells in lipomatous hypertrophy do not form signet ring structures and do not have enlarged, hyperchromatic-indented nuclei. The hyperchromatic, enlarged myocytes are also sometimes mistaken for malignant cells, but the lack of mitotic figures and other features of lipomatous hypertrophy point to the correct diagnosis.

KEY DIAGNOSTIC CRITERIA: Absolute requirements for diagnosis: Presence of interspersed myocytes, often bizarre; occasional fetal fat cells (may not be present in all sections).

Items incompatible with diagnosis: microscopic encapsulation; presence of true lipoblasts; mitotic figures.

LIPOSARCOMA

Entry Author: Allen P. Burke

DEFINITION: Sarcoma that contains lipoblasts.

GROSS FINDINGS: Gross features of cardiac sarcomas are difficult to describe due to their rarity. Reported cases are often in the atrium or on the epicardium.

MICROSCOPIC FINDINGS: Myxoid liposarcoma has a background of branching capillary vessels with few lipoblasts. Pleomorphic liposarcoma may resemble malignant fibrous histiocytoma, but lipoblasts are easily identified. Lipoblasts contain large fat vacuoles that sharply indent or otherwise disturb the outline of the cell nucleus.

SPECIAL PROCEDURES NEEDED FOR DIAGNOSIS: Fat stains demonstrate positivity in a variety of sarcomas. A positive fat stain is, therefore, not diagnostic of liposarcoma. Ultrastructure will demonstrate large fat vacuoles indenting the cell nucleus.

DIFFERENTIAL DIAGNOSIS: Lipomatous hypertrophy of the atrial septum contains fetal-type adipocytes (multivesicular fat) that may be confused for lipoblasts and hypertrophied myocytes. Mitotic figures are absent.

KEY DIAGNOSTIC CRITERIA: Absolute requirements for diagnosis: Lipoblasts.

Items incompatible with diagnosis: Hypertrophic myocytes within tumor, fetal-type fat.

LYMPHOMA

Entry Author: Allen P. Burke

DEFINITION: Lymphoma is a malignant proliferation of lymphoid cells. "Primary cardiac lymphoma" denotes a lymphoma that is primarily intrapericardial, presents as a cardiac tumor, and may have regional lymph node involvement. Previous definitions have been more strict, requiring an absence of lymphoma outside the pericardial sac, demonstrated by a complete autopsy examination. Many cardiac lymphomas diagnosed today occur in immunocompromised patients, arise in potentially reversible benign lymphoid proliferations ("posttransplant lymphoproliferative disorder") and contain episomal Epstein-Barr virus DNA.

GROSS FINDINGS: Multiple masses of firm, white nodules are characteristic of cardiac lymphoma. The heart is usually enlarged, with a mean weight of approximately 700 g. Hemorrhage and necrosis are uncommon, as is significant extension into the ventricular or atrial cavities or valves. The sites of the heart most often affected by lymphoma are the right atrium, followed by the right ventricle, left ventricle, left atrium, atrial septum, and ventricular septum. More than one cardiac chamber is involved in over 75% of cases, although tumors confined to the atria, pericardium, and coronary arteries may occur. Extension onto the pericardial surfaces is typical.

MICROSCOPIC FINDINGS: There is a variety of histologic types, including small noncleaved follicular center cell, intermediate lymphoma, B-immunoblastic, large cell undifferentiated, large cell non-cleaved, and centroblastic/centrocytic (cleaved follicular center cell) lymphoma. To date, every cardiac lymphoma reported with immunophenotypic data has been of B-cell origin.

DIFFERENTIAL DIAGNOSIS: Undifferentiated metastatic carcinoma or melanoma can be distinguished from lymphoma by immunohistochemical stains for epithelial, neural, and melanoma-specific markers, that are generally negative in lymphoma. Polyclonal reactive lymphoid proliferations in immunocompromised patients are polymorphous and lack significant atypia and may regress with restoration of immunity. Severe rejection may be difficult to distinguish from lymphoproliferative disorders. The infiltrate is generally T-cell rich and composed primarily of well-differentiated lymphocytes.

MALIGNANT FIBROUS HISTIOCYTOMA

Entry Author: Allen P. Burke

DEFINITION: Pleomorphic sarcoma showing no distinct line of differentiation.

GROSS FINDINGS: Bulky tumor, usually situated in left atrium. Often endocardium based with infiltration of surrounding myocardium or valves.

MICROSCOPIC FINDINGS: Similar to fibrosarcoma but having a haphazard fascicular arrangement. In addition, pleomorphic areas with xanthoma cells, tumor giant cells, and arborizing vessels may occur. Myxoid areas may occur. A storiform pattern is classically described but frequently absent. Mitotic figures are usually easy to identify and areas of necrosis are typically present. In the heart, the pleomorphic, storiform, and myxoid types of malignant fibrous histiocytoma have been described.

SPECIAL PROCEDURES NEEDED FOR DIAGNOSIS: Immunohistochemical stains are generally negative for epithelial markers although focal staining for cytokeratin may occur. Desmin expression is absent.

DIFFERENTIAL DIAGNOSIS: Fibrosarcoma lacks the degree of pleomorphism and storiform pattern. Metastatic carcinoma will diffusely express epithelial markers.

KEY DIAGNOSTIC CRITERIA: Absolute requirements for diagnosis: Marked cellular pleomorphism.

Incompatible with diagnosis: Evidence of differentiation along a specific cell line, e.g., myogenous, osteosarcomatous.

MALIGNANT PERIPHERAL NERVE SHEATH TUMOR (NEUROFIBROSARCOMA, MALIGNANT SCHWANNOMA)

Entry Author: Allen P. Burke

DEFINITION: Sarcoma with schwann cell differentiation.

GROSS FINDINGS: Epicardial tumors, may grow into the myocardium. Extremely rare in the heart.

MICROSCOPIC FINDINGS: Spindled cell tumors, often with a myxoid background. Nuclei may be irregular (buckled). Areas with rhabdomyoblasts may be present (malignant Triton tumor).

SPECIAL PROCEDURES NEEDED FOR DIAGNOSIS: Immunohistochemical stains may demonstrate nuclear positivity for S-100 protein. Other neural markers may be expressed.

DIFFERENTIAL DIAGNOSIS: Fibrosarcoma is usually intracavitary and S-100-negative.

MESOTHELIAL/MONOCYTIC INCIDENTAL CARDIAC EXCRESCENCE (MICE)

Entry Author: Allen P. Burke

DEFINITION: Avascular collection of detached mesothelial cells, histiocytes, and fat that are presumed artifacts of cardiac bypass.

GROSS FINDINGS: Fragments of tissue that are incidentally found in the atria, on valves, or other cardiac and aortic locations, including attached to neoplasms.

MICROSCOPIC FINDINGS: Detached mesothelial cells, fat cells, and inflammatory cells, the majority of which are histiocytes. The general appearance is that of a cytologic preparation.

SPECIAL PROCEDURES NEEDED FOR DIAGNOSIS: Immunohistochemical stains will demonstrate expression of cytokeratin in the mesothelial cells.

DIFFERENTIAL DIAGNOSIS: Hemangioma of heart may have epithelioid areas in contrast to mesothelial/monocytic incidental cardiac excrescences. These are true tumors that occur within the myocardium.

KEY DIAGNOSTIC CRITERIA: Absolute requirements for diagnosis: Presence of mesothelial cells, monocytes, fat cells. Items incompatible with diagnosis: Tumor stroma or vascularity.

NEUROFIBROMA, NEURILEMOMA

Entry Author: Allen P. Burke

DEFINITION: Neurofibromas and neurilemomas are benign tumors of nerve sheath origin that extremely rarely involve the heart.

GROSS FINDINGS: Well-demarcated mass, usually in the atrium or on the atrial epicardium. May rarely be present within either ventricle.

MICROSCOPIC FINDINGS: Similar to extracardiac nerve sheath tumors.

OSTEOSARCOMA

Entry Author: Allen P. Burke

DEFINITION: Sarcoma where malignant cells produce areas of osteoid with or without cartilage.

GROSS FINDINGS: Endocardial-based tumor of left atrium.

MICROSCOPIC FINDINGS: A portion or a majority of the tumor often resembles fibrosarcoma (see above). There are areas of osteoid produced by atypical cells or chondroid areas resembling chondrosarcoma.

DIFFERENTIAL DIAGNOSIS: Fibrosarcoma: Lack of osteoid or chondroid. Chondrosarcoma: this term may be used if the bulk of tumor is chondrosarcoma, although areas of osteosarcoma are generally present as well. Myxoma with osseous metaplasia: hemosiderosis typical of myxoma will be present. Myxoma cells will be present. Osseous metaplasia will consist of marrow and mature bone.

KEY DIAGNOSTIC CRITERIA: Absolute requirements for diagnosis: Osteoid. Items incompatible with diagnosis: Areas of myxoma.

PAPILLARY ENDOTHELIAL HYPERPLASIA

Entry Authors: Allen P. Burke and Elizabeth A. Montgomery

DEFINITION: Exuberant organizing thrombus, that may be mistaken for neoplasm.

GROSS FINDINGS: Bluish or purplish nodule, generally located within a vein.

MICROSCOPIC FINDINGS: Papillary fronds lined by single layer of endothelial cells. Core of fronds contain organizing fibrin thrombus, and later, collagen. Endothelial cells may be plump but lack significant atypia or mitotic figures. Fronds are often detached and appear to lack connection to the remainder of the lesion. Process is typically confined to an intravascular location.

DIFFERENTIAL DIAGNOSIS: Angiosarcoma is rarely confined to a vascular lumen, will demonstrate significant cellular pleomorphism, generally possesses solid or trabeculated areas, and will often show numerous mitotic figures and necrosis.

KEY DIAGNOSTIC CRITERIA: Absolute requirements for diagnosis: Intravascular location, papillary fronds, single-cell endothelial layer.

Items incompatible with diagnosis: Frequent mitotic figures, trabecular growth, solid, or spindled areas.

PAPILLARY FIBROELASTOMA (FIBROELASTIC PAPILLOMA)

Entry Author: Allen P. Burke

DEFINITION: Papillary tumor resembling Lambl's excrescences. Differ from Lambl's excrescence by large size and location away from nodules of Arantii.

GROSS FINDINGS: Papillary tumor resembling "sea anemone" appreciated best by immersion in water. May occur anywhere on endocardial surfaces, most commonly on valves.

MICROSCOPIC FINDINGS: Avascular papillary structures lined by a single layer of endothelial cells. Core is formed by fibrous tissue, outer lining is myxoid, with scattered smooth muscle cells. Presence of elastic fibers is variable. These are most prominent at base of tumor.

DIFFERENTIAL DIAGNOSIS: Lambl's excrescences are located exclusively in the mid-portion of valve cusps at the line of closure. In the case of the aortic valve, this is usually at the nodule of Arantii. No set size criteria distinguishing Lambl's excrescence from papillary fibroelastoma at this site. Apart from this site, tumor is termed papillary fibroelastoma.

KEY DIAGNOSTIC CRITERIA: Absolute requirements for diagnosis: Papillary fronds, endothelial lining, endocardial location.

Items incompatible with diagnosis: Presence of vessels within tumor.

PARAGANGLIOMA

Entry Author: Allen P. Burke

DEFINITION: Cardiac paraganglioma is a neoplasm of paraganglial cells. Extra-adrenal paragangliomas that secrete catecholamines are generally chromaffin-positive and have been termed "chromaffin" paragangliomas, or "pheochromocytomas." Tumors of similar morphology that occur in the region of the carotid body and aortic body are generally called "chemodectomas." These latter tumors are generally chromaffin-negative or weakly positive, and rarely secrete significant amounts of catecholamines. The terms *pheochromocytoma* and *chemodectoma* have been used for cardiac paragangliomas that are functional or nonfunctional, respectively. Because there are no consistent histologic differences between functioning and nonfunctioning paragangliomas, and because the chromaffin reaction does not reliably separate these tumors, the preferred terms are nonfunctional and functional paraganglioma for cardiac tumors, as has been recommended for extra-adrenal paragangliomas of soft tissue.

GROSS FINDINGS: Cardiac paragangliomas are large, poorly circumscribed masses that are 5–15 cm in greatest dimension. Most are located on the epicardial surface of the base of the heart or atria. Less common locations are the atrial cavity or septum, and rarely, the ventricles.

MICROSCOPIC FINDINGS: Histologic features: Unencapsulated, monomorphous tumors composed of nests of paraganglial cells surrounded by sustentacular cells. The histologic appearance and immunohistochemical profile are identical to extracardiac paragangliomas. Immunohistochemically, they are positive for chromogranin, neuron specific enolase, and often met-enkephalin. The sustentacular cells are positive for S-100 protein. Endocrine polypeptides

have not been demonstrated within tumor cells. Ultrastructurally, both epineph-
rine- and norepinephrine-type granules have been demonstrated, although the
latter predominate.

DIFFERENTIAL DIAGNOSIS: Granular cell tumors are smaller (<3 cm)
and contain granular cells. Spindle cell sarcoma shows mitotic figures, necrosis,
and absence of cell nests surrounded by sustentacular cells.

PRIMARY CARDIAC SARCOMA

Entry Author: Allen P. Burke

SUBTYPES: Angiosarcoma (heart/pericardium), fibrosarcoma, leiomyosarcoma, liposarcoma, lymphoma, malignant fibrous histiocytoma, malignant
peripheral nerve sheath tumor (neurofibrosarcoma, malignant schwannoma),
osteosarcoma, rhabdomyosarcoma, synovial sarcoma.

DEFINITION: Malignant neoplasm of mesenchymal origin.

GROSS FINDINGS: Dominant mass, endocardial- or myocardial-based, may
be bulky and infiltrating, hemorrhagic, cystic, necrotic and calcified areas may
occur. Alternatively, tumor may be relatively circumscribed and homogeneous.

MICROSCOPIC FINDINGS: Histologic findings: There are a variety of
patterns (see entries for specific subtypes). Spindle cells usually predominate,
although small round cell sarcomas and pleomorphic sarcomas may also occur.
Mitotic figures are invariably present. Necrosis is often present. Areas of fibrosis are common in the fibrous subtypes. Myxoid areas are common, especially
in spindled or chondrosarcomatous types. In well-differentiated tumors, spindled
areas may be deceptively bland, although cellular and atypical areas will be
found with extensive tumor sampling.

DIFFERENTIAL DIAGNOSIS: Myxoma may be confused with myxoid
sarcoma. Myxomas have a paucity of mitotic figures, myxoma cells forming
typical structures, and abundant hemosiderin and inflammatory cells. Metastatic
sarcoma must be ruled out clinically, although rarely presents as a cardiac mass.
Metastatic carcinoma and melanoma must be considered and excluded by appropriate immunohistochemical markers.

KEY DIAGNOSTIC CRITERIA: Features incompatible with diagnosis:
Presence of known extracardiac primary sarcoma or spindled or undifferentiated
carcinoma. Diffuse positivity for epithelial markers.

Absolute requirements for diagnosis: Mitotic figures, focal cellular pleomorphism and cell crowding.

PYOGENIC GRANULOMA
(LOBULAR CAPILLARY HEMANGIOMA)

Entry Authors: Allen P. Burke and Elizabeth A. Montgomery

DEFINITION: Lobulated proliferation of capillary-sized vessels with features of granulation tissue and capillary hemangioma. Surface ulceration results in a granulation tissue appearance.

GROSS FINDINGS: Red or violaceous mucosal, cutaneous, or subcutaneous nodule, usually solitary. May be sessile, pedunculated, or polypoid. Range in size from a few millimeters to a few centimeters. Surface ulceration is typical in larger lesions. An intravascular form of pyogenic granuloma has been described.

MICROSCOPIC FINDINGS: Multilobular proliferation of capillary-sized vessels sharply delineated from surrounding tissue (i.e., not invading). Collar of hyperplastic epithelium may occur. Inflammation is associated with surface ulceration.

DIFFERENTIAL DIAGNOSIS: Bacillary angiomatosis contains foci of necrosis and bacilli will be demonstrated by Warthin Starry stains. Angiosarcoma demonstrates infiltrative growth, anastomosing vascular channels, and atypical endothelial cells often with necrosis and atypical mitoses. Kaposi sarcoma, in the early stages, may be difficult to differentiate from pyogenic granuloma, although intracytoplasmic PAS-positive, diastase-resistant hyaline globules and a peripheral plasma cell response are characteristic of early Kaposi sarcoma, and not seen in pyogenic granuloma. Pyogenic granuloma may be considered a form of capillary hemangioma.

KEY DIAGNOSTIC CRITERIA: Absolute requirements for diagnosis: Nodular skin or mucosal lesion (except for intravascular type). Lobulated capillary channels.

Items incompatible with diagnosis: Infiltration, irregular margins, areas of necrosis or cellular atypia.

RHABDOMYOMA

Entry Author: Allen P. Burke

DEFINITION: Cardiac rhabdomyoma is a hamartoma of cardiac myocytes that occurs exclusively in the heart, often as multiple nodules, often in association with tuberous sclerosis.

GROSS FINDINGS: Rhabdomyomas are firm, white, well-circumscribed lobulated nodules that occur in any location in the heart but are more common in the ventricles. When multiple, they can consist of numerous miliary nodules measuring less than 1 mm ("rhabdomyomatosis"). Tumors can measure up to 10 cm, especially in sporadic cases, and average 3–4 cm.

MICROSCOPIC FINDINGS: Cardiac rhabdomyomas are well-demarcated masses composed of enlarged cells with clear cytoplasm and occasional spider cells. There is uniform vacuolization of cells and cytoplasm is relatively sparse. Cells are strongly PAS-positive, reflecting their glycogen content. Spider cells are so named because of their centrally located nucleus, surrounded by cytoplasm with radial extensions from the center of the cell to the periphery. Immunohistochemical studies document the striated muscle characteristics of rhabdomyoma cells, which express myoglobin, desmin, actin, and vimentin.

DIFFERENTIAL DIAGNOSIS: Granular cell tumors are small lesions that are generally present on the epicardial surface and lack the vacuolated cells of rhabdomyoma. Granular cell tumors do not posses myofibers and are S-100-positive and desmin- and myoglobin-negative, unlike rhabdomyomas. Glycogen storage diseases can mimic the vacuolated appearance of cardiac rhabdomyoma, and possess abundant intracytoplasmic glycogen as does cardiac rhabdomyoma. However, they do not form well-circumscribed nodules, and ultrastructurally the cells show intact polar intercalated discs of mature myocytes. Histiocytoid cardiomyopathy has been termed a form of *rhabdomyomatosis*, in contrast to rhabdomyoma. However, tumor nodules are small, and there is fine granularity to the cells without large vacuoles and spider cells.

KEY DIAGNOSTIC CRITERIA: Absolute requirements for diagnosis: Vacuolated cells, presence of abundant glycogen; clearly circumscribed nodule(s).

Features incompatible with diagnosis: Age of more than 25 years at time of presentation; mitotic figures.

RHABDOMYOSARCOMA

Entry Author: Allen P. Burke

DEFINITION: Sarcoma with striated muscle differentiation.

GROSS FINDINGS: Bulky, infiltrative tumor of ventricles or atria. Generally not endocardial based or primarily intracavitary.

MICROSCOPIC FINDINGS: Most, if not all, cardiac rhabdomyosarcomas are of the embryonal or small cell type. Rhabdomyoblasts may be few. These are identified by abundant glycogen (coarse PAS-positivity). Cross-striations are rarely identified. A portion or a majority of the tumor is a small round cell undifferentiated neoplasm. A myxoid background may be present. An alveolar pattern for rhabdomyosarcoma of the myocardium has not been described.

SPECIAL PROCEDURES NEEDED FOR DIAGNOSIS: Immunohistochemistry will demonstrate desmin and/or myoglobin within rhabdomyoblasts. Ultrastructure may demonstrate Z-bands.

DIFFERENTIAL DIAGNOSIS: Small cell undifferentiated sarcoma. Although peripheral neuroectodermal tumors and Ewing sarcoma have not been described in the heart, these are in the theoretical differential diagnosis of embryonal rhabdomyosarcoma. Leiomyosarcoma usually has a more spindled appearance than rhabdomyosarcoma.

KEY DIAGNOSTIC CRITERIA: Absolute requirements for diagnosis: Presence of rhabdomyoblasts.

SPINDLE CELL EMANGIOENDOTHELIOMA

Entry Authors: Allen P. Burke and Elizabeth A. Montgomery

DEFINITION: Cutaneous vascular tumor of indeterminate biologic potential, composed of juxtaposed cavernous vessels set in a spindled stroma containing scattered vacuolated epithelioid endothelial cells.

GROSS FINDINGS: Painless, generally multifocal masses occurring in the dermis or subcutis of the hands, feet, extremities, or trunk.

MICROSCOPIC FINDINGS: Sharply delineated tumor with areas of cavernous hemangioma and spindled cells. Smooth muscle may be present at the periphery and epithelioid endothelial cells with intracytoplasmic lumina may be present within the tumor.

DIFFERENTIAL DIAGNOSIS: Kaposi sarcoma is less circumscribed, does not have admixture of spindled endothelial cells and cavernous spaces, and generally occurs in the immunosuppressed. Epithelioid hemangioendothelioma is an infiltrative tumor without spindling, composed of epithelioid endothelial cells with cytoplasmic lumina. Epithelioid hemangioma occurs generally in the head and neck region, and is often associated with an artery, and generally has an inflammatory component. Spindle cells are absent. Cutaneous angiosarcoma is an infiltrating tumor with cytologically atypical cells lining anastomosing vascular channels.

KEY DIAGNOSTIC CRITERIA: Absolute requirements for diagnosis: Presence of spindled endothelial cells, cavernous spaces, dermal or subcutaneous location.

Incompatible with diagnosis: frequent mitotic figures, necrosis.

SYNOVIAL SARCOMA

Entry Author: Allen P. Burke

DEFINITION: Biphasic or monophasic sarcoma characterized by a typical histologic appearance (see below) and X-18 chromosomal translocations.

GROSS FINDINGS: Infiltrating, firm tan masses, often on the epicardium.

MICROSCOPIC FINDINGS: Biphasic tumor with spindled areas resembling fibrosarcoma and epithelial areas with glandular spaces containing acid mucins. Spindled areas are monomorphous, often have alternating cellular and relatively acellular myxoid areas. May have a sparse lymphocytic infiltrate at the margins. Glands will contain PAS-positive diastase-resistant material. In extracardiac soft tissue, many examples only exhibit the spindled component. These tumors may have a prominent hemangiopericytoma-like vascular pattern. Examples of monophasic cardiac synovial sarcoma have yet to be reported.

SPECIAL PROCEDURES NEEDED FOR DIAGNOSIS: Immunohistochemical staining demonstrates positive staining for cytokeratin and epithelial membrane antigen within epithelial areas and, to a lesser degree, in spindle areas. Cytogenetics will reveal an X-18 chromosomal translocation.

DIFFERENTIAL DIAGNOSIS: Malignant mesothelioma is generally less discrete a mass than synovial sarcoma that diffusely infiltrates the pericardium. The spindled areas are usually poorly demarcated from the epithelioid areas and are more pleomorphic.

KEY DIAGNOSTIC CRITERIA: X-18 chromosomal translocation. Without this may be difficult to distinguish from mesothelioma.

TERATOMA

Entry Author: Allen P. Burke

DEFINITION: Tumor of germ cell origin that contains three cell types: mesodermal, ectodermal, and endodermal.

GROSS FINDINGS: Most teratomas of the heart lie within the pericardial sac. When intramyocardial, they may obstruct the right ventricular outflow tract.

MICROSCOPIC FINDINGS: Similar to teratoma of the gonads. Usually contain only mature elements. Extremely rarely, malignant elements are seen. These include embryonal carcinoma (including yolk sac or endodermal sinus tumor) or choriocarcinoma.

DIFFERENTIAL DIAGNOSIS: Bronchogenic cyst, unlike teratoma, lacks ectodermal elements.

KEY DIAGNOSTIC CRITERIA: Absolute requirements for diagnosis: Three germ cell layers.

VENOUS HEMANGIOMA

Entry Authors: Allen P. Burke and Elizabeth A. Montgomery

DEFINITION: Vascular proliferation consisting of multiple vein-like channels. Are often considered a subset of cavernous hemangioma.

GROSS FINDINGS: These are typically deep-seated lesions which grossly appear as ectatic vessels.

MICROSCOPIC FINDINGS: Blood-filled, endothelium-lined channels with prominent muscular walls typical of veins, i.e., there is disorganization of the muscular bundles and distinct elastic laminae are absent.

SPECIAL PROCEDURES NEEDED FOR DIAGNOSIS: Arteriography will often fail to identify the lesion due to sluggish blood flow. However, venography will demonstrate a vascular tumor.

DIFFERENTIAL DIAGNOSIS: Cavernous hemangioma is a related lesion. Unlike venous hemangioma, the vascular walls are thin, without abundant smooth muscle. Arteriovenous malformation is best demonstrated by angiography and, histologically, will show arteries as well as veins.

KEY DIAGNOSTIC CRITERIA: Absolute requirement for diagnosis: Proliferation of vascular channels resembling veins.

Section 6

Traumatic, Forensic, and Iatrogenic Lesions

Section Editor: Michael D. Bell
Entry Authors: Virginia M. Walley, David A. Chiasson, and
John P. Veinot

AIR EMBOLISM, ARTERIAL

Entry Authors: Michael D. Bell, Virginia M. Walley, David A. Chiasson, and John P. Veinot

DEFINITION: The introduction of air into the pulmonary venous channels (usually traumatic) with its carriage into the superior arterial system of the head, neck, upper extremities, and coronary arteries. Sudden death results when air occludes the coronary or cerebral arteries. Fatal drowning may occur in scuba divers rendered unconscious by nonlethal cerebral occlusion while still in the water.

GROSS FINDINGS: Frothy blood may be present in the left ventricle and aorta if the volume of the arterial air embolism is large. Air bubbles may be seen in the retinal arteries during pre- or postmortem funduscopic examination (done prior to incising the body). The skin of the upper body may appear "marbled" and a small incision into the skin will show "air bleeding." Air emboli may be seen interspersed in the coronary and cerebral arteries. Look for subcutaneous and mediastinal emphysema in scuba divers and victims with chest trauma.

MICROSCOPIC FINDINGS: Not useful.

SPECIAL PROCEDURES NEEDED FOR DIAGNOSIS: Pre- or postmortem funduscopic examination. Cut upper body skin to demonstrate "air bleeding." Postmortem chest and cranial radiography if the volume of air is large enough to be detected. Examine the heart for interatrial or interventricular septal defects in case the air entered through a systemic vein.

DIFFERENTIAL DIAGNOSIS: None, if the gross findings above are present and the clinical history is appropriate. If they are absent, many other causes of sudden death enter the differential diagnosis.

KEY DIAGNOSTIC CRITERIA: The key to diagnosis is anticipating when arterial air embolism may occur and performing those procedures during the autopsy. Arterial air embolism should be anticipated when sudden death occurs during the following procedures or activities:

Scuba diving
Penetrating trauma on the chest (needle puncture, stab wound, gunshot wound, rib fracture)
Open heart surgery with incomplete evacuation of air in the left ventricle
Use of extracorporeal circulation machines

Scuba divers who do not exhale during ascent can overdistend their lungs and develop fistulas among the alveolar air spaces, interstitial spaces, and alveolar capillaries. The amount of air required to produce death can theoretically be very small if the coronary or cerebral arteries are involved. In animal experiments, as little as 0.05 cc of air is required to occlude the coronary artery in dogs.

POTENTIAL PITFALLS: Because the amount of air required to kill may be very small, this diagnosis may be overlooked or impossible to confirm at autopsy. The cerebral and coronary arteries should be tied off before removing the brain and heart to avoid the iatrogenic introduction of air into those vessels during the autopsy.

References

1. Macklin MT, Macklin CC. Malignant interstitial emphysema of the lungs and mediastinum as an important occult complication in many respiratory diseases and other conditions: An interpretation of the clinical literature in the light of laboratory experiment. *Medicine* 1944;23:281–358.
2. Ludwig J. (ed.), *Current methods of autopsy practice, 2nd ed.* Philadelphia, WB Saunders; 1979: 363–366.

AIR EMBOLISM, VENOUS

Entry Authors: Michael D. Bell, Virginia M. Walley, David A. Chiasson, and John P. Veinot

SYNONYM: Pulmonary air embolism.

DEFINITION: The introduction of air (or other gas) into the systemic veins with negative intrathoracic pressure during inspiration pulling the air centrally to obstruct the pulmonary artery and right ventricle. The air trapped in the pulmonary artery and conus arteriosus produces right-sided and left-sided heart failure with cerebral ischemia and death, if untreated.

GROSS FINDINGS: The pulmonary trunk, right ventricle and atrium are distended with fine, foamy blood. The viscera and systemic veins are congested.

Venous injury resulting in air entry is present if diligently sought. If the air embolism is treated, but death from complications occurs hours or days later, no air will be seen at autopsy.

MICROSCOPIC FINDINGS: Not useful.

SPECIAL PROCEDURES NEEDED FOR DIAGNOSIS: Pre- or postmortem chest radiograph (performed prior to opening the body) will show air trapped in the right heart and pulmonary artery. Perform the autopsy as quickly as possible after death to reduce intravascular putrefactive gas formation. Air may be collected and measured with an inverted 300 ml graduated cylinder while incising the right ventricle underwater as described by Spitz. Carefully examine veins for entry site injuries (punctures, stab, or incised wounds, gunshot wounds, lacerations) and document in written report with diagram and photograph. Examine heart for patent fossa ovalis.

DIFFERENTIAL DIAGNOSIS: None, if the gross findings above are present. If they are absent, the differential diagnosis becomes large.

KEY DIAGNOSTIC CRITERIA: The key to diagnosis is anticipating when venous air embolism may occur and perform the procedures described above. Venous air embolism should be anticipated when sudden cardiopulmonary arrest occurs during the following procedures or activities:

Neurosurgical procedures (especially if patient is sitting)
Head and neck surgery or trauma (stab or gunshot wounds)
Orthopedic procedures including arthroscopy, posterior spinal fusion
Surgical procedures involving the uterus (especially if gravid)
Diagnostic, therapeutic, or recreational air insufflation into orifices, cavities, and
  tissue
Central venous catheterization
Pressurized infusion of blood products or intravenous fluids

Premortem signs associated with venous air embolism include a loud, churning sound or "mill wheel" murmur, distended neck veins, cyanosis, hypotension, rapid thready pulse, and syncope. The minimal amount of air necessary to produce death is usually large because obstruction of the pulmonary artery and right ventricle is required. In experimental animal models, the amount of air required to kill is modified by the speed of injection, position of the animal, and effectiveness of the pulmonary excretory mechanism. In man, as little as 100 ml of air produced death in one case report.

POTENTIAL PITFALLS: The presence of air bubbles in the coronary or other small veins is not sufficient evidence for the diagnosis of venous air embolism, because small air bubbles may be introduced during the autopsy or resuscitation. If the diagnosis is not anticipated by the pathologist, it can be easily missed.

References

1. Spitz WU. Selected procedures at autopsy. In: Spitz WU, *Medicolegal investigation of death, 3rd ed.* Springfield IL, Charles C. Thomas; 1993:776–777.
2. Taylor JD. Postmortem diagnosis of air embolism by radiography. *Brit Med J* 1952;1:890–893.
3. Adams VI, Hirsch CS. Venous air embolism from head and neck wounds. *Arch Pathol Lab Med* 1989; 113:498–502.
4. Dudney TM, Elliott CG. Pulmonary embolism from amniotic fluid, fat, and air. *Prog Cardiov Dis* 1994;36:447–474.
5. Durant TM, Long J, Oppenheimer MJ. Pulmonary (venous) air embolism. *Am Heart J* 1947;33: 269–281.

ANAPHYLAXIS TO DIAGNOSTIC/THERAPEUTIC PROCEDURE

Entry Authors: Michael D. Bell, Virginia M. Walley, David A. Chiasson, and John P. Veinot

SYNONYMS: Allergic reaction, contrast agent reaction, anaphylactoid reaction.

DEFINITION: Anaphylaxis is a rapid IgE-mediated hypersensitivity reaction to an allergen associated with a diagnostic or therapeutic reaction. Allergens that incite anaphylaxis are proteins or drug-protein complexes or haptens. They include medications (penicillin), intravenous contrast agents (diatrizoate, iothalamate), and natural rubber (catheters, surgical gloves). Anaphylactoid reactions are identical in findings and outcome but are produced by pharmacological rather than immunological degranulation of mast cells.

GROSS FINDINGS: Laryngeal and epiglottic edema, while prominent during anaphylaxis, may disappear by the time of postmortem examination. This is also true of any facial or tongue swelling. Postmortem examination is often unremarkable.

MICROSCOPIC FINDINGS: Usually nonspecific inflammation in the laryngeal and epiglottic submucosa. Special stains for mast cells are helpful only if there are increased numbers of mast cells with evidence of degranulation.

SPECIAL PROCEDURES NEEDED FOR DIAGNOSIS: Serum tryptase can be useful as a marker of mast cell degranulation. Specific IgE antibodies for the suspect allergen can be helpful to establish prior sensitization. Mast cell stains are used to detect intact and partially degranulated mast cells.

DIFFERENTIAL DIAGNOSIS: Overdose of medication, asthma, natural cardiac disease that may preexist in the victim and cause sudden death.

KEY DIAGNOSTIC CRITERIA: Generalized systemic reaction characterized by allergic symptoms and signs (facial swelling, dyspnea, wheezing, hypotension, gastrointestinal distress) and sudden collapse or death that is temporally related to a diagnostic or therapeutic procedure. Confirm diagnosis with serum tryptase and specific IgE antibodies.

POTENTIAL PITFALLS: Easily overlooked if the premortem history is not available and laryngoedema is absent. This is especially true if there are coexisting diseases at autopsy that could potentially have caused the sudden death.

References

1. Ansari MQ, Zamora JL, Lipscomb MF. Postmortem diagnosis of acute anaphylaxis by serum tryptase analysis. *Am J Clin Path* 1993;99:101–103.
2. Delage C, Orey NS. Anaphylactic death: A clinicopathological study of 43 cases. *J Forensic Sci* 1972; 17:525–540.
3. Edelstein JM. Sudden death following administration of radiocontrast media. *J Forensic Sci* 1988;33: 734–737.
4. James LP Jr., Austen KF. Fatal systemic anaphylaxis in man. *NEJM* 1964;270:597–603.
5. Schwartz LB, Metcalfe DD, Miller JS, Earl H, Sullivan T. Tryptase levels as an indicator of mast cell activation in systemic anaphylaxis and mastocytosis. *NEJM* 1987;316:1622–1626.
6. Slater JE. Rubber anaphylaxis. *NEJM* 1989;320:1126–1130.
7. Yunginger JW, Nelson DR, Squillace DL, Jones RT, Holley KE, Hyma BA, Biedrzycki L, Sweeney KG, Sturner WQ, Schwartz LB. Laboratory investigation of deaths due to anaphylaxis. *J Forensic Sci* 1991;36:857–865.

ANASTOMOTIC DEHISCENCE OF CARDIOVASCULAR DEVICE/GRAFT

Entry Authors: Michael D. Bell, Virginia M. Walley, David A. Chiasson, and John P. Veinot

SYNONYMS: Bland paravalvular leak, paraprosthetic leak, graft failure, nonmechanical valve dysfunction. See related entries: *False aneurysm, Cardiovascular device/graft-related hemolysis.*

DEFINITION: A separation or discontinuity between an implanted cardiovascular device/graft (usually mechanical prosthetic valve) and its implantation site (valve annulus) resulting in a paravalvular leak. With vascular grafts, dehiscence can cause exsanguination or a false aneurysm. Valve dehiscence is usually due to diseased annular tissue (ring abscess, myxomatous, calcification) that is an unsatisfactory anchor for suturing. Slipped sutures and other technical problems can also lead to dehiscence. Valve dehiscence is more likely to occur in mitral than aortic prostheses. Small (<5 mm) dehiscences are due to tissue retraction during healing and are usually not clinically significant.

GROSS FINDINGS: Defect or gap between the valve/graft and the anastomotic tissue. Paravalvular defect may contain bland or infected thrombus. Vascular grafts with dehiscences are surrounded by extravasated blood or false aneurysm. The annular or anastomotic native tissue may show calcification or friable tissue due to infection. Surgical pathology specimens may show only a normal valve or graft.

MICROSCOPIC FINDINGS: Examine annular or anastomosis tissue for infection, myxomatous change.

SPECIAL PROCEDURES NEEDED FOR DIAGNOSIS: Measure the size of the dehiscence (leak) and record location. Examine the annulus and surrounding tissue carefully for pathology. Culture from area of dehiscence, including any thrombi. Review clinical record for evidence of acute hemolysis.

DIFFERENTIAL DIAGNOSIS: Primary graft/device failure, graft disproportion, postoperative (late) ring abscess.

KEY DIAGNOSTIC CRITERIA: Clinical or autopsy evidence that valve/graft has separated from the anchoring tissues. Large paravalvular leaks have a prominent regurgitant murmur and a "dancing or rocking" prosthetic valve on fluoroscopy or echocardiography. There may also be hemolytic anemia.

POTENTIAL PITFALLS: Misinterpreting small paravalvular defects (<5 mm) as being clinically and pathologically significant. Accidentally cutting and disturbing the sutures while examining the valve/graft (this is only a problem when the pathologist examining the valve/graft is different from the person who performed the autopsy or removed the valve/graft).

References

1. Schoen FJ, Levy RJ, Piehler HR. Pathological considerations in replacement cardiac valves. *Cardiovascular Pathol* 1992;1:29–52.
2. Silver MD, Wilson GJ. Pathology of mechanical heart valve prostheses and vascular grafts made of artificial materials. In: Silver MD, ed, *Cardiovascular pathology, 2nd ed*. Churchill Livingstone, New York; 1991:1487–1545.
3. Wesolowski SA. A plea for early recognition of late vascular prosthetic failure. *Surgery* 1978;84:575–576.
4. Yashar JJ, Richman MH, Dyckman J et al. Failure of Dacron prostheses caused by structural defect. *Surgery* 1978;84:659–663.

ARTIFACTUAL CHANGE

Entry Authors: Michael D. Bell, Virginia M. Walley, David A. Chiasson, and John P. Veinot

SYNONYM: Artifact.

DEFINITION: Any change introduced after patient death or specimen resection. In histology or microscopy, any structure or feature that has been introduced during the processing of a tissue.

GROSS FINDINGS: Varies greatly. Examples include:

Introduction of air into blood vessels during autopsy
Introduction of blood into body cavities during autopsy
Tears or defects produced during surgical removal or autopsy

MICROSCOPIC FINDINGS: Varies greatly. Examples include:

Hemoglobin-derived pigment produced by unbuffered formalin
Tissue fragments introduced into tissue blocks during dissection.

SPECIAL PROCEDURES NEEDED FOR DIAGNOSIS: Depends on the artifact.

DIFFERENTIAL DIAGNOSIS: Injury or pathologic change occurring *in vivo* or during the agonal period.

KEY DIAGNOSTIC CRITERIA: Artifact is inconsistent with clinical or other pathologic findings.

POTENTIAL PITFALLS: Misinterpreting artifact as an *in vivo* phenomenon. Myocardial contraction bands can be produced by mechanical trauma (during biopsy, car or plane crash, etc.) and should not be considered an artifact. It should also not be interpreted as resulting from ischemia without clinical correlation.

References

1. Artifacts In: Luna LG, ed. *Manual of histologic staining methods of the AFIP, 3rd ed.* New York, McGraw-Hill; 1968:242–251.
2. Baroldi G. Morphologic forms of myocardial necrosis related to myocardial cell function, Chapter 17. In: Silver MD, ed, *Cardiovascular pathology 2nd ed.* New York: Churchill Livingstone; 1991:642–670.
3. Walley VM, Stinson WA, Upton C, Santerre JP, Mussivand T, Masters RG, Ghadially FN. Foreign materials found in the cardiovascular system after instrumentation or surgery (including a guide to their light microscopic identification). *Cardiovasc Pathol* 1993:157–185.

BAROTRAUMA

Entry Authors: Michael D. Bell, Virginia M. Walley, David A. Chiasson, and John P. Veinot

SYNONYMS: Dysbarism, hypobarism, hyperbarism.
See related entry: *Air embolism, arterial*

DEFINITION: Injury resulting from the failure of a gas-filled body space (lungs, middle ears, sinuses) to equalize its internal pressure to correspond to changes in the surrounding environmental pressure. It is the result of Boyle's Law which states that at a constant temperature, the volume of gas varies inversely with the pressure applied. Barotrauma is usually seen in the setting of underwater diving when insufficient time is allowed during rapid ascent for pressure equilibrium. During ascent, gas in the lungs expands as the ambient pressure decreases. If the diver does not allow the expanding gas to escape by exhalation, the alveoli and respiratory passages distend and rupture. Life-threatening complications include pneumothorax, pneumomediastinum, pneumopericardium, and arterial air embolism as air escapes from the torn alveoli into the surrounding structures or pulmonary veins. These complications kill directly or more often render the diver unconscious or panic-stricken, resulting in drowning. Barotrauma also occurs in hospitalized critically ill patients requiring positive-pressure ventilation. Barotrauma is not synonymous with decompression sickness or caisson disease, although the latter may also occur during ascent from underwater diving.

GROSS FINDINGS: Subcutaneous emphysema, pneumothorax, pneumomediastinum, pneumopericardium, and arterial air embolism may be present. Interstitial pulmonary emphysema in the form of 0.1–0.5 cm subpleural blebs may be seen. Divers may also have hemorrhage in the middle ears and paranasal sinuses.

MICROSCOPIC FINDINGS: Interstitial pulmonary emphysema produces empty spaces in the interlobular septa, subpleural tissue, and around the bronchovascular bundles compressing the adjacent blood vessels and acini.

SPECIAL PROCEDURES NEEDED FOR DIAGNOSIS: Specifically examine body for subcutaneous emphysema, pneumothorax, interstitial pulmonary emphysema, pneumomediastinum, pneumopericardium, and arterial air embolism. Perform chest radiography. Examine the middle ears and paranasal sinuses.

DIFFERENTIAL DIAGNOSIS: Drowning, decompression sickness in divers.

KEY DIAGNOSTIC CRITERIA: Detailed investigation of the circumstances surrounding the death (scuba divers rarely dive alone). Anticipate possibility of barotrauma and perform meticulous examination for subcutaneous emphysema, interstitial pulmonary emphysema, pneumothorax, pneumomediastinum, pneumopericardium, and arterial air embolism.

POTENTIAL PITFALLS: Unfortunately, evidence of barotrauma is often obscured by the signs of drowning. Failure to investigate circumstances of death and not anticipating the possibility of barotrauma.

References

1. Melamed Y, Shupak A, Bitterman H. Medical problems associated with underwater diving. *NEJM* 1992;326:30–35.
2. Open water sport diver manual, 4th ed. Englewood CO: Jeppesen Sanderson; 1989:2–25 to 2–48.
3. Findley TP. An autopsy protocol for skin- and scuba-diving deaths. *Am J Clin Path* 1977;67:440–443.
4. Macklin MT, Macklin CC. Malignant interstitial emphysema of the lungs and mediastinum as an important occult complication in many respiratory diseases and other conditions: An interpretation of the clinical literature in the light of laboratory experiment. *Medicine* 1944;23:281–358.

CARDIOVASCULAR DEVICE/GRAFT-RELATED HEMOLYSIS

Entry Authors: Michael D. Bell, Virginia M. Walley, David A. Chiasson, and John P. Veinot

SYNONYM: Acquired intravascular hemolytic anemia.

DEFINITION: Mechanical lysis of red blood cells after passing through or around an intravascular prosthesis (usually a mechanical heart valve). Hemolysis occurs after the placement of all mechanical heart valves, but is usually compensated. Increased hemolysis in a patient with a prosthetic valve usually indicates damage to the valve or a paravalvular leak. Hemolysis is less likely in prosthetic valves with tilting discs or coated with pyrolytic carbon and more likely in those covered by cloth. Disruption of the red blood cell membrane occurs when sheer stress exceeds 3000 dynes/cm. Hemolysis has also been described in vascular patches for VSD repair.

GROSS FINDINGS: The cardiovascular device (prosthetic heart valve) usually has tears, thromboses, or defects that create turbulence and hemolysis. Paravalvular leaks may be present. Chronic hemolysis may produce brown discoloration of the organs due to hemosiderin deposition. Chronic hemolysis is also associated with the production of cholelithiasis.

MICROSCOPIC FINDINGS: Examine the kidney and other reticuloendothelial tissues (liver, spleen, bone marrow) for hemosiderosis. Chronic hemolytic anemia produces normoblastic hyperplasia of the bone marrow. Peripheral blood smear may show schistocytes and irregularly shaped red blood cells such as helmet and triangular red cells.

SPECIAL PROCEDURES NEEDED FOR DIAGNOSIS: Examine the cardiovascular device/graft carefully for causes of turbulence and hemolysis. Examine the peripheral blood smear. Use iron stain to detect hemosiderin in the affected organs. Examine the gallbladder for gallstones. Review medical record for Coomb's negative normocytic anemia, reticulocytosis, elevated lactate dehydrogenase (LD), reduced haptoglobin, elevated plasma hemoglobin, hemoglobinuria, or hemosiderinuria.

DIFFERENTIAL DIAGNOSIS: Drug or autoimmune hemolytic anemia, hemolysis following crush or thermal injuries, thrombotic thrombocytopenic purpura, hemolytic uremic syndrome.

KEY DIAGNOSTIC CRITERIA: Hemolytic anemia occurring after placement of a prosthetic valve or other cardiovascular device/graft. Laboratory studies can be helpful in ruling out other types of hemolytic anemia.

POTENTIAL PITFALLS: Usually none.

References

1. Silver MD, Wilson GJ. Pathology of mechanical heart valve prostheses and vascular grafts made of artificial materials. In: Silver MD, ed *Cardiovascular pathology, 2nd ed.* New York: Churchill Livingstone; 1991:1516–1517.
2. Marsh GW, Lewis SM. Cardiac haemolytic anaemia. *Semin Hematol* 1969;6:133–149.

CARDIOVASCULAR DEVICE/GRAFT-RELATED HEMORRHAGE

Entry Authors: Michael D. Bell, Virginia M. Walley, David A. Chiasson, and John P. Veinot

SYNONYMS: Device/graft-related bleeding, pseudoaneurysm. See related entries: *False aneurysm, Anastomotic dehiscence of cardiovascular device/graft.*

DEFINITION: The escape of blood from a cardiovascular device or graft (usually an aortic or aortoiliac graft). If unabated, this will produce shock and, eventually, death. On rare occasions, the surrounding tissues limit the blood's egress creating a false aneurysm or pseudoaneurysm. The hemorrhage may occur through the graft itself (primary graft failure) or at the junction of the graft and native tissue (anastomotic leak or dehiscence).

GROSS FINDINGS: Extravasated blood, hematoma, and/or false aneurysm surrounding the cardiovascular device or graft. Examination of the graft and anastomotic site will usually reveal the defect.

MICROSCOPIC FINDINGS: Usually not helpful, unless the leak involves the anastomosis site.

SPECIAL PROCEDURES NEEDED FOR DIAGNOSIS: Examine cardiovascular device/graft and surrounding vascular structure (heart, aorta, artery) for bleeding site and iatrogenic injuries. Check medical record or history for anticoagulation therapy or other predisposing factors for spontaneous hemorrhage (disseminated intravascular coagulation, hereditary clotting disorders).

DIFFERENTIAL DIAGNOSIS: Penetrating stab or gunshot wound, non-penetrating blunt injury, iatrogenic intravascular injury.

KEY DIAGNOSTIC CRITERIA: Nontraumatic hemorrhage at the site of the cardiovascular device or graft. Rule out iatrogenic intravascular catheter injuries.

POTENTIAL PITFALLS: Usually none.

Reference

1. Schoen FJ. *Interventional and surgical cardiovascular pathology: Clinical correlations and basic principles.* Philadelphia, PA: WB Saunders; 1989.

CARDIOVASCULAR DEVICE/GRAFT-RELATED INJURY, NOS

Entry Authors: Michael D. Bell, Virginia M. Walley, David A. Chiasson, and John P. Veinot

SYNONYMS: See related entries: *Anastomotic dehiscence of cardiovascular device/graft, Cardiovascular device/graft-related hemolysis, Cardiovascular device/graft-related hemorrhage, Embolism of foreign body/cardiovascular device/graft, False aneurysm, Iatrogenic infection, Iatrogenic injury, Infection of cardiovascular device/graft, Injury due to suture ligation, Malalignment/disproportion of cardiovascular device/graft, Obstruction of cardiovascular device/ graft, Structural failure of cardiovascular device/graft, Traumatic arrhythmia or conduction disturbance, Traumatic arteriovenous fistula, Traumatic dissection.*

DEFINITION: Injury produced by the surgical placement or malfunction of a cardiovascular device/graft (heart valve, prosthetic patch, aortic or arterial graft, intra-arterial or intracardiac catheter or balloon, etc.) but not otherwise specified.

GROSS FINDINGS: Varies with injury.

MICROSCOPIC FINDINGS: Varies with injury.

SPECIAL PROCEDURES NEEDED FOR DIAGNOSIS: Varies with injury.

DIFFERENTIAL DIAGNOSIS: Varies with injury.

KEY DIAGNOSTIC CRITERIA: Varies with injury.

POTENTIAL PITFALLS: Varies with injury.

COMMOTIO CORDIS

Entry Authors: Michael D. Bell, Virginia M. Walley, David A. Chiasson, and John P. Veinot

SYNONYMS: Cardiac concussion; cardiac commotion. See related entries: *Traumatic arrhythmia or conduction disturbance.*

DEFINITION: Disturbance in cardiac function occurring immediately after a blunt precordial impact in the absence of a morphologically identifiable injury to the heart. The functional disturbance may range from sinus bradycardia to fatal ventricular arrhythmia (cases most likely seen by pathologists). This is a type of blunt injury to the heart. It is the myocardial equivalent of the cerebral concussion, except it is usually fatal. It is the most common cause of traumatic death in youth baseball.

GROSS FINDINGS: No gross abnormalities (including myocardial contusions) of the heart. There may be contusion (bruising) of the precordial chest wall or skin.

MICROSCOPIC FINDINGS: No microscopic abnormalities to which sudden death can be readily attributed. Resuscitation related reperfusion-type myocardial changes may be present (subendocardial hemorrhage with or without contraction bands).

SPECIAL PROCEDURES NEEDED FOR DIAGNOSIS: A complete autopsy must be performed including examination of the brain and spinal cord. Complete toxicology analysis must be done. The cardiac conduction system (sinoatrial node, atrioventricular node, bundle of His, bundle branches) should be sampled even if the heart appears normal.

DIFFERENTIAL DIAGNOSIS: Cocaine or other stimulant drug intoxication. Cardiac conduction system morphologic abnormality (acquired or congenital).

KEY DIAGNOSTIC CRITERIA: History of precordial impact with or without demonstrable chest wall contusion. The cardiac disturbance (usually fatal) must occur within seconds or a few minutes after the impact. No morphologic (gross or microscopic) heart abnormality (excluding resuscitation phenomenon). No drugs detected in toxicology analysis.

POTENTIAL PITFALLS: Ignorance of circumstances surrounding death because of poor communication or unwitnessed death.

References

1. Hirsch CS. Homicidal commotio cordis. *American Society of Pathologists check sample FP 87-6.*
2. Frazer M, Mirchandani H. Commotio cordis, revisited. *Am J Forensic Med Path* 1984;5:249–251.
3. Maron BJ, Poliac LC, Kaplan JA, Mueller FO. Blunt impact to the chest leading to sudden death from cardiac arrest during sports activities. *NEJM* 1995;333:337–342.

CONTUSION

Entry Authors: Michael D. Bell, Virginia M. Walley, David A. Chiasson, and John P. Veinot

SYNONYM: Bruise.

DEFINITION: A blunt mechanical injury causing microvascular tears resulting in the extravasation of red blood cells into the injured tissue. Although the skin is most frequently involved, any vascularized tissue (including the heart) can contuse.

Related Terms: A *hematoma* is a localized collection of clotted and/or unclotted blood that acts as a mass lesion pushing on surrounding tissues as it expands.

GROSS FINDINGS: The acute extravasation of red blood cells produces a dark red gross appearance in the tissue, whether skin or myocardium. With time, the contusion turns gold-brown with the appearance of hemosiderin-laden macrophages. Other colors including green, orange, and yellow may be seen from the skin's surface depending on the extent and depth of the contusion. Other types of blunt injuries (abrasions, lacerations, fractures) are often present in addition to the contusion. Myocardial contusions may affect any layer including the endocardium and epicardium. The location does not necessarily indicate the direction of the blunt force. Subendocardial hemorrhages of the left ventricular septum are often seen after blunt head trauma and shock in the absence of direct chest trauma. Blood vessel contusions are confined to the adventitia.

MICROSCOPIC FINDINGS: In acute contusions, extravasation of red blood cells into the interstitium of the tissue is the only microscopic finding. In the heart, contraction bands may be seen in the myocytes. Polymorphonuclear leukocytes may be seen 8 hours after the injury and reach their peak 24 hours after the injury. Lymphocytes and macrophages replace the polymorphonuclear leukocytes. Hemosiderin-laden macrophages usually appear 3–5 days after the injury. If the contusion is small, hemosiderin may not appear. Fibrosis does not ordinarily occur unless extensive necrosis or laceration is present.

SPECIAL PROCEDURES NEEDED FOR DIAGNOSIS: Microscopic examination may be useful to roughly estimate the age of the contusion. Iron stains can assist in the identification of hemosiderin.

DIFFERENTIAL DIAGNOSIS: Subendocardial hemorrhage in left ventricular septum associated with noncardiac trauma and shock. Circumferential subendocardial hemorrhage associated with reperfusion seen in various settings. Thrombotic thrombocytopenic purpura. Hemorrhagic myocardial infarcts.

KEY DIAGNOSTIC CRITERIA: History of blunt trauma with other types of blunt injuries (abrasions, lacerations, fractures) present. Coronary artery and microscopic examination will exclude TTP and myocardial infarction.

POTENTIAL PITFALLS: Cannot reliably correlate the presence of myocardial contusion with its functional and clinical sequelae. Most myocardial contusions are asymptomatic and produce no clinically significant ECG or CK-MB changes. Conversely, ECG and cardiac enzyme determinations do not accurately diagnose myocardial contusions (as defined above). Confusing the subendocardial hemorrhage associated with blunt head trauma, shock, reperfusion injury, etc. with blunt myocardial contusion.

ELECTRICAL INJURY, HIGH-VOLTAGE

Entry Authors: Michael D. Bell, Virginia M. Walley, David A. Chiasson, and John P. Veinot

SYNONYM: Electrocution.

DEFINITION: An injury produced by the flow of electrons through the body in which the voltage is greater than 1,000 volts. In all cases of electrocution, the person must be in contact with the circuit or flow of electrons. High-voltage electrocutions kill by causing hyperthermia and always produce skin burns. The 7,620 volt transmission lines found along roads and lightning are the most common sources of high voltage electrocution.

GROSS FINDINGS: High-voltage electrocution always produces skin burns at the points of direct contact and/or arcing, if it occurs. The classic electrical burn is a round or oval crater with central charring or redness, surrounded by an area of pallor and then surrounded by a rim of red, hyperemic, blistered skin. This stereotypic electrical burn is produced by the heat generated by electricity. The amount of heat produced (as measured in calories) increases with the square of the voltage and with the amount of time in contact with the electrical source. In survivors of high-voltage electrocutions, blood vessel thrombosis may occur resulting in gangrene or myocardial infarction. Reversible ECG, conduction disturbances, and CK-MB changes have been reported in survivors. Lightning produces a dendritic tree-like pattern of lividity on the skin in a third of the fatal cases. Tympanic membrane laceration is seen in most fatal cases. Myocardial contusions and pericardial laceration have been described in 9% of victims killed by lightning.

MICROSCOPIC FINDINGS: The electrical (actually thermal) injury in skin is characterized by vacuolization of the keratin layer, subepidermal vesicles, hyperchromasia and streaming of the epidermal nuclei, and coagulation of the dermal collagen. Myocardial contraction band necrosis with fiber rupture and intercellular dehiscence has been described in all four chambers as well as the conduction system. Contraction band necrosis has also been described in the tunica media of arteries along with endothelial cell swelling.

SPECIAL PROCEDURES NEEDED FOR DIAGNOSIS: Premortem history and death scene investigation required. Careful examination of arms, hands, legs, and feet is necessary to document electrical burns. Careful heart and brain examination necessary to rule out natural disease.

DIFFERENTIAL DIAGNOSIS: Usually none, if premortem history is known.

KEY DIAGNOSTIC CRITERIA: Premortem history, scene investigation, and thorough autopsy.

POTENTIAL PITFALLS: Failure to get premortem history. Failure to examine extremities carefully for electrical burns.

References

1. Wright RU, Gantner GE. Electrical injuries and lightning. In: Froede RC, ed. *Handbook of forensic pathology.* Northfield, IL: CAP Press; 1990:149–157.
2. James TN, Riddick L, Embry JH. Cardiac abnormalities demonstrated postmortem in four cases of accidental electrocution and their potential significance relative to nonfatal electrical injuries of the heart. *Am Heart J* 1990:120:143–157.

ELECTRICAL INJURY, LOW-VOLTAGE

Entry Authors: Michael D. Bell, Virginia M. Walley, David A. Chiasson, and John P. Veinot

SYNONYM: Electrocution.

DEFINITION: An injury produced by the flow of electrons through the body in which the voltage is less than 1,000 volts. In all cases of electrocution, the person must be in contact with a source of electrons and grounded. Low-voltage electrocutions kill by causing ventricular fibrillation. Ventricular fibrillation occurs when current is between 0.1 and 1.0 amps, typical of a household 120 volt AC outlet. At that current range, the heart attempts (usually unsuccessfully!) to match the cycling electron flow of alternating current, 60 times per second or 3,600 times per minute in the US and Canada.

GROSS FINDINGS: Low-voltage electrocutions produce burns on the skin that are in contact with the electrical source in only 50% of the cases. The other 50% have no gross abnormalities. Only 3 calories of heat are produced by a quick contact with a 120 volt source, so skin burns will not occur unless the contact is prolonged. The classic electrical burn is a round or oval crater with central charring or redness, surrounded by an area of pallor and then surrounded by a rim or red, hyperemic, blistered skin. This stereotypic burn is more likely to be encountered in books and exams than real life. The myocardium and blood vessels are usually grossly normal.

MICROSCOPIC FINDINGS: Electrical burns of the skin are seen in only 50% of low-voltage electrocutions and are usually due to prolonged contact with the electrical source. The electrical (actually thermal) injury in skin is characterized by vacuolization of the keratin layer, subepidermal vesicles, hyperchromasia and streaming of the epidermal nuclei, and coagulation of the dermal collagen. Despite death by ventricular fibrillation, the heart usually shows no abnormalities. Reversible nonlethal cardiac arrhythmias and ECG changes may occur in survivors.

SPECIAL PROCEDURES NEEDED FOR DIAGNOSIS: Premortem history and death scene investigation is absolutely essential. The scene must be examined for electrical tools, extension cords, and other electrical devices, and they must all be tested. Careful examination of arms, hands, legs, and feet is necessary to document electrical burns. Careful heart and brain examination is necessary to rule out natural disease.

DIFFERENTIAL DIAGNOSIS: If the premortem history is not known, the death scene not examined, and no skin burns are seen, the diagnosis of electrocution will never enter the pathologist's differential diagnosis. Instead, the differential diagnosis will be centered around any minuscule autopsy finding.

KEY DIAGNOSTIC CRITERIA: The diagnosis must be anticipated if a person is found dead near any electrical device. The electrical device must be tested in a nondestructive manner (in other words, do not take it apart). Premortem history, scene investigation, and thorough autopsy are absolutely essential.

POTENTIAL PITFALLS: Failure to get premortem history. Failure to examine scene or electrical devices. Failure to examine extremities carefully for electrical burns. Failure to thoroughly examine the heart and brain.

Reference

1. Wright RK, Gantner GE. Electrical injuries and lightning. In: Froede RC, ed, *Handbook of forensic pathology*. Northfield, IL: CAP Press; 1990:149–157.

EMBOLISM OF FOREIGN BODY/CARDIOVASCULAR DEVICE/GRAFT

Entry Authors: Michael D. Bell, Virginia M. Walley, David A. Chiasson, and John P. Veinot

SYNONYM: Foreign body embolism.

DEFINITION: A foreign object or cardiovascular device that travels and eventually impacts in the vascular tree. The foreign body may gain entrance into the vasculature by a gunshot wound (bullet), explosion (shrapnel), or a medical procedure (catheter tip, guide wire, needle). Intravenous drug abusers can also introduce foreign material (insoluble filler and adulterants, needle tips) into their vessels. The foreign body may also permanently reside in the vasculature and break loose (heart valve or part, suture). The clinical, gross, and microscopic findings will vary with the foreign object(s) and whether the object enters the venous or arterial circulation.

GROSS FINDINGS: The object is usually grossly visible, if one knows where to look for it. An exception is foreign material introduced during intravenous drug use. This insoluble material (talc, starch, fillers in oral medications) impacts in the pulmonary arteries and capillaries inciting a granulomatous reaction. This produces firm nodular lungs and if present, signs of pulmonary hypertension (right ventricular hypertrophy, chronic passive congestion of liver).

MICROSCOPIC FINDINGS: Not useful, since only macroscopic objects are likely to produce symptoms or death. The exception is the intravenous drug abuser who injects insoluble material into his veins that later impact in the pulmonary arteries inciting a granulomatous reaction. The pulmonary vessels are occluded by vascular and perivascular foreign-body granulomas containing birefringent foreign material. Plexiform lesions may be seen as well as interstitial inflammation and fibrosis.

SPECIAL PROCEDURES NEEDED FOR DIAGNOSIS: Radiology will often aid in locating the foreign object.

DIFFERENTIAL DIAGNOSIS: Primary pulmonary hypertension, plexiform type, and sarcoidosis versus granulomatous vasculitis in intravenous drug abusers.

KEY DIAGNOSTIC CRITERIA: Appropriate clinical history with signs and symptoms of acute vascular insufficiency due to the impacted foreign object. Granulomatous vasculitis in intravenous drug abusers often presents insidiously with signs and symptoms of pulmonary hypertension.

POTENTIAL PITFALLS: Failure to use radiography to find a bullet embolus which has evidentiary value.

References

1. Davis PK, Myers JL, Pennock JL, Thiele BL. Strut fracture and disc embolization in Bjork-Shiley mitral valve prostheses: Diagnosis and management. *Ann Thorac Surg* 1985;40:65–68.
2. Kabbani SS, Bashour TT, Ellertson DG, Crew JR, Hanna ES. Mechanical valve occluder dislodgement. *Am Heart J* 1984;108:1374–1377.
3. Michelassi F, Pietrabissa A, Ferrari M, Mosca F, Vargish T, Moosa HH. Bullet emboli to the systemic and venous circulation. *Surgery* 1990;107:239–245.
4. Odell JA, Durandt J, Shama DM, Vythilingum S. Spontaneous embolization of a St. Jude prosthetic mitral valve leaflet. *Ann Thorac Surg* 1985;39:569–572.

FALSE ANEURYSM

Entry Authors: Michael D. Bell, Virginia M. Walley, David A. Chiasson, and John P. Veinot

SYNONYM: Pseudoaneurysm. See entries for: *Cardiovascular device/graft-related hemorrhage, Anastomotic dehiscence of cardiovascular device/graft, Posttraumatic aneurysm.*

DEFINITION: A false aneurysm is an organized extravascular hematoma that communicates with the intravascular space (heart chamber, aorta, large artery). Its walls are formed by adjacent tissues (pericardium, retroperitoneum) and the organized blood clot. There is no myocardial or arterial structures (myocytes, parallel elastic fibers) in the false aneurysm wall. The communication or defect in the vascular structure can be caused by natural disease (ruptured myocardial infarction, mycotic aneurysm), failure of a cardiovascular graft/device (primary or at the anastomotic site), or trauma (stab or gunshot wound, needle or catheter injury, blunt trauma). The aneurysm may cause symptoms by rupturing (producing shock and death) or impinging on adjacent structures including the true lumen. Mural thrombi within the aneurysm may embolize. In addition to vascular grafts, false aneurysm have also occurred with ventricular patches and extracardiac conduits in the surgical repair of congenital heart disease.

GROSS FINDINGS: Saccular or fusiform shape, surrounding the defect in the cardiovascular structure. Often contains a mural thrombus because of stagnant blood flow. If a prosthetic graft or patch is involved, examine it for defects, dehiscence at the anastomotic sites.

MICROSCOPIC FINDINGS: The false aneurysm wall is formed by the organizing hematoma and surrounding tissues (pericardium, retroperitoneum, mediastinum, etc). No myocytes or elastic lamina are seen in the false aneurysm wall. Chronic false aneurysms have dense fibrotic walls.

SPECIAL PROCEDURES NEEDED FOR DIAGNOSIS: Careful gross examination will reveal the defect site and thorough sampling of the aneurysm wall can help differentiate a true and false aneurysm. Elastic and trichrome stains are helpful. In mycotic aneurysm, special stains may help to detect microorganisms.

DIFFERENTIAL DIAGNOSIS: True ventricular, aortic, or arterial aneurysm due to transmural myocardial infarction or aortic and arterial atherosclerosis, rarely syphilis.

KEY DIAGNOSTIC CRITERIA: Wall of the false aneurysm does not contain normal elements of myocardial, aortic, or arterial wall. Usually occurs after trauma or at the site of a cardiovascular graft/device.

POTENTIAL PITFALLS: Confuse with a true aneurysm (unlikely).

References

1. Ersek RA, Chesler E, Korns ME, Edwards JE. Spontaneous rupture of a false left ventricular aneurysm following myocardial infarction. *Am Heart J* 1969;77:677–680.
2. Jamshidi A, Berry RW. Left ventricular pseudoaneurysm secondary to cardiac stab wound: Successful repair in a thirteen year old girl. *Am J Cardiol* 1965;16:601–604.
3. Merrill WH, Achuff SC, White RI et al. Late false aneurysm following replacement of ascending aorta: The problem of the teflon graft in combination with silk suture anastomosis. *Ann Thoracic Surg* 1985; 39:271–274.

GUNSHOT WOUND

Entry Authors: Michael D. Bell, Virginia M. Walley, David A. Chiasson, and John P. Veinot

SYNONYMS: Bullet wound; firearm injury.

DEFINITION: A mechanical injury produced by the discharge and passage of a bullet or projectile through the body. The firearms used to fire the projectile include handguns, rifles, and shotguns.

Related Terms: A penetrating gunshot wound of the heart passes into the heart but not out. A perforating gunshot wound of the heart passes completely through the heart producing an entrance and exit site. A bullet embolus is a gunshot wound in which the bullet enters the vascular system and is carried, by blood flow or gravity, to another location within the vascular tree. The entrance site is usually the heart and the bullet (usually small caliber) usually travels to the lower extremities.

GROSS FINDINGS: Gunshot wounds through the body can vary greatly in their appearance from small narrow wound tracks to large destructive wound cavities. Bullets disrupt tissue by direct contact and a kinetic energy wave dependent on the bullet's mass and velocity. This kinetic energy wave can cause bursting wounds of the heart or aorta if these structures are hit while maximally distended with blood.

MICROSCOPIC FINDINGS: In acute gunshot wounds of the heart, there is tissue disruption with localized extravasated red blood cells in the myocardium alongside the wound track. Contraction bands are also seen in adjacent myocytes. Uncomplicated gunshot wounds of the heart (if the person survives) heal leaving only a small indistinct cicatrix through the myocardium and focal fibrous patches over the epicardial and endocardial ends.

SPECIAL PROCEDURES NEEDED FOR DIAGNOSIS: Always perform postmortem radiology to locate the projectile and/or its fragments. This test is usually the first indicator of bullet embolus. The gunshot wound track through the body should be carefully dissected and described. The gunshot wound of the skin should be photographed. Never mark a projectile for identification—put it in an envelope and mark that instead.

DIFFERENTIAL DIAGNOSIS: Usually none if performed by or under the supervision of a forensic pathologist. Contact gunshot wound over the head can resemble lacerations. Gunshot wounds with .22 caliber ammunition can resemble puncture wounds.

KEY DIAGNOSTIC CRITERIA: All autopsies with gunshot wounds should be done by or under the direction of a forensic pathologist. The key to identifying a gunshot wound is by its appearance on the skin and the presence of a projectile within the body on postmortem radiograph.

POTENTIAL PITFALLS: Failure to document the appearance and mistakenly identify the direction of the gunshot wound. May confuse gunshot wound with lacerations or puncture wounds.

References

1. DiMaio VJM. *Gunshot wounds*. Elsevier, New York; 1985.
2. Hirsch CS, Zumwalt RE. Forensic pathology. In: Damjanov I, Linder J, eds *Anderson's pathology, 10th ed.* Mosby, St. Louis, MO; 1996:89–96.
3. Spitz WU. Injury by gunfire. In: Spitz WU, ed, *Spitz and Fisher's medicolegal investigation of death, 3rd ed.* Charles C. Thomas, Springfield, IL; 1993:311–412.

HEMOPERICARDIUM

Entry Authors: Michael D. Bell, Virginia M. Walley, David A. Chiasson, and John P. Veinot

SYNONYMS: Bloody pericardial effusion, sanguinous pericardial effusion.

DEFINITION: An effusion or escape of blood into the pericardial cavity.

RELATED TERMS: Cardiac tamponade is the development of hemodynamic changes (ending in shock and death, if untreated) resulting from the accumulation of pericardial fluid (or rarely air) at a rate that exceeds the distensibility of the pericardium. Whether or not a pericardial fluid (hemopericardium) causes pericardial tamponade depends on the amount of fluid and how quickly it accumulates in the pericardial cavity. As little as 150 ml of fluid can cause death if it accumulates within minutes to hours. As much as several hundred milliliters of fluid can be accommodated without symptoms if it accumulates slowly over days, weeks, or months.

GROSS FINDINGS: Liquid blood with or without clots in the pericardial cavity. Liquid blood with large clots is the rule in cardiac rupture from injury (gunshot wound, stab wound, blunt force laceration) or myocardial infarction. This is also true with injury or nontraumatic dissection of the ascending aorta with blood dissecting into the pericardial cavity. Pericardial neoplasia, tuberculosis, radiation, postpericardiotomy syndrome produce pericardial fluid that is usually serosanguinous or blood diluted in a larger volume of serous fluid. This is in striking contrast with the dark red blood and clots seen with myocardial or aortic rupture.

MICROSCOPIC FINDINGS: Varies widely depending on the etiology of the hemopericardium. Pericardial neoplasms are usually metastatic from the lungs or breast. Hematologic malignancies and mesothelioma are also relatively common.

SPECIAL PROCEDURES NEEDED FOR DIAGNOSIS: Cultures and special stains if infectious agent is suspected. Cytology of the serosanguinous effusion can detect malignancy. Measure the amount of blood (including clots) present.

DIFFERENTIAL DIAGNOSIS: Serous effusion with blood contamination during dissection of the chest plate, mediastinum, and pericardium (This only occurs when the pathologist allows someone else to perform the autopsy). Blood introduced during final resuscitation efforts by pericardiocentesis or open heart message.

KEY DIAGNOSTIC CRITERIA: Note if it is true blood or serosanguinous fluid. Note the amount of blood and if clots are present. The presence of blood clots and a large amount of blood (usually 100 ml or more) indicates that the rupture occurred while the person was alive. The blood produced by pericardiocentesis during final resuscitation efforts is always liquid without clots and usually measures less than 100 ml.

POTENTIAL PITFALLS: Allowing someone else to open the chest and pericardium, thus depriving you of direct observation of the pericardial contents before any possible contamination. Overlooking the history of terminal pericardiocentesis and ascribing the hemopericardium to another cause.

HYPERSENSITIVITY MYOCARDITIS, DRUG-RELATED

Entry Authors: Michael D. Bell, Virginia M. Walley, David A. Chiasson, and John P. Veinot

SEE ALSO: *Myocarditis, hypersensitivity,* in Section 1, Diseases of the Myocardium.

DEFINITION: An idiosyncratic inflammation of the myocardium associated with drugs. The myocarditis is caused by a delayed hypersensitivity immunologic reaction to chemically reactive metabolites of the offending drug. The drugs include (*account for 75% of cases of hypersensitivity myocarditis):

*sulfonamides
*penicillin
*methyldopa
acetazolamide
amitriptyline
amphotericin B
carbamazepine
chloramphenicol
diphenylhydantoin
diphtheria toxin
hydrochlorothiazide
indomethacin
isoniazid
p-aminosalicylic acid
phenindione
phenylbutazone
smallpox vaccine
spironolactone
streptomycin
sulfonylureas
tetanus toxoid
tetracycline

Drug-induced hypersensitivity myocarditis is self-limiting and does not result in cardiac fibrosis or cardiomyopathy.

GROSS FINDINGS: Varies from no gross abnormalities to patchy areas of pallor involving all four chambers.

MICROSCOPIC FINDINGS: There is a patchy interstitial inflammatory infiltrate consisting of eosinophils, plasma cells, and atypical lymphocytes. Isolated giant cells are infrequently seen. The inflammation is predominantly perivascular. If a vasculitis is present, it is non-necrotizing and no microthrombi or hemorrhage is seen. Myocyte necrosis is absent, although myocytolysis is seen (see entry for *Myocytolysis I* in Section 1). Fibroblasts and collagen are absent because necrosis is absent. All of the lesions appear of the same age.

SPECIAL PROCEDURES NEEDED FOR DIAGNOSIS: None.

DIFFERENTIAL DIAGNOSIS: Toxic myocarditis, viral myocarditis, giant cell myocarditis (+myocyte necrosis), hypereosinophilic myocarditis (has persistent peripheral eosinophilia >1500 eosinophils/ml^3 for >6 months).

KEY DIAGNOSTIC CRITERIA: Diagnosis should be considered in any patient with peripheral eosinophilia and the new appearance of ECG changes, CK elevation, mild cardiomegaly, or unexplained tachycardia.

POTENTIAL PITFALLS: May be overlooked if sampling is limited (endomyocardial biopsy). Can be confused with other causes of myocarditis.

References

1. Billingham ME. Morphologic changes in drug-induced heart disease. In: Bristow MR, ed. *Drug-induced heart disease*. Elsevier-North-Holland Biomedical Press, Amsterdam; 1980:127.
2. Edwards WD. Pathology of endomyocardial biopsy. In: Waller BF, ed. *Pathology of the heart and great vessels*. Churchill-Livingstone, New York; 1988:217–232.
3. Fenoglio JJ, Mcallister HA, Mullick FG. Drug-related myocarditis: I. Hypersensitivity myocarditis. *Human Pathol* 1981;12:900–907.
4. Fenoglio JJ, Silver MD. Effects of drugs on the cardiovascular system. In: Silver MD, ed. *Cardiovascular pathology, 2nd ed*. Churchill-Livingstone, New York; 1991:1205–1229.
5. Lewin D, d'Amati G, Lewis W. Hypersensitivity myocarditis: Findings in native and transplanted hearts. *Cardiovasc Pathol* 1992;1:225–229.
6. Talierco CP, Olney BA, Lie JT. Myocarditis related to drug hypersensitivity. *Mayo Clin Proc* 1985;60:463–468.

HYPERTHERMIA, SYSTEMIC

Entry Authors: Michael D. Bell, Virginia M. Walley, David A. Chiasson, and John P. Veinot

SYNONYMS: Heat stroke, heat exhaustion, environmental hyperthermia, heat pyrexia.

DEFINITION: Injury or death from an increase in core body temperature greater than 105°F (40.6°C) due to prolonged exposure to environmental heat. The rise in core body temperature occurs when the high environmental temperature (and humidity) overwhelms the victim's compensatory heat loss mechanisms primarily evaporation through sweating. This definition does not include hyperthermia caused by infection or drugs. A rise in the circulating blood temperature to 42.5°C or higher leads to generalized vasodilation with resulting effective blood volume reduction due to the disparity between the newly expanded circulatory capacity and the unchanged amount of blood to fill it. There is also tachycardia and heart dilation with impaired cardiac efficiency. Finally, there is stimulation of the respiratory centers with tachypnea initially and followed by irregular breathing and finally cessation of respiration. Thus the mechanisms of death can involve cardiac arrhythmias, seizures or hypovolemic shock with circulatory collapse.

GROSS FINDINGS: No specific gross findings at autopsy.

MICROSCOPIC FINDINGS: No specific microscopic findings. There are no microscopic findings in victims found dead due to the heat. Victims surviving for more than 24 hours after recovery from the hot environment may show skeletal and/or cardiac muscle necrosis, acute tubular necrosis, centrilobular hepatic necrosis, and other nonspecific findings.

SPECIAL PROCEDURES NEEDED FOR DIAGNOSIS: Measure core body temperature at the time of or within a few hours of death. Unfortunately, those persons most at risk live alone and are not discovered until days after death making any core body temperature useless. Toxicology should always be done.

DIFFERENTIAL DIAGNOSIS: Malignant hyperthermia due to halogenated anesthetic agents and succinylcholine. Neuroleptic malignant syndrome. Hyperthermia due to cocaine, phencyclidine, amphetamines.

KEY DIAGNOSTIC CRITERIA: Deaths are classified as heat related if 1 of the 3 criteria is met:
1. Core body temperature of victim is >105°F at the time of death or immediately after death.
2. Substantial environmental or circumstantial evidence of heat as a contributor to death is present.
3. Decomposed body is found without evidence of another cause of death and the victim was last seen alive during the heat wave time period.

POTENTIAL PITFALLS: Lack of a uniform definition for heat-related deaths. Failing to perform toxicology examination. There are no pathognomonic gross or microscopic findings.

References

1. CDC. Heat-related mortality—Chicago, July 1995. *MMWR* 1995;44:577–579.
2. DiMaio DJ, DiMaio VJM. The effects of heat and cold: Hyperthermia and hypothermia. In: DiMaio DJ, Dimaio VJM, eds. *Forensic pathology*. New York, Elsevier Science; 1989:377–384.
3. Hirsch CS, Zumwalt RE. Forensic Pathology. In: Damjanov I, Linder J, eds. *Anderson's pathology 10th ed.* Mosby, St. Louis, MO; 1996:104–105.

HYPOTHERMIA, SYSTEMIC

Entry Authors: Michael D. Bell, Virginia M. Walley, David A. Chiasson, and John P. Veinot

SYNONYMS: Systemic hypothermic injury, exposure, cold immersion injury.

DEFINITION: Systemic injury caused by a core body temperature less than 35°C (95°F) after exposure to cold environment. Hypothermia is graded mild (core body temperature is 35.0–32.2°C, 95–90°F), moderate (32.2–28.0°C, 90–82.4°), or severe (less than 28.0°C, 82.4°F). Hypothermia can also be subclassified as dry or cold or immersion type. Death occurs within hours when immersed in water less than 20°C (68°F). The mechanism of death in systemic hypothermia involves depressed myocardial conduction with the emergence of an ectopic pacemaker followed by ventricular fibrillation. In addition to cardiac dysfunction, systemic hypothermia produces microvascular injury that is usually seen only if there is a period of survival after the exposure. This injury may vary from transudation of fluid and edema to vascular occlusion and gangrene. Intracellular ice formation plays a relatively small role in the pathophysiology of hypothermic injury.

GROSS FINDINGS: Systemic hypothermia shows no pathognomonic gross findings, especially if the victim is found dead in the cold environment. Paradoxical undressing by the victim may be seen at the death scene. Postmortem lividity (livor mortis) is often cherry-red, thus mimicking the livor mortis seen in carbon monoxide and cyanide fatalities. Right ventricular dilation and pulmonary edema are other nonspecific findings. Acute hemorrhagic pancreatitis, visceral and extremity infarction, patchy cutaneous erythema, and gastric erosions (Wischewski ulcers) have been reported in hypothermia victims but are more likely found in survivors who later die of complications. Postmortem vitreous humor glucose is elevated (mean = 82.6 mg/dL) in systemic hypothermia fatalities compared with nondiabetic, nonhypothermic deaths (mean = 37 mg/dL).

MICROSCOPIC FINDINGS: There are no pathognomonic microscopic findings in systemic hypothermia. Antemortem freezing of pig skin produces dermal edema, dilated congested superficial dermal capillaries, and vacuolated keratinocytes. These changes are not seen in a dead pig that is later frozen. Vascular thromboses and gangrene may be seen in survivors but are not usually seen in victims who die in the cold environment. One author reported observable myocardial fiber degeneration (foci of broken or curly homogeneous fibers, exudation and occasional red cell extravasation) in fatal hypothermia, but this is the exception rather than the rule. Histologic preservation of tissues is excellent since postmortem autolysis by intracellular enzymes is retarded by the cold.

SPECIAL PROCEDURES NEEDED FOR DIAGNOSIS: Know the circumstances of death and examine the death scene, if possible. Do a complete autopsy to identify any other cause of death (NOT every body that is found out in the cold is a HYPOTHERMIC death). Submit specimens for toxicology, because failure to escape the cold is often the result of alcohol or drug intoxication. Submit postmortem vitreous humor for glucose determination.

DIFFERENTIAL DIAGNOSIS: In a dead body found outside in the cold, differentiating between systemic hypothermia and other causes of sudden death, including cardiovascular, cerebrovascular, and drug etiologies as well as strangulation.

KEY DIAGNOSTIC CRITERIA: Thorough knowledge of the circumstances surrounding the death, death scene examination, and complete autopsy, including microscopic examination of the skin (look for red areas).

POTENTIAL PITFALLS: Automatically ascribing hypothermia as the cause of death in a body (especially children or young women) found outside in the cold without a complete police investigation and autopsy.

References

1. Danzi DF, Pozos RS. Accidental hypothermia. *NEJM* 1994;331:1756–1760.
2. Hirvonen J. Necropsy findings in fatal hypothermia cases. *Forensic Sci* 1976;8:155–164.
3. Mant AK. Autopsy diagnosis of accidental hypothermia. *J Forensic Med* 1969;16:126–129.
4. Coe JI. Hypothermia: Autopsy findings and vitreous glucose. *J Forensic Sci* 1984;29:389–395.
5. Schoning P. Frozen cadaver: Antemortem versus postmortem. *Am J Forensic Med Path* 1992;13: 18–20.
6. Graham MA, Gantner GE. Heat and cold. In: Froede RC, ed. *Handbook of forensic pathology.* Northfield, IL, CAP; 1990:165–169.

IATROGENIC INFECTION

Entry Authors: Michael D. Bell, Virginia M. Walley, David A. Chiasson, and John P. Veinot

SYNONYMS: See related entry: *Infection of cardiovascular device/graft.*

DEFINITION: A cardiovascular infection (endocarditis, myocarditis, vasculitis, or mycotic aneurysm) caused by a diagnostic or therapeutic procedure. The specific infection depends on the site of entry, the pathogenicity of the organism, host defense, the presence of an intravascular device, and preexisting cardiovascular structural abnormalities. Examples include bacterial endocarditis seeded from an intravascular catheter, postoperative ring abscess involving a prosthetic valve, myocardial microabscesses from hematogenous spread of a postsurgical wound infection, postoperative purulent pericarditis, infected thrombosis or mycotic aneurysm from an intravascular catheter.

GROSS FINDINGS: Varies with the type of infection.

MICROSCOPIC FINDINGS: Varies with the type of infection, usually acute inflammation with abundant polymorphonuclear leukocytes. The causative bacteria may be seen singly or in small groups within the leukocytes or in large extracellular groups. Fungi may be seen with and without special stains. Degenerating bacteria and inflammatory cells may undergo mineralization.

SPECIAL PROCEDURES NEEDED FOR DIAGNOSIS: Aerobic and anaerobic cultures should be taken from blood, affected tissue, and contaminated intravascular device or prosthetic valve. Special stains for bacterial, fungi, mycobacterium, and other microbes should be done when suspected.

DIFFERENTIAL DIAGNOSIS: Noniatrogenic infections.

KEY DIAGNOSTIC CRITERIA: A cardiovascular infection that can be traced directly or temporally to a diagnostic or therapeutic procedure or intravascular device.

POTENTIAL PITFALLS: Because numerous diagnostic and therapeutic procedures are performed routinely on critically ill patients, it may be difficult or impossible to distinguish an iatrogenic from a noniatrogenic cardiovascular infection.

IATROGENIC INJURY

Entry Authors: Michael D. Bell, Virginia M. Walley, David A. Chiasson, and John P. Veinot

SYNONYMS: Iatrogenic trauma, complication of diagnostic or therapeutic procedure.

DEFINITION: An injury occurring as the result of diagnostic or therapeutic procedure by a physician or health care worker but not otherwise specified. The injury may directly cause morbidity or mortality (catheter perforates right ventricle) or set into motion a series of events (thromboembolism, infection, disseminated intravascular coagulation) that eventually result in death.

GROSS FINDINGS: Varies with the type of iatrogenic injury.

MICROSCOPIC FINDINGS: Varies with the type of iatrogenic injury.

SPECIAL PROCEDURES NEEDED FOR DIAGNOSIS: Varies with the type of iatrogenic injury.

DIFFERENTIAL DIAGNOSIS: Varies with the type of iatrogenic injury.

KEY DIAGNOSTIC CRITERIA: Varies with the type of iatrogenic injury.

POTENTIAL PITFALLS: Varies with the type of iatrogenic injury.

INFECTION OF CARDIOVASCULAR DEVICE/GRAFT

Entry Authors: David A. Chiasson, Michael D. Bell, Virginia M. Walley, and John P. Veinot

SYNONYMS: Prosthetic valve endocarditis; annular/perigraft abscess; mycotic false aneurysm.

DEFINITION: *In vivo* growth of microorganisms, most commonly bacteria and fungi on or around a device or graft which may occur as a result of implantation of an infected graft/device, colonization during surgical implantation or subsequent seeding, during an episode of septicemia. Prosthetic valve endocarditis is classified as early (within 60 days of valve replacement) when it is related to perioperative valve contamination or bacteremia or late (after 60 days) when it is due to bacteremic seeding. Common etiologic organisms include staphylococcus (especially epidermidis and aureus), streptococci, gram-negative bacilli and fungi. Early infection of vascular grafts is most often initiated by intraoperative contamination or wound complications whereas hematogenous seeding following bacteremia is usually responsible for late infections. Common etiological organisms include staphylococcus and gram-negative bacteria. Fungal infections of vascular grafts are rare.

GROSS FINDINGS: Infections associated with prosthetic valves may present with abundant infected thrombotic material adherent to the valve components or as infection/abscess involving the annulus, the latter sometimes associated with perivalvular dehiscence/leaks or with fistulas between the cardiac chambers or great vessels. Infection of bioprosthetic valves may manifest as cuspal tears or more characteristically as large central perforations. Infection of vascular grafts may be associated with perigraft seromas and fistulas, for example, between the aorta and small bowel.

MICROSCOPIC FINDINGS: Characteristically, histologic examination shows microorganisms within device/graft thrombi or perigraft tissues associated with tissue necrosis and mixed inflammatory infiltration. Microorganisms may not be readily apparent on routine histologic stains. Degenerating bacterial and inflammatory cells within cuspal vegetations may undergo mineralization.

SPECIAL PROCEDURES NEEDED FOR DIAGNOSIS: Special histologic stains for microorganisms, such as Gram and Grimelius methanine silver (GMS) are mandatory. The former may not readily stain bacteria if there has been previous antibiotic therapy. The GMS stain will aid in the morphologic assessment of bacteria in such cases as well as stain fungal organisms. Cultures of thrombi and perigraft tissues are indicated to establish a specific microbiologic diagnosis. At autopsy, postmortem blood cultures may also be useful.

DIFFERENTIAL DIAGNOSIS: Noninfective thrombosis; degenerative cuspal tears and perforations; dehiscence or pseudoaneurysm due to technical problems; florid foreign body reactions.

KEY DIAGNOSTIC CRITERIA: Histologic demonstration of microorganisms within adherent thrombus or perigraft tissues, supported by microbiologic cultures.

POTENTIAL PITFALLS: Not histologically examining thrombi and perigraft tissues; not performing special stains for microorganisms because of absence or paucity of inflammatory reaction confusing degenerative micro-calcifications with microorganisms on routine or special stains.

References

1. Zussac C, Galloni MR, Zattera GF et al. Endocarditis in patients with bioprostheses: Pathology and clinical correlations. *Intl J Cardiol* 1984;6:719–732.
2. Anderson DJ, Bulkley BH, Hutchins GM. A clinicopathologic study of prosthetic valve endocarditis in 22 patients. Morphologic basis for diagnosis and therapy. *Am Heart J* 1977;94:325–332.

INJURY, BLUNT FORCE

Entry Authors: Michael D. Bell, Virginia M. Walley, David A. Chiasson, and John P. Veinot

SYNONYMS: Blunt force trauma. See related entries: *Contusion* and *Commotio cordis.*

DEFINITION: A mechanical injury produced by a blunt object. The blunt force injuries include abrasions (scrapes), contusions (bruises), lacerations (tears), and fractures (breaks). Abrasion, contusion, laceration, and fracture refer to blunt force injuries and should NOT be used to describe stab or gunshot wounds.

GROSS FINDINGS: Varies with the type of blunt injury.

MICROSCOPIC FINDINGS: Varies with the type of blunt injury.

SPECIAL PROCEDURES NEEDED FOR DIAGNOSIS: Not applicable.

DIFFERENTIAL DIAGNOSIS: Blunt injuries can be confused with stab or incised wounds and gunshot wounds. Contusions can be confused with livor mortis or postmortem lividity.

KEY DIAGNOSTIC CRITERIA: Autopsies with blunt or other types of injuries should be performed by or under the supervision or a forensic pathologist.

POTENTIAL PITFALLS: Varies with the type of blunt injury. Contusions can be confused with postmortem lividity. Lacerations can be confused with stab or incised wounds and rarely gunshot wounds.

References

1. Hirsch CS, Zumwalt RE. Forensic pathology. In: Damjanov I, Linder J, eds. *Anderson's pathology, 10th ed.* Mosby, St. Louis, MO; 1996:84–87.
2. Spitz WU. Blunt force injury. In: Spitz WU, ed. *Spitz and Fisher's medicolegal investigation of death, 3rd ed.* Charles C. Thomas, Springfield, IL; 1993:199–251.

INJURY DUE TO SUTURE LIGATION

Entry Authors: Michael D. Bell, Virginia M. Walley, David A. Chiasson, and John P. Veinot

SYNONYM: Suture encroachment.

DEFINITION: Tissue injury due to inadvertent tying or binding with a suture(s). This is an iatrogenic or accidental injury and can occur during valve replacement or surgery for congenital heart disease (see reference below).

GROSS FINDINGS: Varies. Examples include coronary artery ligation by sewing ring suture from valve prostheses or conduction system injury by sutures during closure of membranous septum defects.

MICROSCOPIC FINDINGS: Not useful except to identify portion of conduction system or other microscopic structure injured.

SPECIAL PROCEDURES NEEDED FOR DIAGNOSIS: Specimen angiography may be helpful to demonstrate coronary (or other) artery occlusion by the suture. Examination of the cardiac conduction system may be helpful if an injury is suspected from suture penetration.

DIFFERENTIAL DIAGNOSIS: None.

KEY DIAGNOSTIC CRITERIA: Demonstrate suture in injured tissue.

POTENTIAL PITFALLS: Overlooking the sutures within the injured tissue.

Reference

1. Bharati S, Lev M, Kirklin JW. *Cardiac surgery and the conduction system.* 2nd rev ed. Futura, Mount Kisco, NY; 1992.

INJURY, NOT OTHERWISE SPECIFIED (NOS)

Entry Authors: Michael D. Bell, Virginia M. Walley, David A. Chiasson, and John P. Veinot

SYNONYMS: Damage, trauma, wound.

DEFINITION: Any damage to a body, organ, tissue, or cell. The damage may be macroscopic or microscopic, reversible or irreversible, and involve the object's function, structure, or both. Injury that alters function alone need not be visible macro- or microscopically (e.g., commotio cordis).

GROSS FINDINGS: Varies with the type of injury.

MICROSCOPIC FINDINGS: Varies with the type of injury.

SPECIAL PROCEDURES NEEDED FOR DIAGNOSIS: Varies with the type of injury.

DIFFERENTIAL DIAGNOSIS: Varies with the type of injury.

KEY DIAGNOSTIC CRITERIA: Varies with the type of injury.

POTENTIAL PITFALLS: Failure to recognize that some injury (and death) produces only functional alterations with no morphologic changes. Varies with the type of injury.

INJURY, TRAUMATIC CARDIOVASCULAR

Entry Authors: Michael D. Bell, Virginia M. Walley, David A. Chiasson, and John P. Veinot

SYNONYM: Wound.

DEFINITION: Any injury or wound of the heart or blood vessels resulting typically from mechanical, thermal, or electrical forces. The most common injuries are due to mechanical force and include contusions, lacerations, stab and puncture wounds, and gunshot wounds.

GROSS FINDINGS: Varies with the specific type of injury.

MICROSCOPIC FINDINGS: Varies with the specific type of injury.

SPECIAL PROCEDURES NEEDED FOR DIAGNOSIS: Varies with the specific type of injury.

DIFFERENTIAL DIAGNOSIS: Varies with the specific type of injury.

KEY DIAGNOSTIC CRITERIA: Be able to recognize each type of injury.

POTENTIAL PITFALLS: Varies with the specific type of injury.

LACERATION

Entry Authors: Michael D. Bell, Virginia M. Walley, David A. Chiasson, and John P. Veinot

SYNONYM: Tear.

DEFINITION: A tear in an organ produced by blunt force injury. While the skin is most commonly involved, deeper structures such as the heart and blood vessels can also lacerate. Severe force is necessary to lacerate the heart or great vessels such as the force seen in motor vehicle accidents or great falls (>1 story tall).

Related terms: Myocardial rupture is the bursting or breaking open of the heart producing hemopericardium. Myocardial rupture may result from a laceration (blunt force injury), an intravascular catheter puncture (sharp force injury), or from weakening of the wall from myocardial infarction and necrosis (disease). A transection injury is that which is made transversely across the long axis of an object dividing it. It may be produced by a laceration, incision or stab wound, or gunshot wound.

GROSS FINDINGS: The laceration edges are irregular and ragged. Within the laceration, tissue traverses or bridges the sides of the wound in contrast to stab wounds. There is often bruising within and surrounding the laceration depending on the tissue involved. Myocardial lacerations may involve the endocardium or the entire wall resulting in rupture. Isolated lacerations of the pericardium, valve leaflets, or chordae tendineae are rare. Aortic lacerations are common in motor vehicle accidents and are usually located at the isthmus, the site of the ligamentum arteriosum insertion. Lacerations of the heart or arteries may result in pseudoaneurysm formation, if the person survives the initial injury.

MICROSCOPIC FINDINGS: With acute injuries, there is tissue disruption with extravasated red blood cells. In the heart, myocytes may contain contraction bands. In the heart, lacerations, like gunshot and stab wounds, heal as unimpressive cicatricial scars with endocardial and epicardial fibrous patches, if the person survives.

SPECIAL PROCEDURES NEEDED FOR DIAGNOSIS: None.

DIFFERENTIAL DIAGNOSIS: Stab and shrapnel wounds may produce similar-appearing injuries to the neophyte. When a myocardial or aortic rupture is found at autopsy in a person involved in a car accident, the question of which came first (the rupture or the crash) is often asked.

KEY DIAGNOSTIC CRITERIA: All deaths involving trauma should be done by or under the supervision of a forensic pathologist. A premortem history and death scene investigation is essential in resolving whether the rupture caused or was caused by the car accident. The coronary arteries and adjacent myocardium should be examined for atherosclerosis, coronary thrombosis, and myocardial infarction. Traumatic myocardial rupture is usually accompanied by other blunt force injuries (abrasions, contusions, lacerations, fractures) in other organs—it is rarely an isolated injury. Spontaneous aortic ruptures usually show media dissection before breaking through the adventitia. Aortic rupture due to blunt injury typically shows no dissection.

POTENTIAL PITFALLS: Confusing lacerations with stab or gunshot wounds. Ascribing myocardial lacerations in children to cardiopulmonary resuscitation or minor blunt force rather than intentional injury—remember, myocardial lacerations require severe forces.

References

1. Hirsch CS, Zumwalt RE. Forensic pathology. In: Damjanov I, Linder J, eds. *Anderson's pathology 10th ed.* Mosby, St. Louis, MO; 1996:84–87.
2. Spitz WU. Blunt force injury. In: Spitz WU, ed. *Spitz and Fisher's medicolegal investigation of death, 3rd ed.* Charles C. Thomas, Springfield, IL; 1993:199–251.

MALALIGNMENT/DISPROPORTION OF CARDIOVASCULAR DEVICE/GRAFT

Entry Authors: David A. Chiasson, Michael D. Bell, Virginia M. Walley, and John P. Veinot

SYNONYMS: Malposition; abnormal prosthesis lie; kinking of graft.

DEFINITION: Abnormal positioning of a device or graft such that blood flow is inappropriately directed or otherwise disturbed; disproportion refers specifically to placement of a valvular prostheses or vascular graft which is too large or too small for annulus/heart chamber or vessel into which it is inserted.

GROSS FINDINGS: The degree of malalignment and disproportion can vary from minimal (clinically insignificant) to severe, the latter including insertion of a valve in the "upside-down" position. Malpositioning of a prosthetic valve at the aortic site may result in obstruction of a coronary ostium by the ring or one of the stents. Abnormal angulation of a valve can result in blood flow impacting upon surrounding tissues, causing mural thrombosis and eventually a fibrous reaction at the site of impaction. Weakening of the native wall and development of an aneurysm may occur in vessels. Disproportion of a heart valve prostheses in the early postoperative period may be associated with ulceration and thrombosis of the chamber or vessel wall on which it impinges. Chronic effects of disproportion include endocardial thickening or indentation caused by impingement of the struts which may become incorporated into the wall of the chamber or vessel and interfere within graft function.

MICROSCOPIC FINDINGS: Histologic evaluation of mural thrombus is indicated in order to rule out infection.

SPECIAL PROCEDURES NEEDED FOR DIAGNOSIS: Specimen radiography may be useful.

DIFFERENTIAL DIAGNOSIS: Other causes of valvular dysfunction including impingement by residual long sutures and native valvular elements and graft/device thrombosis.

KEY DIAGNOSTIC CRITERIA: Evidence of mechanical impingement or abnormal hemodynamic flow identified on careful *in situ* evaluation of the prosthetic device or graft.

POTENTIAL PITFALLS: Not performing a careful inspection of the device/graft *in situ* before fixation that may result in distortion of tissue/graft relationships; overinterpreting the significance of minor degrees of malalignment and disproportion.

References

1. Wally VM, Masters RG. Complications of cardiac valve surgery and their autopsy interpretation. *Cardiovascular Pathol* 1995;4:269–286.
2. Silver MD, Butany J. Mechanical heart valves: Methods of examination, complications and modes of failure. In: Virmani R, Atkinson JB, Fenoglio JJ, eds. *Cardiovascular Pathology*. WB Saunders, Philadelphia; 1991:354–372.

OBSTRUCTION OF CARDIOVASCULAR DEVICE/GRAFT

Entry Authors: David A. Chiasson, Michael D. Bell, Virginia M. Walley, and John P. Veinot

SYNONYMS: Stenosis, occlusion, thrombosis, kinking, suture/tissue impingement. See entry: *Malalignment/disproportion of cardiovascular device/ graft.*

DEFINITION: Decreased blood flow/pressure gradient resulting from stenosis or occlusion of a prosthesis orifice or graft lumen. Common causes of obstruction include prosthesis/graft thrombosis, degenerative calcification, kinking, and suture or tissue impingement. The obstruction may be associated with hemolytic anemia caused by local turbulence.

GROSS FINDINGS: Obstruction of a valvular prostheses is most commonly due to thrombus. Tilting disk prostheses are particularly susceptible, with thrombus most commonly involving the minor orifice. Even small amounts of thrombus may significantly affect occluder function and result in obstruction. Although bioprostheses are less prone to thrombosis, obstruction due to large, sometimes calcified, thrombotic deposits within the prosthesis sinuses does occur as a late postoperative complication, often with no demonstrable underlying pathology of tissue cusps. Heavily calcified, native valve remnants, and/or masses of pledgetted sutures may also stenose the orifice of a valve prosthesis. Fibrous tissue pannus may encroach into tissue cusps or extend into the orifice of a prosthetic valve obstructing blood flow. Long residual suture ends or native valve remnants may protrude into the orifice and cause occluder "sticking." Intrascuspal hematomas and inward bending of struts (stent creep) are infrequent causes of stenosis.

In the early postoperative period, vascular graft thrombosis is generally associated with technical problems at the anastomoses, such as twisting or kinking of the graft or poor run-off secondary to distal native vessel disease. With time, progressive extension of mural thrombus may lead to stenosis of the graft itself. Late postoperative kinking of a vascular conduit may result from fibrous adherence to a local fixed structure such as the sternum.

MICROSCOPIC FINDINGS: Examine thrombi and large calcific masses for evidence of infection.

SPECIAL PROCEDURES NEEDED FOR DIAGNOSIS: Culture thrombi and large calcific masses; consider specimen radiography to document extent of calcification; at autopsy, consider angiography to document location and severity of obstruction.

DIFFERENTIAL DIAGNOSIS: Device/graft disproportion or malalignment; infective endocarditis; artefactual protrusion of tissue fragments into valve orifice during surgical resection; adherence of postmortem clot or prosthesis/graft.

KEY DIAGNOSTIC CRITERIA: Presurgical/premortem clinical/radiologic evidence of valvular or graft stenosis with or without evidence of hemolytic anemia.

POTENTIAL PITFALLS: Inadequate clinical information and findings at surgery; misinterpreting artefactually produced distortion of surgically excised prostheses or grafts; confusing postmortem blood clot with premortem thrombus at autopsy; misinterpretation of significance of long residual sutures and tissue encroachment.

References

1. Schoen FJ. *Interventional and surgical cardiovascular pathology: Clinical correlations and basic principles.* WB Saunders, Philadelphia; 1989:124–172, 249–280.
2. Silver MD, Wilson GJ. Pathology of mechanical heart valve prostheses and vascular grafts made of artificial materials. In: Silver MD, ed. *Cardiovascular pathology, 2nd ed.* Churchill Livingstone, New York; 1991:1487–1545.

PNEUMOPERICARDIUM

Entry Authors: Michael D. Bell, Virginia M. Walley, David A. Chiasson, and John P. Veinot

SYNONYM: Air pericardial tamponade.

DEFINITION: Pneumopericardium is the accumulation of air within the pericardial sac. If there is sufficient pericardial air compressing the heart to produce hemodynamic changes, then this is called air pericardial tamponade or air tamponade. Pneumopericardium is usually produced by chest trauma or presence of a fistula between the pericardium and adjacent organs (usually lung or gut).

Related terms: Pneumomediastinum is entrapped air in the mediastinal soft tissues and is usually seen in the setting of chest and lung injury. The entrapped air produces crepitus or crackling of the affected tissues. Pneumomediastinum is not the same as pneumopericardium.

GROSS FINDINGS: Air pericardial tamponade can be seen on premortem and postmortem chest radiology. It can also be demonstrated by echocardiography. At autopsy, the distended pericardium sac will produce an audible hiss as the pericardium is incised. In the absence of trauma, a fistula between the pericardium and lungs or gut is usually demonstrable. Pneumothorax and pneumomediastinum may also be present.

MICROSCOPIC FINDINGS: Not helpful.

SPECIAL PROCEDURES NEEDED FOR DIAGNOSIS: Chest radiography, prior to opening the body, is helpful and shows separation of the parietal and visceral pericardium by air with more distention on the left side. The heart appears small in air tamponade.

DIFFERENTIAL DIAGNOSIS: None.

KEY DIAGNOSTIC CRITERIA: Pneumopericardium is rare. When it does occur it is usually following chest trauma with injuries to the lungs and pericardium. The incidence of air tamponade among individuals with pneumopericardium is up to 37%. In the absence of trauma, look for a bronchopericardial fistula in the setting of a bronchogenic infection (i.e., tuberculosis) or cancer. Communications can also occur between the pericardium and esophagus or stomach.

POTENTIAL PITFALLS: Not documenting the pneumopericardium with chest radiography.

References

1. Costo IVI, Soto B, Diethelm L, Zarco P. Air pericardial tamponade. *Am J Cardiol* 1987;60:1421–1422.
2. Cummings RG, Wesley RLR, Adams DH, Lowe JE. Pneumopericardium resulting in cardiac tamponade. *Ann Thorac Surg* 1989;37:511–518.
3. Levin S, Maldonado I, Rehm C, Ross S, Weiss RL. Cardiac tamponade without pericardial effusion after blunt chest trauma. *Am Heart J* 1996;131:198–200.
4. Macklin CC. Transport of air along sheathes of pulmonary blood vessels from alveoli to mediastinum: Clinical applications. *Arch Intern Med* 1939;64:913–921.

POSTTRAUMATIC ANEURYSM

Entry Authors: Michael D. Bell, Virginia M. Walley, David A. Chiasson, and John P. Veinot

SYNONYMS: Traumatic aneurysm. See related entry: *False aneurysm.*

DEFINITION: Any localized dilation of a cardiovascular structure (heart chamber, aorta, artery) produced by trauma (stab or gunshot wound, nonpenetrating blunt trauma, needle, or catheter injury). These may be true or false aneurysms. A false aneurysm rarely results from a penetrating injury of the heart or aorta (they are usually fatal). If the injury interrupts the blood supply (example: traumatic coronary artery thrombosis) to the cardiovascular structure (usually the heart) rather than penetrating it, ischemia and infarction may occur. Healing and fibrosis then results in weakening of the wall producing a true aneurysm.

GROSS FINDINGS: Depends on whether a true or false aneurysm is produced and how long it has been present. There is vessel/chamber wall thinning with variable external protrusion. A mural thrombus is often seen in the aneurysm. Rupture may be present.

MICROSCOPIC FINDINGS: False aneurysms show discontinuity of the normal vessel/chamber wall.

SPECIAL PROCEDURES NEEDED FOR DIAGNOSIS: Elastic stains highlight elastic fibers and are therefore helpful in determining if there is discontinuity in a large artery or aortic wall. Trichrome stain is more helpful when the heart is involved.

DIFFERENTIAL DIAGNOSIS: Atherosclerotic, syphilitic, or mycotic aneurysms are usually easily distinguished from posttraumatic aneurysms. The differential diagnosis in the heart would be a postmyocardial infarction aneurysm due to nontraumatic coronary occlusion (atherosclerosis).

KEY DIAGNOSTIC CRITERIA: There must be a clinical history of previous trauma (stab or gunshot wound, blunt trauma, iatrogenic injury).

POTENTIAL PITFALLS: Confusion with nontraumatic aneurysms (atherosclerotic, luetic, postmyocardial infarction).

References

1. Fleming AW, Green DC. Traumatic aneurysms of the thoracic aorta: Report of 43 patients. *Ann Thoracic Surg* 1974;18:91–101.
2. Jamsidi A, Berry RW. Left ventricular pseudoaneurysm secondary to cardiac stab wound: Successful repair in a thirteen year old girl. *Am J Cardiol* 1965;16:601–604.

RADIATION INJURY

Entry Authors: Michael D. Bell, Virginia M. Walley, David A. Chiasson, and John P. Veinot

SYNONYM: Ionizing radiation injury.

DEFINITION: Injury produced by ionizing radiation. Ionizing radiation injures cells by directly damaging DNA, membranes, and enzymes and indirectly damaging those structures through free radical formation. Cardiac muscle should be resistant to radiation because it is a nonproliferating tissue. However, the myocardial microcirculation (endothelial cells) and mesothelium-lined pericardium can be damaged leading to secondary myocardial and pericardial injury.

Most cardiac injury occurs after focal radiation exposure confined to the thorax for the treatment of Hodgkin's disease, breast cancer, and other malignancies. Treatment often involves total doses of 36–44 Gy or 3600–4400 rads, fractionated and administered over 4–5 weeks. Rarely, injury results from whole-body exposure (Uranium miners, Chernobyl disaster).

GROSS FINDINGS: Acutely, pericardial effusion with or without fibrinous pericarditis may be seen. This may progress to fibrous adhesions obliterating the pericardial cavity. The myocardium is usually grossly normal. In acute cases, nonspecific punctate hemorrhages may be seen and later patchy fibrosis may be present. The endocardium is typically uninvolved.

MICROSCOPIC FINDINGS: In acute injury, there may be a thickened epicardium with fibrinous pericarditis. This may progress to fibrosis. The lymphatic vessels are dilated and there is usually no inflammatory reaction. The small arteries and arterioles in the myocardium and epicardium may have swollen endothelial cells, smudgy and discontinuous intima, and enlarged vacuolated smooth muscle cells. In severe injury, there may be segmental vasculitis with fibrinoid change. One may also see extravasated red cells, granulocytes, and edema adjacent to the affected vessels. The myocytes appear normal. This may progress to endothelial proliferation and collagenous thickening of the artery wall causing lumen narrowing. This may contribute to the interstitial fibrosis seen as a late complication.

SPECIAL PROCEDURES NEEDED FOR DIAGNOSIS: Complete autopsy with careful examination of the heart, pericardium, and mediastinum. Document the type of radiation involved, dose range, and schedule, and treatment field.

DIFFERENTIAL DIAGNOSIS: Acute uremic pericarditis.
Metastatic tumor to pericardium and/or myocardium.
Pericardial or myocardial infection (direct extension or hematogenous spread).
Autoimmune heart disease (rheumatoid arthritis, SLE).

KEY DIAGNOSTIC CRITERIA: The gross and microscopic findings in radiation injury are nonspecific, therefore, more common etiologies must be excluded first:
1. Sequelae of prior intrathoracic surgery.
2. Inflammation of contiguous structures.
3. Infiltration of the heart or pericardium by tumor.
4. Autoimmune response associated with destruction of tumor by chemotherapy or radiotherapy.
5. Exacerbation of preexistent heart disease or the development of cardiac manifestations of systemic disease (uremic pericarditis).

Valvular, endocardial, and coronary artery disease should be ascribed to radiation injury with great caution.

POTENTIAL PITFALLS: Ascribing cardiac findings to radiation injury without considering alternative etiologies.

References

1. White DC. *An atlas of radiation histopathology.* Springfield VA, US Dept. of Commerce National, Technical Information Service TID-26676; 1975:93–105.
2. Benoff LJ, Schweitzer P. Radiation therapy-induced cardiac injury. *Am Heart J* 1995;129:1193–1196.
3. Radiation injury. In: Cotran RS, Kumar V, Robbins SL, *Robbins pathologic basis of disease.* WB Saunders, Philadelphia, PA; 1989:504–511.
4. Pope AM, Rall DP, ed. *Environmental medicine.* National Academy Press, Washington, DC; 1995: 641–668.

STAB WOUND

Entry Authors: Michael D. Bell, Virginia M. Walley, David A. Chiasson, and John P. Veinot

SYNONYMS: Knife wound; sharp force injury.

DEFINITION: A mechanical injury produced by a sharp-edged (knife, scalpel) or pointed weapon (ice pick, needle) or instrument in which the wound track that is deeper than it is long. The heart and all blood vessels can be injured by a stab wound. An incised wound or cut is a mechanical injury produced by a sharp-edged weapon or instrument with a wound track that is longer than it is deep. The heart and other deeply located vessels are rarely injured by incised wounds, except in the neck. Stab and incised wounds are both examples of sharp force injury. A penetrating stab wound of the heart passes into the heart, but not out. A perforating stab wound of the heart passes completely through the heart producing an entrance and exit site.

GROSS FINDINGS: Stab wounds are recognized best by their appearance on and through the skin. Stab wounds have sharp, straight edges with no undermining. The lack of crushing and tearing by stab wounds is the reason why there is no contusion or bruising around the stab wound. There are no abrasions at the edges of a stab wound except when the knife is plunged completely into the body and its handle scrapes against the skin producing a "hilt mark." There is no "tissue bridging" within the wound because the sharp edge cuts through blood vessels and nerves within the wound track. Stab wounds through the heart similarly produce sharp, straight wound tracks with no crushing or tearing of the adjacent myocardium. Adjacent extravasated blood may be seen in the epicardial fat around the entrance site.

MICROSCOPIC FINDINGS: Not useful. Acute stab wounds of the heart typically show only extravasated red blood cells in the epicardial fat next to the wound entrance site and along the wound track. Uncomplicated stab wounds (as well as gunshot wounds and lacerations) heal leaving only a small indistinct scar through the myocardium and focal fibrous plaques over the epicardial and endo-cardial ends.

SPECIAL PROCEDURES NEEDED FOR DIAGNOSIS: Any autopsy in which stab wounds are involved should be performed by or under the supervision of a forensic pathologist. The wound should be described in detail in the autopsy report as well as diagrammed and photographed (a ruler must be in the photograph). The wound track's direction through the body should be described after careful dissection. Avoid using a probe or finger to delineate the wound track because it will often produce a false track instead. Postmortem radiography of the wound area rarely shows a retained knife tip or blade that has broken off the weapon.

DIFFERENTIAL DIAGNOSIS: None, if the autopsy is done by or under the supervision of a forensic pathologist. Others may confuse stab wounds of the skin with lacerations, gunshot wounds, or distant shotgun wounds caused by buckshot pellets. Ice pick wounds may be confused with .22 caliber gunshot wounds.

KEY DIAGNOSTIC CRITERIA: Skin wounds show sharp, smooth edges with no tissue bridging within the wound. The same applies to heart wounds.

POTENTIAL PITFALLS: Performing an autopsy involving stab wounds without any experience or supervision by a forensic pathologist. Stab wounds of the skin can be confused with lacerations, gunshot, and shotgun wounds. Failure to adequately document the wound and its track through the body can lead to medicolegal problems and a good deal of personal embarrassment. Small stab wounds and punctures can be easily overlooked.

Reference

1. Spitz WU. Sharp force injury. In: Spitz WU, ed. *Medicolegal investigation of death, 3rd ed.* Charles C. Thomas, Springfield, IL; 1993:252–310.

STRUCTURAL FAILURE OF CARDIOVASCULAR DEVICE/GRAFT

Entry Authors: David A. Chiasson, Michael D. Bell, Virginia M. Walley, and John P. Veinot

SYNONYMS: Graft/device material tear/loss; housing fracture; cuspal degeneration, calcification, or tearing.

DEFINITION: Dysfunction of a device or graft due to: intrinsic defects related to the design, manufacture, assembly, shipping or storage; damage during surgical implantation; biological or physical degradation associated with *in situ* functioning. Failure may manifest itself suddenly, usually after a prolonged period of wear, stress, or tissue degeneration. Failure of vascular grafts most commonly occurs at anastomotic sites where deterioration of the graft material may result in graft-native vessel dehiscence.

GROSS FINDINGS: The findings vary depending on the nature of the prosthetic valve or vascular graft. With mechanical valves, there may be complete fracture of a strut with escape of the poppet. Materials such as teflon, which coat valve components, may show evidence of wear in areas of contact with the occluder. The surface of a ball occluder may show splits or cracks. Wearing of the edges of disk-type occluders from contact with the struts of the cage also occurs. The most common causes of tissue valve failure are degenerative tears or perforations of the cusps which are often associated with calcification. Most commonly, tears extend from the free margin. Central perforations of varying size and configuration also are seen, some of which result from contact of excessively long sutures with the cusp. Explanted vascular grafts may show degeneration of the graft material, most notably near the anastomoses. At autopsy this may be associated with rupture and formation of a false aneurysm.

MICROSCOPIC FINDINGS: Degenerative changes seen in bioprosthetic valve cusps include: loss of the layered architectural definition with collagen bundle separation, fluid insudation, loss of connective tissue cell staining (best assessed with the Movat stain); and degenerative calcification (von Kossa stain helpful).

SPECIAL PROCEDURES NEEDED FOR DIAGNOSIS: Radiography of tissue valves is useful in documenting the extent and distribution of calcific degeneration. X-rays of the body can help locate fractured components and occluders of mechanical valves. Scanning electronic microscopy may demonstrate evidence of wear and fatigue of metallic components and may also be useful in the assessment of primary vascular graft failure.

DIFFERENTIAL DIAGNOSIS: Anastomotic dehiscence of device/graft; artefactual distortion of the prostheses during surgical removal; infective endocarditis.

KEY DIAGNOSTIC CRITERIA: Adequate clinical information including results of preoperative evaluation and findings at surgery; demonstration of structural defects on gross examination.

POTENTIAL PITFALLS: Certain structural abnormalities, most notably tearing of tissue valve cusps and vascular grafts may occur as a result of surgical excision and subsequent handling; similarly scratches and other marks may be artefactually created on mechanical valve components.

References

1. Silver MD, Butany J. Mechanical heart valves: Methods of examination, complications and modes of failure. In: Virmani R, Atkinson JB, Fenoglio JJ, eds. *Cardiovascular pathology*. WB Saunders, Philadelphia; 1991:354–372.
2. Schoen FJ. Approach to the analysis of cardiac valve prostheses as surgical pathology or autopsy specimens. *Cardiovascular Pathol* 1995:241–255.
3. Schoen FJ, Hobson CE. Anatomic analysis of removed prosthetic heart valves: Causes of failure of 33 mechanical valves and 58 bioprostheses, 1980 to 1983. *Human Pathol* 1985:16:549–559.

THERMAL INJURY

Entry Authors: Michael D. Bell, Virginia M. Walley, David A. Chiasson, and John P. Veinot

SYNONYMS: Burn, fire injury, scald injury.

DEFINITION: Injury resulting from the direct application of heat to the body or by indirect radiant heat. The usual heat sources include fire (produces flames and indirect radiant heat), heated objects, high-voltage electricity, hot liquids (scalding), chemical, and microwave. Because the heat source is exogenous, the skin is usually affected and burns are classified by the depth of skin involvement as 1st, 2nd, and 3rd degree burns. Forensic pathologists see 4th degree burns with charring and severe loss of tissue and even limbs.

GROSS FINDINGS: First degree burns of the skin show only redness with no blisters. Second degree burns show moist red skin with epidermal blisters that may or may not result in scarring. Third degree burns have a dry, white leathery appearance, and extend through the epidermis to involve the dermis resulting in dried eschars. Healing results in scarring. Severely burned bodies are often black from carbonization or charring. Burned bodies assume a pugilistic pose due to muscle contracture and coagulation. Charred bodies often show tearing of the soft tissues and muscle (the tears should run parallel with the muscle fibers) with extrusion of the bowel. Peculiar curved fractures are seen in bones exposed to high temperatures, especially in the extremities. Skull fractures and epidural blood clot may result from severe heat and the production of steam inside the calvarium. Despite severe charring of the body, the internal contents are often unaffected, contain blood and other fluids for toxicology, and can be examined for other injuries. Soot (black particles) within the lower respiratory tract and stomach indicates that the victim was alive when the fire started. Victims who survived the fire but die later of its complications usually show the nonspecific findings of shock and may have pneumonia.

MICROSCOPIC FINDINGS: First degree burns are limited to the superficial epidermis and show no characteristic microscopic changes except for focal nuclear pyknosis and cytoplasmic vacuolization. The dermal blood vessels are congested and dilated. Second degree burns show destruction of the upper epidermal layers with blister formation. The blister occurs at the dermal–epidermal junction with sparing of the dermal appendages. Third degree burns show coagulative necrosis of the epidermis, dermis, and often the subcutaneous fat. The dermal appendages are necrotic. The dermal collagen is swollen into strap-like bands or solid masses. The collagen stains pink-red rather than blue with trichrome stain.

SPECIAL PROCEDURES NEEDED FOR DIAGNOSIS: Radiologic examination of severely charred bodies for bullets (a body is occasionally set on fire to coverup the original homicide). Toxicology examination for carbon monoxide to aid in determining if the victim was alive prior to the start of the fire.

DIFFERENTIAL DIAGNOSIS: Localized thermal burns with blisters must be distinguished from electrocution burns, barbiturate blisters, friction blisters, putrefactive bullae, and the usual bullous diseases. Radiant heat injury can mimic dried abrasions (blunt injury).

KEY DIAGNOSTIC CRITERIA: History of thermal exposure. Severely burned bodies should be autopsied by or under the supervision of a forensic pathologist.

POTENTIAL PITFALLS: Automatically assuming that a severely charred body found in a fire died from the fire or smoke inhalation. Confusing the effects of severe heat with premortem injuries (epidural hematoma, skull fracture, lacerations).

References

1. Spitz WU. Thermal injuries. In: Spitz WU, ed. *Medicolegal investigation of death, 3rd ed.* Charles C. Thomas, Springfield, IL; 1993:413–443.
2. Gantner GE, Graham MA. Deaths associated with fire and burns. In: Froede RC, ed. *Handbook of forensic pathology.* Northfield, IL, College of American Pathologists; 1990:159–163.
3. Sevitt S. *Burns: Pathology and therapeutic applications.* London, Butterworth; 1957:18–27.
4. Moritz AR. Studies of thermal injury. III, The pathology and pathogenesis of cutaneous burns—An experimental study. *Am J Path* 1947;23:915–941.

TOXIC MYOCARDITIS, DRUG-RELATED

Entry Authors: Michael D. Bell, Virginia M. Walley, David A. Chiasson, and John P. Veinot

SYNONYM: Drug-induced myocarditis.

DEFINITION: A necrotizing myocarditis caused directly by a drug. Both myocyte necrosis and inflammation are seen. A toxic myocarditis is also characterized by multifocal areas of myocyte injury of different ages. The drugs most commonly associated with toxic myocarditis include:

5-fluorouracil	lithium
daunorubicin	antimony
arsenicals	phenothiazine
catecholamines	plasmocid
cocaine	cyclophosphamide
emetine	

GROSS FINDINGS: The cardiac chambers may be dilated and the myocardium pale and soft. No hypertrophy is seen.

MICROSCOPIC FINDINGS: The myocardium shows patchy areas of myocyte necrosis and repair with a nongranulomatous lymphocytic infiltrate. No eosinophils or giant cells are seen. Healing myocarditis is characterized by proliferating fibroblasts and sparse macrophages. Endothelial injury and microthrombi may be seen, but the large arteries and veins are normal and no true vasculitis is seen.

SPECIAL PROCEDURES NEEDED FOR DIAGNOSIS: None.

DIFFERENTIAL DIAGNOSIS: Viral myocarditis, hypersensitivity myocarditis.

KEY DIAGNOSTIC CRITERIA: The presence of necrosis and myocyte injury of varying ages along with the absence of eosinophils differentiates toxic myocarditis from hypersensitivity myocarditis. Viral myocarditis may be difficult to differentiate from toxic myocarditis by morphology alone. Clinical history and viral cultures or titers will aid in the diagnosis.

POTENTIAL PITFALLS: Distinguishing between viral and toxic myocarditis based on morphologic features alone.

References

1. Billingham ME. Morphologic changes in drug-induced heart disease. In: Bristow MR, ed. *Drug-induced heart disease*. Elsevier-North-Holland Biomedical Press, Amsterdam, 1980:127.
2. Edwards WD. Pathology of endomyocardial biopsy. In: Waller BF, ed. *Pathology of the heart and great vessels*. Churchill-Livingstone, New York; 1988:217–232.
3. Fenoglio JJ, Silver MD. Effects of drugs on the cardiovascular system. In: Silver MD, ed. *Cardiovascular pathology, 2nd ed.* Churchill-Livingstone, New York; 1991:1205–1229.

TRAUMATIC ARRHYTHMIA OR CONDUCTION DISTURBANCE

Entry Authors: Michael D. Bell, Virginia M. Walley, David A. Chiasson, and John P. Veinot

SYNONYMS: Injury-related arrhythmia. See related: *Commotio cordis.*

DEFINITION: Cardiac arrhythmia (bradycardia to ventricular tachycardia) or conduction disturbance (hemiblock, complete heart block) caused by trauma. The injury may involve the cardiac conduction system or induce arrhythmias by other mechanisms (local ischemia, vasovagal reflex). The injury may occur during open heart surgery (often for congenital heart or valvular repair), cardiac catheterization, or after penetrating or nonpenetrating heart injury. The arrhythmia or conduction disturbance may be asymptomatic, symptomatic but nonfatal, or symptomatic and fatal. Fortunately, conduction system injury after heart surgery is often asymptomatic, transitory, and reversible.

GROSS FINDINGS: There may be no gross abnormalities. There may be hemorrhage or pallor in acute injuries. Fibrosis or calcification may be seen in old healed injuries. There may be overlying endocardial thickening in old injuries. The type of conduction disturbance depends on the location of the trauma.

MICROSCOPIC FINDINGS: There may be no microscopic findings (commotio cordis). Hemorrhage, coagulative necrosis, fibrosis, calcification may all be seen at the site of injury.

SPECIAL PROCEDURES NEEDED FOR DIAGNOSIS: Electrocardiography is required to diagnose this type of injury unless death is sudden and unexpected (commotio cordis). Examination of the cardiac conduction system may reveal the location of the conduction injury; however, it will not explain all arrhythmias or conduction disturbances.

DIFFERENTIAL DIAGNOSIS: Nontraumatically produced cardiac arrhythmia or conduction disturbance such as occur with myocardial infarction, hyperkalemia, or hypokalemia, etc.

KEY DIAGNOSTIC CRITERIA: There must be a change in the heart rhythm or conduction (demonstrated by electrocardiography or clinically) after cardiac trauma (injury or surgery). There can be no nontraumatic causes for the rhythm change.

POTENTIAL PITFALLS: Patients with preexisting heart disease and complex medical problems are likely to have nontraumatic causes for the arrhythmia or conduction disturbance, making the diagnosis of traumatic-induced arrhythmia difficult or impossible.

References

1. Bharati S, Lev M. The cardiac conduction system in unexplained sudden death. Futura, Mount Kisco, NY; 1990:375–376.
2. Finn WF, Byrum KE. Fatal traumatic heart block as a result of apparently minor trauma. *Ann Emerg Med* 1988;17:59–62.
3. Hudson REB. The conducting system: Anatomy, histology, and pathology in acquired heart disease. In: Silver MD, ed. *Cardiovascular pathology, 2nd ed.* Churchill-Livingstone, New York; 1991:1408–1410.

4. Maron BJ, Poliac LC, Kaplan JA, Mueller FO. Blunt impact to the chest leading to sudden death from cardiac arrest during sports activities. *NEJM* 1995;333:337–342.

5. Steinberg C, Levin AR, Engle MA. Transient complete heart block following percutaneous balloon pulmonary valvuloplasty: Treatment with systemic corticosteroids. *Pediatr Cardiol* 1992;13: 181–183.

TRAUMATIC ARTERIOVENOUS FISTULA

Entry Authors: Michael D. Bell, Virginia M. Walley, David A. Chiasson, and John P. Veinot

SYNONYM: Traumatic fistula.

DEFINITION: A traumatically produced communication between an artery and a vein that bypasses the normal capillary bed. The arterial pressure forces blood into the vein, dilating it. Ninety-six percent of traumatic arteriovenous fistulas are produced by penetrating wounds (gunshot wounds, stab wounds, needle punctures), whereas 4% are produced by nonpenetrating blunt injury. Vertebral arteriovenous fistulas are common because of the close relationship between the vertebral arteries and the paravertebral venous plexus. They commonly present as a continuous thrill and murmur with systolic accentuation over the fistula site. Arteriovenous fistula is also suspected in a patient with increased systemic arterial pulse pressure in the absence of aortic regurgitation. Congestive heart failure occurs only when large arteries (subclavian, femoral, common carotid, iliac) or the aorta are involved. Traumatic arteriovenous fistulas are usually easily diagnosed and treated and rarely produce significant morbidity or mortality.

GROSS FINDINGS: Initially, a hematoma forms around the artery and vein preventing blood from escaping into the remaining tissues and allowing communication between the lumen of each vessel. The arterial pressure produces venous dilation and wall hypertrophy or venous "arterialization." Gross enlargement of the fistula may produce pressure effects on adjacent structures. Increased blood flow through the artery proximal to the fistula slowly produces dilation and wall hypertrophy with degenerative changes. The tissues or organ(s) supplied by the affected artery may show ischemic changes distal to the fistula. Cardiac hypertrophy may be seen if the arteriovenous fistula is sufficiently large to produce high cardiac output heart failure.

MICROSCOPIC FINDINGS: Vascular structures surrounded by a recent or organizing hematoma with the venous side dilated and its wall thickened like an artery.

SPECIAL PROCEDURES NEEDED FOR DIAGNOSIS: Selective angiography will demonstrate the arteriovenous fistula.

DIFFERENTIAL DIAGNOSIS: Traumatic versus nontraumatic arteriovenous fistula (congenital or acquired such as a complication of mycotic aneurysm).

KEY DIAGNOSTIC CRITERIA: A history of trauma at the site of the fistula permits distinction of a traumatic from a nontraumatic fistula.

POTENTIAL PITFALLS: Diagnosis is often delayed (up to years) because signs and symptoms are produced only after the fistula enlarges over time. Other life-threatening injuries can also overshadow the vascular injury during the initial hours and days after the trauma leading to delayed diagnosis.

References

1. Robbs JV, Carrim AA, Kadwa AM, Mars M. Traumatic arteriovenous fistula: Experience with 202 patients. *Brit J Surg* 1994;81:1296–1299.

TRAUMATIC DISSECTION

Entry Authors: Michael D. Bell, Virginia M. Walley, David A. Chiasson, and John P. Veinot

SYNONYM: None.

DEFINITION: Longitudinal splitting of the aortic or arterial wall by blood as a result of intimal injury. Blunt force injury and puncture wounds are the usual causes. Stab or gunshot wounds are unlikely to produce traumatic dissection because damage to the adventitia and media allows blood to escape rather than dissect. The carotid and vertebral arteries are common sites for dissection, thrombosis, or laceration after a blunt impact to the head or neck by a punch, kick, or fall. Angioplasty is a common iatrogenic cause of dissection because the technique deliberately fractures the atherosclerotic plaque potentially allowing blood to enter the media.

GROSS FINDINGS: Blunt force impact of the artery produces intimal and inner medial lacerations resulting in traumatic dissection. The dissection extends for only a short distance from the intimal defect. The intimal flap can protrude into the lumen causing obstruction and thrombosis. The vascular catheter that produced the dissection may be found within the dissection track or false lumen.

MICROSCOPIC FINDINGS: There is hemorrhage dissecting through the media, which may track through to the adventitia. Luminal thrombosis may also be seen. Medial degenerative changes seen in hypertension or Marfan's disease are not seen.

SPECIAL PROCEDURES NEEDED FOR DIAGNOSIS: In iatrogenic injuries, review of the premortem angiographic films is often helpful. In iatrogenic fatalities, it is best to examine the body with the catheter or device undisturbed, but frequently it has been removed prior to postmortem examination.

DIFFERENTIAL DIAGNOSIS: Nontraumatic or "spontaneous" aortic or arterial dissections.

KEY DIAGNOSTIC CRITERIA: History of trauma or vascular catheterization. Iatrogenic vascular injuries are more likely to occur if the patient has severe atherosclerosis of the affected vessel or if catheterization was "difficult."

POTENTIAL PITFALLS: Inadequate information about the events that occurred before death. Traumatic dissections of the carotid and vertebral arteries can be mistakenly diagnosed as spontaneous because there is often a delay (hours) between the injury (which can be a simple punch, kick, or fall, and therefore, forgotten) and the symptoms.

TRAUMATIC RUPTURE

Entry Authors: Michael D. Bell, Virginia M. Walley, David A. Chiasson, and John P. Veinot

SYNONYMS: Cardiac laceration, vascular laceration.
Related terms: See *Hemopericardium, Laceration,* and *Injury, blunt force.*

DEFINITION: Transmural disruption of a heart chamber, vessel, or associated structure (valve, papillary muscle) due to blunt force injury. The blunt force is usually applied externally to the chest. Vascular or valvular rupture can also occur from over inflation of an intravascular balloon in a vessel or valve that is too small or too rigid to accommodate it.

GROSS FINDINGS: Irregular defect in the heart wall, blood vessel, or associated structures (heart valve, papillary muscle). Rupture of the heart (free wall) or ascending aorta results in hemopericardium. Rupture of the descending thoracic aorta results in hemothorax. Abdominal aortic rupture produces retroperitoneal hemorrhage with or without hemoperitoneum.

MICROSCOPIC FINDINGS: Disrupted myocardium with clotted blood in the wound track and extravasated red blood cells in the adjacent myocardium. There may be contraction bands in adjacent myocytes. There is no inflammation unless the victim survives the rupture. No coagulative necrosis or coronary artery thrombus is seen.

SPECIAL PROCEDURES NEEDED FOR DIAGNOSIS: Identify the rupture site and examine grossly and microscopically. Examine the coronary artery supplying the ruptured wall carefully. Selective angiography may help identify and document arterial rupture. In aortic rupture, measure the circumference of the aorta at the rupture site.

DIFFERENTIAL DIAGNOSIS: Rupture following acute myocardial infarction. Nontraumatic aortic dissection and rupture. Ruptured aortic aneurysm (atherosclerotic, luetic, mycotic).

KEY DIAGNOSTIC CRITERIA: History of trauma (usually severe blunt force is required for cardiac or aortic rupture). History of sudden death during or after inflation of an intravascular balloon (coronary) angioplasty, pulmonary artery catheter balloon, balloon valvuloplasty, or aortoplasty).

POTENTIAL PITFALLS: Attributing the rupture to a natural or nontraumatic etiology. This has serious medicolegal consequences because natural death is treated differently from an accident or homicide.

Appendix: SNOMED Codes for Cardiovascular Pathology

SNOMED coding is complex, and the following listing is necessarily incomplete. A more complete discussion is available in *SNOMED International: Microglossary for Pathology*, published by the College of American Pathologists. There are many ways to code a single lesion, and it is often best to use more than one code designation. SNOMED employs modules that reflect different aspects or qualities of a given specimen. The modules are identified by an alpha prefix, and some key examples are:

Topography	T
Morphology	M
Function	F
Living Organisms	L
Chemicals, Drugs and Biological Products	C
Physical Agents, Forces, and Activities	A
Diseases/Diagnoses	D
Procedures	P
General Linkage/Modifiers	G

Below are examples of SNOMED codes for a variety of conditions or specimens relevant to cardiovascular pathology. Two lists are given. The first shows conditions arranged alphabetically. The second is ordered according to the SNOMED code.

SNOMED codes listed alphabetically by condition:

Aneurysm	M-32400
Aneurysm, A-V	M-32220
Aneurysm, congenital, NOS	M-24610
Aneurysm, false	M-32590
Aneurysm, dissecting	M-32270
Aneurysm, mycotic	M-32520
Aneurysm, NOS	M-32200
Aneurysm, ruptured, NOS	M-32201
Annular thrombus	M-35120
Anomalies, congenital	D4-F0000
Anomalies, multiple	M-20080
Aorta	T-42000
Aorta, abdominal	T-42500
Aorta, aneurysm, NOS	D3-83300

Aorta, aneurysm, ruptured, NOS	D3-83310
Aorta, atherosclerosis	D3-83200
Aortic valve	T-35400
Aortic valve, prosthesis	A-04116
Aortic valve, rheumatic disease	D3-17640
Arteriolar nephrosclerosis	D7-13120
Arteriosclerosis	M-52000
Arteriolosclerosis, NOS	M-52200
Arteriosclerotic vascular disease	D3-81100
Arteritis, NOS	D3-81600
Artery, cerebral	T-45510
Artery, carotid, NOS	T-45010
Artery, disease, NOS	D3-81000
Artery, femoral, NOS	T-47400
Artery, NOS	T-41000
Artery, of extremity, NOS	T-47000
Atheroma, artery	D3-81202
Atheroma, artery, NOS	M-52100
Atheromatous embolus	M-35360
Atheromatous plaque, calcified	M-52101
Atheromatous plaque, NOS	M-52100
Atheromatous plaque, ulcerated	M-52103
Atherosclerosis, NOS	M-52110
Atrial thrombosis, NOS	D3-81500
Atrium, NOS	T-32100
Atrophy, NOS	M-58000
Biopsy procedure code, biopsy, NOS	Pl-03100
Biopsy procedure code, heart, NOS	Pl-31310
Bodies, Aschoff	M-44070
Bodies, asteroid	M-55065
Bodies, Schaumann	M-55060
Buerger's disease	D3-81510
Calcific stenosis	M-34210
Calcification, dystrophic	M-55430
Calcification, medial	M-52420
Calcification, metastatic	M-55440
Calcification, NOS	M-55400
Calcified atheromatous plaque	M-52101
Capillaries, disease of, NOS	D3-85000
Capillary hemangioma	M-91310
Capillary telangiectasis	M-32441
Cardiac	T-32000
Cardiac atrium	T-32100
Cardiac dilation	D3-16180

Granulation tissue, hypertrophic	M-45022
Granuloma, calcified	M-44001
Granuloma, caseating	M-44700
Granuloma, foreign body	M-44140
Granuloma, giant cell, NOS	M-44110
Granuloma, histiocytic	M-44000
Granuloma, noncaseating	M-44200
Granuloma, NOS	M-44000
Granuloma, sarcoid type	M-44210
Granulomatosis, Wegener's	D3-81690
Gross diagnosis	M-09320
Gunshot wound, NOS	M-14500
Heart	T-32000
Heart, aortic valve (see *aortic valve*)	T-35400
Heart, hypertensive heart disease, NOS	D3-02500
Heart, microinfarct	D3-15010
Heart, mitral valve (see *mitral valve*)	T-35300
Heart, papillary muscle, acute infart	D3-11140
Heart, papillary muscle, ruptured	D3-11110
Heart, papillary muscle, ventricle, NOS	T-32400
Heart, papillary muscle, ventricle, left, NOS	T-32621
Heart, papillary muscle, ventricle, right, NOS	T-32521
Heart, pulmonic valve	T-35200
Heart, rheumatic disease of valve, NOS	D3-17600
Heart, rheumatic disease, NOS	D3-17400
Heart, transplant cardiectomy	Pl-31838
Heart, tricuspid valve, NOS	T-35100
Heart valve prosthesis	A-04110
Heart valve prosthesis, artificial	A-04112
Heart valve prosthesis, biologic	A-04114
Hemangioma, arteriovenous	M-91230
Hemangioma, capillary	M-91310
Hemangioma, cavernous	M-91210
Hemangioma, NOS	M-91200
Hemangioma, venous	M-91420
Hemangiopericytoma, NOS	M-91501
Hemangiopericytoma, benign	M-91500
Hemangiopericytoma, malignant	M-91503
Hematoidin pigmentation	M-57420
Hemochromatosis, NOS	D6-31210
Hemofuscin pigmentation	M-57440
Hemorrhage due to ruptured berry aneurysm	D3-89130
Hemorrhage, NOS	M-37000
Hemorrhagic infarct	M-54730

Hemorrhagic inflammation, NOS	M-40790
Hemorrhagic necrosis	M-54040
Hemosiderin deposition, NOS	M-57500
Hemosiderin pigmentation, NOS	M-57500
Hemosiderin-laden macrophages	M-57570
Hepatic vein thrombosis	D3-87520
Hydropic change	M-50070
Hydropic degeneration	M-50070
Hypercholesterolemia, NOS	D6-60030
Hyperemia, NOS	M-36110
Hyperlipidemia, NOS	D6-60010
Hypertension, primary, pulmonary	D3-40310
Hypertensive cardiomegaly	D3-02500
Hypertensive heart disease, NOS	D3-02500
Hypertrophy, cardiac	D3-16170
Hypertrophy, concentric	M-71040
Hypertrophy, NOS	M-71000
Hypoplasia, NOS	M-75300
Incompetence, valvular	F-32400
Infarct, acute	M-54720
Infarct, cystic	M-54800
Infarct, full thickness	M-54860
Infarct, healed	M-54750
Infarct, hemorrhagic	M-54730
Infarct, lacunar	M-54830
Infarct, microscopic	M-54701
Infarct, multiple	M-54706
Infarct, NOS	M-54700
Infarct, old	M-54750
Infarct, old and recent	M-54790
Infarct, recent	M-54720
Infarction, acute, bowel	D5-41370
Infarction, acute, myocardial, NOS	D3-15100
Infarction, cerebral, NOS	D3-89400
Infarction, myocardial, NOS	D3-15000
Infarction, NOS	M-54700
Infarction, old myocardial	D3-15200
Infarction, pulmonary	D3-40210
Infarction, renal	D7-13150
Infarction, splenic	DC-80160
Infarction, thrombotic mesenteric	D5-41404
Infiltration, acute, inflammatory, NOS	M-41000
Infiltration, chronic, inflammatory, NOS	M-43000
Infiltration, eosinophilic, NOS	M-43040

Infiltration, fatty	M-55201
Infiltration, inflammatory, NOS	M-40000
Infiltration, plasma cell, NOS	M-43060
Infiltration, subacute inflammation, NOS	M-42000
Inflammation, active chronic	M-42000
Inflammation, acute and chronic	M-42000
Inflammation, acute exudative	M-41100
Inflammation, acute fibrinous	M-41300
Inflammation, acute gangrenous	M-41700
Inflammation, acute hemorrhagic	M-41790
Inflammation, acute necrotizing	M-41700
Inflammation, acute, NOS	M-41000
Inflammation, chronic exudative, NOS	M-43100
Inflammation, chronic gangrenous, NOS	M-43700
Inflammation, chronic, NOS	M-43000
Inflammation, chronic, lymphocytic	M-43010
Inflammation, chronic, necrotizing	M-43700
Inflammation, chronic, ulcerative	M-43750
Inflammation, exudative, NOS	M-40100
Inflammation, gangrenous, NOS	M-40700
Inflammation, necrotizing, NOS	M-40700
Inflammation, NOS	M-40000
Inflammation, perivascular, NOS	M-40800
Inflammation, plasma cell, NOS	M-43060
Inflammation, pseudomembranous, NOS	M-41780
Inflammation, pseudopolyp	M-76820
Inflammation, purulent, NOS	M-40600
Inflammation, ulcerative, NOS	M-40750
Inflammation, with fat necrosis, NOS	M-45600
Inflammation, with fibrosis, NOS	M-45000
Inflammation, with repair, NOS	M-45000
Inflammation, gummatous, NOS	M-44740
Ischemia, NOS	F-39340
Ischemic bowel disease, NOS	D5-41200
Ischemic colitis, NOS	D5-41210
Ischemic enteritis, NOS	D5-41220
Ischemic enterocolitis, NOS	D5-41230
Ischemic necrosis	M-54200
Ischemic ulcer, NOS	DO-60104
Juvenile hemangioma	M-91310
Kawasaki disease	D3-81660
Keshan disease	D6-38420
Leaflet, mitral valve	T-35320
Lupus erythematosus, systemic	Dl-10100

Lymphatic	T-09010
Macrophage, hemosiderin-laden	M-57570
Marfan's syndrome	D6-90800
Mineralization, NOS	M-55400
Mitral valve	T-35300
Mitral valve, prolapse	M-31050
Mitral valve prosthesis	A-04118
Mitral valve, rheumatic disease of mitral and aortic valves	D3-17650
Mitral valve, rheumatic disease, NOS	D3-17630
Mönckeberg's medial calcification	M-52430
Morphologic abnormality	M-01000
Multinucleated giant cell, NOS	M-62500
Mummification	M-54360
Mural thrombus	M-35130
Myocardial abscess	M-41610
Myocarditis, acute	D3-26001
Myocarditis, bilateral, direct	L-10000
Myocarditis, catecholamine-induced	L-68000
Myocarditis, chlamydial	L-2A900
Myocarditis, chronic interstitial	D3-26003
Myocarditis, cocaine-induced	LCB720
Myocarditis, collagen vascular disease-associated	D1-10000
Myocarditis, coxsackie virus-associated	L-30400
Myocarditis, diphtheria-associated	L-14401
Myocarditis, drug-induced, general	D3-26400
Myocarditis, eosinophilic, hypereosinophilia syndrome	D3-20130 M-43040
Myocarditis, eosinophilic, necrotizing	M-41700 M-43040
Myocarditis, fungal	L-40000
Myocarditis, giant cell	D3-26010
Myocarditis, granulomatous	D3-26007 M-44000
Myocarditis, hypersensitivity	D3-26100
Myocarditis, Lyme disease-associated	L2A003
Myocarditis, NOS	D3-26000
Myocarditis, rheumatic	D3-17420 M-40000
Myocarditis, rickettsial	L2A000
Myocarditis, sarcoidosis-associated	L-00004 DE-A1420
Myocarditis, spirochetal	L-24700
Myocarditis, subacute interstitial	D3-17420
Myocarditis, toxic	D3-26300
Myocarditis, *Toxoplasma ghondii*-associated	L-52801
Myocarditis, viral	L-30000

Myocardium, NOS	T-32020
Myofibroma	M-88900
Necrosis, acute	M-54001
Necrosis, coagulative	M-54060
Necrosis, cystic medial	M-52470
Necrosis, fat	M-54110
Necrosis, fibrinoid	M-54090
Necrosis, focal	M-54004
Necrosis, hemorrhagic	M-54040
Necrosis, ischemic	M-54200
Necrosis, liquefactive	M-54050
Necrosis, NOS	M-54000
Necrotizing inflammation, NOS	M-40700
Necrotizing inflammation, NOS, acute	M-41700
Necrotizing inflammation, NOS, chronic	M-43700
Necrotizing inflammation, NOS, fibrinoid	M-44750
Necrotizing inflammation, NOS, granulomatous	M-44700
Nephrosclerosis	D3-02703
Nephrosclerosis, arteriolar, NOS	D7-13120
Nephrosclerosis, arteriolar, NOS, benign	D7-13124
Nephrosclerosis, arteriolar, NOS, malignant	D7-13128
No diagnostic abnormality	M-00110
Normal tissue, NOS	M-00100
Obliterative pericarditis	D3-91020
Obstruction, NOS	M-34000
Organizing hematoma	M-35061
Organizing inflammation, NOS	M-45000
Papillary muscle, NOS	T-32421
Parasitic cyst	M-33700
Passive chronic P congestion	M-36142
Passive chronic P congestion, of liver	D5-81212
Passive congestion	M-36140
Passive hyperemia	M-36140
Pericarditis, NOS	D3-91000
Perivascular inflammation, NOS	M-40800
Phlebitis, NOS	D3-87700
Polyarteritis nodosa	D3-81630
Prosthesis, aortic valve	A-04116
Prosthesis, cardiac valve, artificial	A-04112
Prosthesis, cardiac valve, biologic	A-04114
Prosthesis, mitral valve	A-04118
Prosthesis, NOS	A-04000
Prosthesis, valve, NOS	A-38100

Rejection, graft, NOS	F-CC300
Repair, changes of	M-67054
Repair, NOS	M-78000
Repeat study suggested	M-09490
Rheumatic heart diseases, chronic (healed)	T-32000 M-43000 D3-17500
Rheumatic heart disease, NOS	D3-17400
Rheumatic valvulitis	D-7150 M-40900
Rupture, NOS	M-14400
Sarcoidosis, NOS	DE-A1420
Scleroderma	Dl-10200
Septic embolus	M-35390
Septic infarct	M-54760
Stenosis, NOS	M-34200
Sternum, NOS	T-11210
Syphilis, NOS	DE-14300
Thromboembolism	M-35310
Thrombophlebitis, NOS	D3-87710
Thrombosis, NOS	M-35100
Thrombus, canalized	M-35140
Thrombus, NOS	M-35100
Thrombus, obstructive	M-35110
Thrombus, occlusive	M-35110
Thrombus, propagating	M-35180
Tissue lost in processing	M-09150
Tissue, no diagnostic abnormality	M-00110
Tissue, normal, NOS	M-00100
Tissue not received	M-09100
Toxemia, NOS	D8-11205
Transplanted organ, NOS	M-15500
Traumatic abnormality	M-10000
Tricuspid valve	T-35100
Valve, nonrheumatic dz, heart, NOS	D3-29000
Valve prosthesis, NOS	A-04100
Valve prosthesis, NOS, biologic	A-04114
Valve, rheumatic dz, heart, NOS	D3-17600
Valvular insufficiency	F-32400
Varices	M-32600
Varices, esophageal, NOS	D5-30830
Varicose vein	M-32600
Varicose vein, lower extremity, NOS	D3-87020
Vascular dz, arteriosclerotic, NOS	D3-81100
Vasculitis, skin, NOS	D0-00520
Vein, femoral	T-49410
Vein, NOS	T-48000

Vena cava, superior	T-48610
Wegener's granulomatosis	D3-81690
Wound, biopsy	M-14020
Wound, gunshot, NOS	M-14500
Wound, NOS	M-14000
Wound, stab	M-14070

SNOMED codes and conditions arranged
in order of the SNOMED code:

Prosthesis, NOS	A-04000
Valve prosthesis, NOS	A-04100
Heart valve prosthesis	A-04110
Prosthesis, cardiac valve, artificial	A-04112
Heart valve prosthesis, artificial	A-04112
Prosthesis, cardiac valve, biologic	A-04114
Heart valve prosthesis, biologic	A-04114
Valve prosthesis, NOS, biologic	A-04114
Prosthesis, aortic valve	A-04116
Aortic valve, prosthesis	A-04116
Mitral valve prosthesis	A-04118
Prosthesis, mitral valve	A-04118
Prosthesis, valve, NOS	A-38100
Rheumatic valvulitis	D-7150
Vasculitis, skin, NOS	D0-00520
Ischemic ulcer, NOS	D0-60104
Myocarditis, collagen vascular disease-associated	D1-10000
Lupus erythematosus, systemic	D1-10100
Scleroderma	D1-10200
Disease, cardiovascular system, NOS	D3-00000 T-30000
Hypertensive cardiomegaly	D3-02500
Hypertensive heart disease, NOS	D3-02500
Heart, hypertensive heart disease, NOS	D3-02500
Nephrosclerosis	D3-02703
Heart, papillary muscle, ruptured	D3-11110
Heart, papillary muscle, acute infarct	D3-11140
Coronary artery disease, NOS	D3-13000
Coronary atherosclerosis	D3-13010
Coronary artery thrombosis	D3-13210
Coronary artery embolism	D3-13220
Infarction, myocardial, NOS	D3-15000
Heart, microinfarct	D3-15010
Infarction, acute, myocardial, NOS	D3-15100
Infarction, old myocardial	D3-15200
Cardiomegaly	D3-16170

 APPENDIX

Hypertrophy, cardiac	D3-16170
Dilation, cardiac	D3-16180
Cardiac dilation	D3-16180
Rheumatic heart disease, NOS	D3-17400
Heart, rheumatic disease, NOS	D3-17400
Disease, rheumatic, heart	D3-17400
Myocarditis, rheumatic	D3-17420 M-40000
Myocarditis, subacute interstitial	D3-17420
Heart, rheumatic disease of valve, NOS	D3-17600
Disease, rheumatic, heart valve	D3-17600
Valve, rheumatic dz, heart, NOS	D3-17600
Mitral valve, rheumatic disease, NOS	D3-17630
Aortic valve, rheumatic disease	D3-17640
Mitral valve, rheumatic disease of mitral and aortic valves	D3-17650
Cardiomyopathy, NOS	D3-20000 T-32020
Myocarditis, eosinophilic, hypereosinophilia syndrome	D3-20130 M-43040
Myocarditis, NOS	D3-26000
Myocarditis, acute	D3-26001
Myocarditis, chronic interstitial	D3-26003
Myocarditis, granulomatous	D3-26007 M-44000
Myocarditis, giant cell	D3-26010
Myocarditis, hypersensitivity	D3-26100
Myocarditis, toxic	D3-26300
Myocarditis, drug-induced, general	D3-26400
Endocarditis, acute, NOS	D3-28001
Endocarditis, subacute, NOS	D3-28002
Endocarditis, chronic, NOS	D3-28003
Endocarditis, acute, bacterial	D3-28101 T-32060
Valve, nonrheumatic dz, heart, NOS	D3-29000
Congenital anomaly of cardiovascular system, NOS	D3-30000
Infarction, pulmonary	D3-40210
Embolism, pulmonary	D3-40230
Hypertension, primary, pulmonary	D3-40310
Artery, disease, NOS	D3-81000
Arteriosclerotic vascular disease	D3-81100
Vascular dz, arteriosclerotic, NOS	D3-81100
Atheroma, artery	D3-81202
Atrial thrombosis, NOS	D3-81500
Buerger's disease	D3-81510
Disease, Buerger's	D3-81510
Arteritis, NOS	D3-81600

Polyarteritis nodosa	D3-81630
Giant cell arteritis	D3-81640
Kawasaki disease	D3-81660
Granulomatosis, Wegener's	D3-81690
Wegener's granulomatosis	D3-81690
Aorta, atherosclerosis	D3-83200
Aorta, aneurysm, NOS	D3-83300
Aorta, aneurysm, ruptured, NOS	D3-83310
Capillaries, disease of, NOS	D3-85000
Varicose vein, lower extremity, NOS	D3-87020
Hepatic vein thrombosis	D3-87520
Phlebitis, NOS	D3-87700
Thrombophlebitis, NOS	D3-87710
Hemorrhage due to ruptured berry aneurysm	D3-89130
Infarction, cerebral, NOS	D3-89400
Pericarditis, NOS	D3-91000
Obliterative pericarditis	D3-91020
Congenital anomalies of fetus, NOS	D4-F0000
Anomalies, congenital	D4-F0000
Varices, esophageal, NOS	D5-30830
Ischemic bowel disease, NOS	D5-41200
Ischemic colitis, NOS	D5-41210
Ischemic enteritis, NOS	D5-41220
Ischemic enterocolitis, NOS	D5-41230
Infarction, acute, bowel	D5-41370
Infarction, thrombotic mesenteric	D5-41404
Chronic passive congestion, liver	D5-81212
Congestion, chronic, passive, liver	D5-81212
Passive chronic P congestion, of liver	D5-81212
Hemochromatosis, NOS	D6-31210
Keshan disease	D6-38420
Hyperlipidemia, NOS	D6-60010
Hypercholesterolemia, NOS	D6-60030
Marfan's syndrome	D6-90800
Nephrosclerosis, arteriolar, NOS	D7-13120
Arteriolar nephrosclerosis	D7-13120
Nephrosclerosis, arteriolar, NOS, benign	D7-13124
Nephrosclerosis, arteriolar, NOS, malignant	D7-13128
Infarction, renal	D7-13150
Toxemia, NOS	D8-11205
Eclampsia	D8-11250
Infarction, splenic	DC-80160
Syphilis, NOS	DE-14300
Cysticercosis of the heart	DE-65200

Sarcoidosis, NOS	DE-A1420
Valvular insufficiency	F-32400
Incompetence, valvular	F-32400
Ischemia, NOS	F-39340
Graft, reaction, NOS	F-CC200
Graft versus host reaction	F-CC240
Graft rejection, NOS	F-CC300
Rejection, graft, NOS	F-CC300
Graft rejection, mild	F-CC310
Graft rejection, moderate	F-CC320
Graft rejection, acute cellular	F-CC330
Graft rejection, hyperacute	F-CC340
Graft rejection, chronic, NOS	F-CC400
Myocarditis, sarcoidosis-associated	L-00004 DE-A1420
Myocarditis, bilateral, direct	L-10000
Myocarditis, diphtheria-associated	L-14401
Myocarditis, spirochetal	L-24700
Myocarditis, viral	L-30000
Myocarditis, coxsackie virus-associated	L-30400
Myocarditis, fungal	L-40000
Myocarditis, parasitic, immunologic	L-5000
Myocarditis, parasitic, direct	L-50000
Myocarditis, *toxoplasma ghondii*-associated	L-52801
Myocarditis, catecholamine-induced	L-68000
Myocarditis, rickettsial	L2A000
Myocarditis, Lyme disease-associated	L2A003
Myocarditis, chlamydial	L2A900
Myocarditis, psittaci	L2A902
Myocarditis, cocaine-induced	LCB720
Normal tissue, NOS	M-00100
Tissue, normal, NOS	M-00100
Tissue, no diagnostic abnormality	M-00110
No diagnostic abnormality	M-00110
Morphologic abnormality	M-01000
Tissue not received	M-09100
Tissue lost in processing	M-09150
Gross diagnosis	M-09320
Repeat study suggested	M-09490
Traumatic abnormality	M-10000
Effect	M-11120
Effect, cryotherapy	M-11220
Effect, radiation	M-11600
Wound, NOS	M-14000
Wound, biopsy	M-14020

Wound, stab	M-14070
Rupture, NOS	M-14400
Chordal rupture	M-14430
Wound, gunshot, NOS	M-14500
Gunshot wound, NOS	M-14500
Transplanted organ, NOS	M-15500
Graft, NOS	M-15500
Anomalies, multiple	M-20080
Coarctation, NOS	M-20310
Aneurysm, congenital, NOS	M-24610
Foreign body, NOS	M-30400
Mitral valve, prolapse	M-31050
Aneurysm, NOS	M-32200
Aneurysm, ruptured, NOS	M-32201
Aneurysm, A-V	M-32220
Aneurysm, dissecting	M-32270
Aneurysm	M-32400
Capillary telangiectasis	M-32441
Aneurysm, mycotic	M-32520
Aneurysm, false	M-32590
Varices	M-32600
Varicose vein	M-32600
Parasitic cyst	M-33700
Obstruction, NOS	M-34000
Coarctation, atypical	M-34100
Stenosis, NOS	M-34200
Calcific stenosis	M-34210
Clot, blood, NOS	M-35000
Coagulum, blood, NOS	M-35000
Clot, fibrin, blood	M-35050
Fibrin blood clot	M-35050
Organizing hematoma	M-35061
Thrombosis, NOS	M-35100
Thrombus, NOS	M-35100
Thrombus, obstructive	M-35110
Thrombus, occlusive	M-35110
Annular thrombus	M-35120
Mural thrombus	M-35130
Thrombus, canalized	M-35140
Fibrin thrombus	M-35150
Thrombus, propagating	M-35180
Embolism, NOS	M-35300
Embolus, NOS	M-35300
Embolus, saddle	M-35301

Thromboembolism	M-35310
Embolus, air	M-35320
Embolus, marrow	M-35330
Foreign body, embolus, NOS	M-35350
Atheromatous embolus	M-35360
Embolus, atheromatous	M-35360
Embolus, septic	M-35390 L-10000
Septic embolus	M-35390
Embolus, fat	M-35450
Fat embolus	M-35450
Embolus, microembolus	M-35480
Congestion, NOS	M-36100
Hyperemia, NOS	M-36110
Congestion, venous	M-36140
Passive congestion	M-36140
Passive hyperemia	M-36140
Passive chronic P congestion	M-36142
Chronic passive congestion	M-36142
Congestion, chronic passive	M-36142
Hemorrhage, NOS	M-37000
Inflammation, NOS	M-40000
Infiltration, inflammatory, NOS	M-40000
Inflammation, exudative, NOS	M-40100
Inflammation, purulent, NOS	M-40600
Inflammation, necrotizing, NOS	M-40700
Inflammation, gangrenous, NOS	M-40700
Necrotizing inflammation, NOS	M-40700
Inflammation, ulcerative, NOS	M-40750
Hemorrhagic inflammation, NOS	M-40790
Inflammation, perivascular, NOS	M-40800
Perivascular inflammation, NOS	M-40800
Rheumatic valvulitis	M-40900
Infiltration, acute, inflammatory, NOS	M-41000
Inflammation, acute, NOS	M-41000
Inflammation, acute exudative	M-41100
Inflammation, acute fibrinous	M-41300
Fibrinopurulent inflammation, acute, NOS	M-41300
Myocardial abscess	M-41610
Necrotizing inflammation, NOS, acute	M-41700
Inflammation, acute gangrenous	M-41700
Myocarditis, eosinophilic, necrotizing	M-41700 M-43040
Inflammation, acute necrotizing	M-41700
Inflammation, pseudomembranous, NOS	M-41780
Inflammation, acute hemorrhagic	M-41790

Inflammation, acute and chronic	M-42000
Inflammation, active chronic	M-42000
Chronic and acute inflammation	M-42000
Infiltration, subacute inflammation, NOS	M-42000
Inflammation, chronic, NOS	M-43000
Infiltration, chronic, inflammatory, NOS	M-43000
Chronic inflammation, NOS	M-43000
Inflammation, chronic, lymphocytic	M-43010
Infiltration, eosinophilic, NOS	M-43040
Inflammation, plasma cell, NOS	M-43060
Infiltration, plasma cell, NOS	M-43060
Inflammation, chronic exudative, NOS	M-43100
Inflammation, chronic, necrotizing	M-43700
Inflammation, chronic gangrenous, NOS	M-43700
Necrotizing inflammation, NOS, chronic	M-43700
Inflammation, chronic, ulcerative	M-43750
Granuloma, histiocytic	M-44000
Granuloma, NOS	M-44000
Granuloma, calcified	M-44001
Bodies, Aschoff	M-44070
Granuloma, giant cell, NOS	M-44110
Granuloma, foreign body	M-44140
Granuloma, noncaseating	M-44200
Granuloma, sarcoid type	M-44210
Caseating granuloma	M-44700
Necrotizing inflammation, NOS, granulomatous	M-44700
Granuloma, caseating	M-44700
Inflammation, gummatous, NOS	M-44740
Necrotizing inflammation, NOS, fibrinoid	M-44750
Inflammation, with repair, NOS	M-45000
Organizing inflammation, NOS	M-45000
Inflammation, with fibrosis, NOS	M-45000
Granulation tissue, NOS	M-45020
Granulation tissue, hypertrophic	M-45022
Inflammation, with fat necrosis, NOS	M-45600
Degeneration	M-50000
Degeneration, cystic	M-50030
Hydropic degeneration	M-50070
Change, hydropic	M-50070
Hydropic change	M-50070
Degeneration, hydropic	M-50070
Change, fatty	M-50080
Degeneration, myxoid	M-50151

Arteriosclerosis	M-52000
Atheroma, artery, NOS	M-52100
Degeneration, atheromatous	M-52100
Atheromatous plaque, NOS	M-52100
Calcified atheromatous plaque	M-52101
Atheromatous plaque, calcified	M-52101
Atheromatous plaque, ulcerated	M-52103
Atherosclerosis, NOS	M-52110
Arteriolosclerosis, NOS	M-52200
Fibrinoid necrosis (or degenerations) in arteriolosclerosis	M-52210
Calcification, medial	M-52420
Mönckeberg's medial calcification	M-52430
Necrosis, cystic medial	M-52470
Cystic medionecrosis (of artery)	M-52470
Necrosis, NOS	M-54000
Cellular necrosis, NOS	M-54000
Necrosis, acute	M-54001
Necrosis, focal	M-54004
Necrosis, hemorrhagic	M-54040
Hemorrhagic necrosis	M-54040
Necrosis, liquefactive	M-54050
Necrosis, coagulative	M-54060
Caseous necrosis	M-54080
Fibrinoid necrosis	M-54090
Necrosis, fibrinoid	M-54090
Necrosis, fat	M-54110
Necrosis, ischemic	M-54200
Ischemic necrosis	M-54200
Mummification	M-54360
Infarct, NOS	M-54700
Infarction, NOS	M-54700
Infarct, microscopic	M-54701
Infarct, multiple	M-54706
Infarct, recent	M-54720
Infarct, acute	M-54720
Infarct, hemorrhagic	M-54730
Hemorrhagic infarct	M-54730
Infarct, old	M-54750
Infarct, healed	M-54750
Septic infarct	M-54760
Infarct, old and recent	M-54790
Infarct, cystic	M-54800
Infarct, lacunar	M-54830

Infarct, full thickness	M-54860
Fibrin deposition	M-55040
Bodies, Schaumann	M-55060
Bodies, asteroid	M-55065
Infiltration, fatty	M-55201
Mineralization, NOS	M-55400
Calcification, NOS	M-55400
Calcification, dystrophic	M-55430
Calcification, metastatic	M-55440
Hematoidin pigmentation	M-57420
Hemofuscin pigmentation	M-57440
Hemosiderin pigmentation, NOS	M-57500
Hemosiderin deposition, NOS	M-57500
Hemosiderin-laden macrophages	M-57570
Macrophage, hemosiderin-laden	M-57570
Atrophy, NOS	M-58000
Foam cell	M-62030
Multinucleated giant cell NOS	M-62500
Giant cell, NOS	M-62500
Repair, changes of	M-67054
Hypertrophy, NOS	M-71000
Hypertrophy, concentric	M-71040
Hypoplasia, NOS	M-75300
Inflammation, pseudopolyp	M-76820
Repair, NOS	M-78000
Chronic fibrosis	M-78003
Fibrous adhesion	M-78430
Embolus, tumor	M-80006
Myofibroma	M-88900
Hemangioma, NOS	M-91200
Hemangioma, cavernous	M-91210
Hemangioma, arteriovenous	M-91230
Juvenile hemangioma	M-91310
Hemangioma, capillary	M-91310
Capillary hemangioma	M-91310
Hemangioma, venous	M-91420
Hemangiopericytoma, benign	M-91500
Hemangiopericytoma, NOS	M-91501
Hemangiopericytoma, malignant	M-91503
Biopsy procedure code, biopsy, NOS	Pl-03100
Biopsy procedure code, heart, NOS	Pl-31310
Heart, transplant cardiectomy	Pl-31838
Lymphatic	T-09010
Sternum, NOS	T-11210

Cardiac	T-32000
Heart	T-32000
Rheumatic heart diseases, chronic (healed)	T-32000 M-43000 D3-17500
Myocardium, NOS	T-32020
Cardiac muscle	T-32020
Cardiac atrium	T-32100
Atrium, NOS	T-32100
Cardiac ventricle	T-32400
Heart, papillary muscle, ventricle, NOS	T-32400
Papillary muscle, NOS	T-32421
Heart, papillary muscle, ventricle, right, NOS	T-32521
Heart, papillary muscle, ventricle, left, NOS	T-32621
Cardiac valve	T-35000
Cardiac valve leaflet, NOS	T-35002
Heart, tricuspid valve, NOS	T-35100
Tricuspid valve	T-35100
Heart, pulmonic valve	T-35200
Heart, mitral valve (see *mitral valve*)	T-35300
Mitral valve	T-35300
Leaflet, mitral valve	T-35320
Aortic valve	T-35400
Heart, aortic valve (see *aortic valve*)	T-35400
Artery, NOS	T-41000
Aorta	T-42000
Aorta, abdominal	T-42500
Artery, carotid, NOS	T-45010
Artery, cerebral	T-45510
Artery, of extremity, NOS	T-47000
Artery, femoral, NOS	T-47400
Vein, NOS	T-48000
Vena cava, superior	T-48610
Vein, femoral	T-49410

Subject Index

Page numbers followed by t indicate tables.

A

Abdominal coarctation, 167
Abnormal lie, of cardiovascular device/graft,
　　310–311
Abscess
　annular
　　of heart valve, 108110
　　of perigraft, 305–306
　myocardial, 52–53
ACI (arterial calcification of infancy), 160–161
Acommissural valves, 130, 131
Acquired immunodeficiency syndrome. *See*
　　AIDS
Acute myocardial infarct (AMI), 60–61
Adriamycin cardiomyopathy, 15
Adventitial cystic disease (ACD), 151–152
Age-related calcification
　medial, of artery, 199–200
　of mitral valve, 140–141
Aging, heart valve changes with, 120–123
AIDS-associated pericarditis, 228–229
AIDS cardiomyopathy, 22–23
Air embolism
　arterial, 278–279
　pulmonary, 279–281
　venous, 279–281
Air pericardial tamponade, 313–314
Alcohol-associated cardiomyopathy, 12–13
ALHE (angiolymphoid hyperplasia with
　　eosinophilia), 157–158, 194
Allergic granulomatosis, and angiitis, 174
Allergic myocarditis, 75–76
Allergic reaction, to diagnostic/therapeutic
　　procedure, 281–282
Allergic vasculitis, 188–189
Allograft rejection, cardiac, 7–10
　acute, 7–8
　chronic, 8
　humoral, 9
　hyperacute, 9–10
　"Quilty" effect, 10
Allograft transplant arteriopathy, 152
AMI (acute myocardial infarct), 60–61
Amiodarone-associated cardiomyopathy, 13–14
Amphetamine-associated cardiomyopathy,
　　14
Amyloid deposits, in heart valves, 121, 122
Amyloidosis, 3–5
Anabolic steroid cardiomyopathy, 35–36
Anaphylactoid purpura, 212–213
Anaphylactoid reaction, 281–282

Anaphylaxis, related to diagnostic/therapeutic
　　procedure, 281–282
Anastomotic dehiscence, of cardiovascular
　　device/graft, 282–283
Anderson's disease, 43–44
Anemia, acquired intravascular hemolytic,
　　286–287
Aneurysm
　annulo-aortic, 101–102
　aortic
　　abdominal, 153–154
　　ascending, 154–155
　　atherosclerotic, 153–154
　　dissecting, 159–160, 177–178
　　inflammatory, 153–154
　　thoracic, 154–155
　　　descending, 154–155
　of aortic arch, 154–155
　arteriovenous, 245–246
　berry, 168–169
　cirsoid, 245–246
　congenital intracranial, 168–169
　false, 152–153, 287–288, 295–296
　　mycotic, 305–306
　infective, 201–202
　mycotic, 191, 201–202
　　false, 305–306
　post-traumatic, 314–315
　racemose, 245–246
　sinus of Valsalva, 101–102
　true, 155–156
　ventricular, 5–6
Angiitis
　allergic granulomatosis and, 174
　disseminated visceral giant cell, 178–179
　hypersensitivity, 188–189
　primary, of CNS, 207
Angioblastoma, 242–243
Angiodysplasia, 156–157
Angioendothelioma, malignant endovascular
　　papillary, 252–253
Angioendotheliomatosis, malignant, 197
Angiohamartomas, 156–157
Angiokeratoma corporis diffusum universale,
　　93–94
Angiolymphoid hyperplasia with eosinophilia
　　(ALHE), 157–158, 194
Angioma, acquired tufted, 242–243
Angiomatosis, bacillary, 246
Angiosarcoma, 243–244
　of heart or pericardium, 244–245, 270